Machine Learning in Medicine

Chapman & Hall/CRC Healthcare Informatics Series

Series Editors:
Christopher Yang,
Drexel University, USA

RECENTLY PUBLISHED TITLES

Process Modeling and Management for Healthcare
Carlo Combi, Giuseppe Pozzi, Pierangelo Veltri

Statistics and Machine Learning Methods for EHR Data: From Data Extraction to Data Analytics
Hulin Wu, Jose-Miguel Yamal, Ashraf Yaseen, Vahed Maroufy

For more information about this series, please visit: https://www.routledge.com/Chapman—HallCRC-Healthcare-Informatics-Series/book-series/HEALTHINF

Machine Learning in Medicine

Edited by
Ayman El-Baz
Jasjit S. Suri

CRC Press
Taylor & Francis Group
Boca Raton London New York

CRC Press is an imprint of the
Taylor & Francis Group, an **informa** business
A CHAPMAN & HALL BOOK

First Edition published 2021
by CRC Press
6000 Broken Sound Parkway NW, Suite 300, Boca Raton, FL 33487-2742

and by CRC Press
2 Park Square, Milton Park, Abingdon, Oxon, OX14 4RN

CRC Press is an imprint of Taylor & Francis Group, LLC

Library of Congress Cataloging-in-Publication Data
Names: El-Baz, Ayman S., editor. | Suri, Jasjit S., editor.
Title: Machine learning in medicine / edited by Ayman El-Baz, Jasjit S. Suri.
Description: First edition. | Boca Raton : CRC Press, 2021. |
Series: Chapman & Hall/CRC healthcare informatics series | Includes bibliographical references and index.
Identifiers: LCCN 2021006004 | ISBN 9781138106901 (hardback) | ISBN 9781032039855 (paperback) | ISBN 9781315101323 (ebook)
Subjects: LCSH: Medical informatics. | Machine learning. | Medicine—Data processing.
Classification: LCC R858 .M32 2021 | DDC 610.285—dc23
LC record available at https://lccn.loc.gov/2021006004

ISBN: 978-1-138-10690-1 (hbk)
ISBN: 978-1-032-03985-5 (pbk)
ISBN: 978-1-315-10132-3 (ebk)

Typeset in Minion
by codeMantra

With love and affection to my mother and father, whose loving spirit sustains me still

- Ayman El-Baz

To my late loving parents, immediate family, and children

- Jasjit S. Suri

Contents

Preface

THIS BOOK COVERS THE STATE-OF-THE-ART TECHNIQUES OF MACHINE learning and their applications in the medical field. Computer-aided diagnosis (CAD) systems have played an important role in the diagnosis of several diseases in the past decade, e.g., cancer detection, resulting in developing several successful systems. However, the robustness of these systems does not meet the requirements of real-world diagnostic situations and still requires significant improvement. The rapid progress in the development of machine learning algorithms makes it promising to have machines in the near future that are capable of completely performing tasks that currently cannot be completed without human aid, especially in the medical field. For example, the application of Convolutional Neural Network (CNN) methods in biomedical image analysis has recently resulted in the development of some CAD systems that aim towards the automatic early detection of several diseases. This will be covered in the book. Among the topics discussed in the book are CNNs with different activation functions for small- to medium-size biomedical datasets, detection of abnormal activities stemming from cognitive decline, thermal dose modeling for thermal ablative cancer treatments, dermatological machine learning clinical decision support system, artificial intelligence-powered ultrasound for diagnosis, practical challenges with possible solutions for machine learning in medical imaging, epilepsy diagnosis from structural MRI, Alzheimer's disease diagnosis, classification of left ventricular hypertrophy, and intelligent medical language understanding.

In summary, the main aim of this book is to help advance scientific research within the broad field of machine learning in the medical field. The book focuses on major trends and challenges in this area, and it presents work aimed to identify new techniques and their use in biomedical analysis.

Ayman El-Baz
Jasjit S. Suri

Acknowledgements

THE COMPLETION OF THIS BOOK COULD NOT HAVE BEEN POSSIBLE without the participation and assistance of so many people whose names may not all be enumerated. Their contributions are sincerely appreciated and gratefully acknowledged. However, the editors would like to express their deep appreciation and indebtedness particularly to Dr. Ali H. Mahmoud and Hisham Abdeltawab for their endless support.

Ayman El-Baz
Jasjit S. Suri

Editors

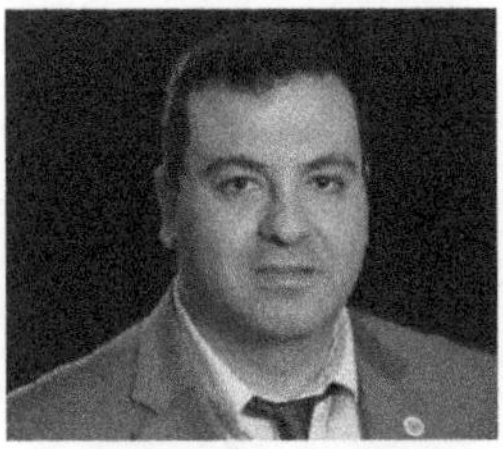

Ayman El-Baz is a Distinguished Professor at the University of Louisville, Kentucky, United States, and the University of Louisville at AlAlamein International University (UofL-AIU), New Alamein City, Egypt. Dr. El-Baz earned his BSc and MSc degrees in electrical engineering in 1997 and 2001, respectively. He earned his PhD in electrical engineering from the University of Louisville in 2006. Dr. El-Baz was named as a Fellow for Coulter, AIMBE, and NAI for his contributions to the field of biomedical translational research. Dr. El-Baz has almost two decades of hands-on experience in the fields of bio-imaging modeling and non-invasive computer-assisted diagnosis systems. He has authored or coauthored more than 700 technical articles (168 journals, 44 books, 91 book chapters, 256 refereed-conference papers, 196 abstracts, and 36 US patents and Disclosures).

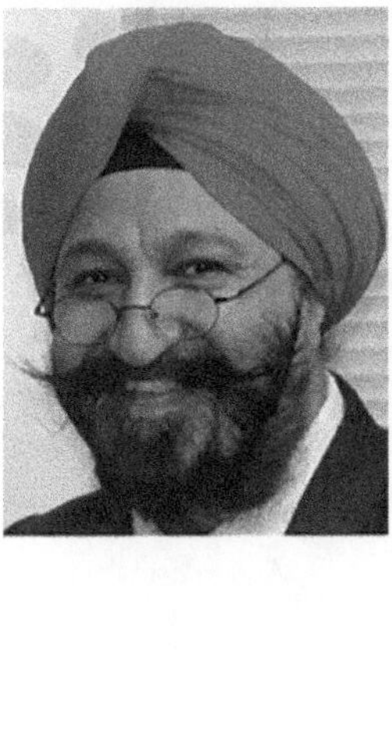

Jasjit S. Suri is an innovator, scientist, visionary, industrialist, and an internationally known world leader in biomedical engineering. Dr. Suri has spent over 25 years in the field of biomedical engineering/devices and its management. He received his PhD from the University of Washington, Seattle, and his Business Management Sciences degree from Weatherhead, Case Western Reserve University, Cleveland, Ohio. Dr. Suri was crowned with the President's Gold medal in 1980 and made a Fellow of the

American Institute of Medical and Biological Engineering for his outstanding contributions. In 2018, he was awarded the Marquis Life Time Achievement Award for his outstanding contributions and dedication to medical imaging and its management.

Contributors

Nabila Abraham
Ryerson Multimedia Research Laboratory
Electrical, Computer, and Biomedical Engineering
Ryerson University
Toronto, Canada

Pushkar Aggarwal
University of Cincinnati College of Medicine
Cincinnati, Ohio

Muhammad Ali Akbar
Department of Surgery
University of Toronto
Toronto, Canada

Zeynettin Akkus
Cardiovascular Research
Mayo Clinic
Rochester, Minnesota

Damla Arifoglu
Department of Computer Science
Faculty of Engineering Science
University College London
London, United Kingdom

Jetan H. Badhiwala
Department of Surgery
University of Toronto
Toronto, Canada

Filippo Berno
Department of Information Engineering
University of Padua
Padua, Italy

Mohini Bindal
Baylor College of Medicine
Houston, Texas

Abdelhamid Bouchachia
Department of Computing and Informatics
Faculty of Science and Technology
Bournemouth University
Poole, United Kingdom

Sheryl Brahnam
Information Technology and Cybersecurity
Missouri State University
Springfield, Missouri

Sunita Chauhan
Department of Mechanical and Aerospace Engineering
Monash University
Clayton, Australia

Wa Cheung
Department of Radiology
The Alfred Hospital
Melbourne, Australia

Esmaeil Davoodi-Bojd
Radiology Image Analysis Laboratory
Henry Ford Health System
Detroit, Michigan

Amy C. Dwyer
Kidney Transplantation — Kidney Disease Center
University of Louisville
Louisville, Kentucky

Maryam El-Baz
Bioengineering Department
University of Louisville
Louisville, Kentucky

Mohamed Abou El-Ghar
Radiology Department
Urology and Nephrology Center
University of Mansoura
Mansoura, Egypt

Ingy El-Torgoman
Department of Basic Sciences
Faculty of Engineering
Pharos University in Alexandria
Alexandria, Egypt

Michael G. Fehlings
Department of Surgery
University of Toronto
Toronto, Canada
and
Spinal Program
Toronto Western Hospital
University Health Network
Toronto, Canada

Mohammed Ghazal
Department of Electrical and Computer Engineering
Abu Dhabi University
Abu Dhabi, United Arab Emirates

Guruprasad Giridharan
Bioengineering Department
University of Louisville
Louisville, Kentucky

Arnulfo González-Cantú
Hospital Clínica Nova de Monterrey
San Nicolás de los Garza
Nuevo León, Mexico
and
Especialidades Médicas
Escuela de Medicina
Universidad de Monterrey
San Pedro Garza García, Mexico

Marcia Hon
Ryerson Multimedia Research Laboratory
Electrical, Computer, and Biomedical Engineering
Ryerson University
Toronto, Canada

Fahmi Khalifa
Bioengineering Department
University of Louisville
Louisville, Kentucky

Naimul Khan
Ryerson Multimedia Research Laboratory
Electrical, Computer, and Biomedical Engineering
Ryerson University
Toronto, Canada

Omar Khan
Department of Surgery
University of Toronto
Toronto, Canada

Gianluca Maguolo
Department of Information Engineering
University of Padua
Padua, Italy

Ali Mahmoud
Bioengineering Department
University of Louisville
Louisville, Kentucky

Loris Nanni
Department of Information Engineering
University of Padua
Padua, Italy

Girijesh Prasad
Intelligent Systems Research Centre
School of Computing, Engineering and Intelligent Systems
Ulster University
Londonderry, United Kingdom

Stuart K. Roberts
Department of Gastroenterology
The Alfred Hospital
Melbourne, Australia

Maria Elena Romero-Ibarguengoitia
Hospital Clínica Nova de Monterrey
San Nicolás de los Garza
Nuevo León, Mexico
and
Especialidades Médicas
Escuela de Medicina
Universidad de Monterrey
San Pedro Garza García, Mexico

Baidya Nath Saha
Concordia University of Edmonton
Alberta, Canada

Jose Sanchez-Bornot
Intelligent Systems Research Centre
School of Computing, Engineering and Intelligent Systems
Ulster University
Londonderry, United Kingdom

Shams Shaker
Bioengineering Department
University of Louisville
Louisville, Kentucky

Ahmed Shalaby
Bioengineering Department
University of Louisville
Louisville, Kentucky

Seyedmohammad Shams
Radiology Image Analysis Laboratory
Henry Ford Health System
Detroit, Michigan

Mohamed Shehata
Bioengineering Department
University of Louisville
Louisville, Kentucky

Ahmed Soliman
Bioengineering Department
University of Louisville
Louisville, Kentucky

Hamid Soltanian-Zadeh
Radiology Image Analysis Laboratory
Henry Ford Health System
Detroit, Michigan
and
CIPCE School of Electrical and Computer Engineering
University of Tehran
Tehran, Iran

Anika Tabassum
Ryerson Multimedia Research Laboratory
Electrical, Computer, and Biomedical Engineering
Ryerson University
Toronto, Canada

KongFatt Wong-Lin
Intelligent Systems Research Centre
School of Computing, Engineering and Intelligent Systems
Ulster University
Londonderry, United Kingdom

Su Yang
University of West London
London, United Kingdom

Jinao Zhang
Department of Mechanical and Aerospace Engineering
Monash University
Clayton, Australia

CHAPTER 1

Another Set of Eyes in Anesthesiology

Pushkar Aggarwal

University of Cincinnati College of Medicine
Cincinnati, Ohio

CONTENTS

1.1 INTRODUCTION/HISTORY

When one thinks of machine learning and artificial intelligence in healthcare, the overwhelming thought is about their applicability in radiology for diagnosing pathologies through chest X-rays/computed tomography or their applicability in dermatology for diagnosing pathologies using skin images. These are logical applications, because we expect that by seeing numerous normal and pathological images, the machine/neural network can decipher the salient features that define each pathology and then use these features to predict pathology in unseen images. The above applications are also the first to come to mind because significant progress has been made in these areas. For example, in May 2019, Google developed a deep learning algorithm for the detection of lung cancer by computed tomography. The deep learning model achieved an area under the receiver operating curve of 94.4% and the model outperformed six radiologists in the diagnosis while at the same time having an absolute reduction of 11% in false positives and 5% in false negatives [1].

Often anesthesiology is not associated with machine learning because the use of images to detect pathology plays a much smaller role in this field than in other healthcare fields. However, machine learning encompasses far more than just image analysis. Machine learning involves a system that is able to perform a task without being explicitly programmed but rather based on algorithms, statistical models, regression, and/or pattern recognition. In addition, the machine learning system is able to learn and improve from experience. This experience is often gained through data, which could include tabular data or pixilated data. In anesthesia, there is a plethora of tabular data. This data could be individual case data, which may consist of variables including gender, age, height, weight, medications, allergies, heart rate, respiratory rate, blood pressure, and temperature. These types of variables, especially those that are monitored and can fluctuate, such as vital signs, can be provided to a machine learning model in combination with another variable of interest such as hypotension. With enough information, the machine learning model can analyze the data in order to develop an association between the dependent variables and the independent outcome variable. After the creation of this type of regression model, the neural network can be provided with new cases/data and can predict the outcome variable based on the association it developed from the training data. In addition, as the neural network is provided with more data, it will continue to update the association between the variables it developed before. As such, this model is performing the task of predicting an independent variable without any explicit algorithm or brute force mechanism being implemented by a user, and the model is learning and improving from experience. The above theoretical example provides some of the underlying information as to how machine learning can be utilized in anesthesiology. Later in this chapter, concrete examples of machine learning in action in anesthesia are provided.

Automation in the field of anesthesiology is not new. One of the earliest recorded implementations of automation includes Bickford's efforts in 1950 [2]. Bickford recognized a relationship between the summated value of brain potentials and the degree to which the central nervous system was depressed by the anesthetic agent. With this information, Bickford designed an apparatus to automate the maintenance of anesthesia.

Since 1950, new variables and new combinations of these variables have been identified that more accurately correlate to the depth of anesthesia. Integrating this information into machines led the Food and Drug Administration to approve Sedasys computer-assisted personalized sedation [3]. This machine was designed to integrate propofol delivery to the patient with monitoring of the patient through measures including pulse oximetry, electrocardiogram, and patient response to auditory and tactile stimuli [4]. There were limitations to its use: only for mild to moderate sedation and only for either a colonoscopy or an esophagogastroduodenoscopy [5]; however, the Sedasys machine is a great example of how automation and the use of algorithm have been used to aid anesthesiologists.

In general, much of the automation that has been developed in anesthesiology requires a programmer to input an algorithm that the machine uses in order to solve a task. The identification of this algorithm is very much still dependent on a human. Furthermore, with new information, it is up to the human to update the algorithm, which often takes time and leads to delay in implementation. This can be compared to machine learning in which the neural network identifies the algorithm and continuously updates it as new data are provided.

1.2 MACHINE LEARNING IMPLEMENTATION IN ANESTHESIA

In the last few years, several applications of machine learning have been implemented in anesthesia including preoperative, perioperative, and postoperative applications.

1.2.1 Hypotension

Two research studies have involved the prediction of hypotension after anesthesia induction. Hatib and colleagues used the dependent variable, high-fidelity arterial pressure waveform, in order to predict the onset of hypotension prior to its actual onset [6]. For training, 545,959 minutes of arterial waveform recording and 25,461 episodes of hypotension were included. In addition, for validation, 33,326 minutes of arterial waveform recording and 1,923 episodes of hypotension were included. Even though on the surface it seems that there was only one dependent variable being analyzed, in fact, over 3,000 individual features were selected from the arterial pressure waveform and each one was run in the analysis in order to generate a receiver operating curve. Afterward, 51 features were selected based on having an area under the curve (AUC) on the receiver operative curve of greater than 0.85. These 51 features/variables with their reciprocal and squared terms and in combination generated a total of over 2.6 million total variables. The model was then able to calculate linear and nonlinear relationships between these variables and hypotension. In the end, the model used 3,022 individual features and achieved a sensitivity, specificity, and AUC of 88%, 87%, and 0.95, respectively, when predicting a hypotensive event 15 minutes before its onset. In predicting a hypotensive event 5 minutes before its onset, these values increased to 92%, 92%, and 0.97, respectively. In addition, Kendale and colleagues implemented machine learning in the prediction of postinduction hypotension [7]. However, in this analysis, the dependent variables included additional characteristics, such as demographics, preoperative medications, medical comorbidities, induction medications, and intraoperative vital signs. In addition, eight different supervised machine-learning classification techniques (logistic regression, support vector machines, naïve Bayes, K-nearest neighbor, linear discriminant analysis, random forest, neural network, and gradient boosting machine) were compared for their performance. Gradient boosting was found to have the highest AUC and the final model had an AUC of 0.77. The better performance of gradient boosting aligns with the type of data as it performs well with class imbalance. Finally, the dependent variables were compared for their importance in the prediction of postinduction hypotension. The top five in importance were first mean arterial pressure, age, BMI, mean peak inspiratory pressure, and maximum sevoflurane concentration. In addition, the model uncovered a high importance of the medications- levothyroxine and bisphosphonates, which would likely not have been expected. Predicting hypotension is a very challenging task and if machine learning and artificial intelligence continue to progress as in the above two studies, anesthesiologists will be less likely to be caught off guard and therefore will be able to provide treatment more quickly and more effectively, possibly even providing preventive treatment in some cases.

1.2.2 Hypoxia

Another study performed a gradient boosting machine model in order to predict hypoxemia during surgery [8]. Some of the features/variables included were patient demographics (e.g. BMI), BP, respiration rate, O_2 flow, medications, SpO_2, and time since the start of the procedure. The machine learning system was utilized for initial risk prediction and for real-time hypoxemia prediction. In both cases, the combination of an anesthesiologist and the machine learning system led to a statistically significant ($P<0.0001$) increase in the AUC. With the amount of data that is available prior to surgery and during surgery, machine learning can provide clinicians with a support system to help them predict life-threatening cases before they occur.

1.2.3 Depth of Anesthesia

Monitoring the depth of anesthesia during a surgical procedure is crucial for patient safety and patient comfort. A high depth of anesthesia can lead to delayed recovery time, hypotension, and decreased perfusion to vital organs. On the other hand, a low depth of anesthesia can lead to post-traumatic stress. Saadeh and colleagues designed a machine learning-based EEG processor that estimated the depth of anesthesia [9]. Six features were extracted from the EEG (spectral edge frequency, beta ratio, and four bands of spectral energy) and were then used in the machine learning system to classify the depth of anesthesia as deep, moderate, light, or awake. During testing, the system achieved 92.2% accuracy in classifying the depth of anesthesia, again highlighting the benefit of machine learning in the operating room.

1.2.4 Mortality Prediction

Predicting mortality is often a task left up to a higher power. In clinical practice, risk scores have been developed that help to quantify the risk such as with the American Society of Anesthesiologists Physical Status Classification or the surgical Apgar score. However, there are some limitations to these. The American Society of Anesthesiologists Physical Status Classification is subjective and has a high inter-rater variability. The surgical Apgar score provides a fast way for clinicians to predict postoperative risks; however, this quickness is also a drawback as only three features/variables are included in its calculation. Lee and colleagues developed a deep neural network that uses 45 features/variables from the end of the surgery and combined it with preoperative information from the American Society of Anesthesiologists (ASA) Physical Status Classification in order to predict postoperative in-hospital mortality [10]. This deep neural network had an AUC of 0.91, which was higher than the AUC for surgical Apgar (AUC=0.58) or ASA (AUC=0.84) alone. Although research on the implementation of machine learning in anesthesia lags behind that in other health care fields, the above research studies demonstrate the tremendous benefit it can provide to anesthesiologists and patients.

1.3 LIMITATIONS

Machine learning and artificial intelligence do not come without limitations, especially in the healthcare field. While there is a large amount of data available preoperatively, intraoperatively, and postoperatively in the anesthesia field, much of the data exists in raw format and has not been processed or analyzed. Furthermore, much of the machine learning research in this field is done in one hospital or hospitals in a network that are typically in one geographic region. This presents a significant challenge for real-world application of the machine learning model as there are significant differences in the patient demographics between hospitals. One of the main limitations would likely be that the machine learning model would have seen data predominantly from one ethnicity in that geographic region and so it would not understand or would not be able to account for the inter-ethnic differences. In addition, while anesthesiology is a data-driven field and large amounts of data are monitored, there are few publically available databases. This is a major difference as compared to the field of radiology or pathology where such publically available databases exist. The lack of this public database in anesthesia hinders programmers from testing the machine learning system and developing methods for improving its accuracy. Another challenge in anesthesiology as compared to other healthcare fields is that anesthesiologists have to quickly recognize problems and even more quickly fix the problem. Fields like dermatology have the luxury that typically a skin condition is unlikely to cause severe health consequences in seconds to minutes. The dermatologist can take a picture of the skin condition and then run it through the machine learning algorithm to help identify the cause. However, in the surgical room, seconds can make the difference between recovery and tragedy. As such, the machine learning system that is implemented in anesthesia has to be seamless and must not require significant input from the anesthesiologist during the surgery. Furthermore, with the addition of a new technology in the hospital, the security risk will grow immensely. The machine learning software is provided a large amount of patient data. The data would need to be de-identified and security measures would have to be in place to prevent the hacking of the infrastructure. The latter is especially important in automated technology. Earlier it was mentioned that the Sedasys computer-assisted personalized sedation machine assisted in the administration of propofol. If this device is not secured from potential attacks, it could lead to disastrous consequences for the patient. Although the

Sedasys computer-assisted personalized sedation machine was approved by the Food and Drug Administration and was being tested in a couple of hospitals, the parent company - Johnson and Johnson - pulled the machine from the market due to slow sales [11]. The specific reason for the slowing down of sales was not provided, but it can be predicted that hospitals and patients are not yet comfortable with automation in potentially life-threatening situations like the administration of anesthesia.

1.4 CONCLUSION

In the last few years, research on the use of machine learning to improve patient health has skyrocketed. This research in the anesthesia field is no different, albeit slower than in other fields in healthcare. The field of anesthesiology contains a huge amount of data, which presents the perfect opportunity for machine learning implementation.

REFERENCES

[1] Ardila D, Kiraly AP, Bharadwaj S, Choi B, Reicher JJ, Peng L, et al. End-to-end lung cancer screening with three-dimensional deep learning on low-dose chest computed tomography. *Nat Med.* 2019;25: 954–961. doi:10.1038/s41591-019-0447-x

[2] Bickford RG. Automatic electroencephalographic control of general anesthesia. *Electroencephalogr Clin Neurophysiol.* 1950;2: 93–96. doi:10.1016/0013-4694(50)90014-9

[3] Boggs S. Computer-Assisted Personalized Sedation (CAPS): Will it Change the Way Moderate Sedation is Administered? In: Anesthesia Business Consultants [Internet]. [cited 19 Dec 2019]. Available: https://www.anesthesiallc.com/publications/communiques/83-communique/past-issues/fall-2014/698-computer-assisted-personalized-sedation-caps-will-it-change-the-way-moderate-sedation-is-administered

[4] Pambianco DJ, Vargo JJ, Pruitt RE, Hardi R, Martin JF. Computer-assisted personalized sedation for upper endoscopy and colonoscopy: a comparative, multicenter randomized study. *Gastrointest Endosc.* 2011;73: 765–772. doi:10.1016/j.gie.2010.10.031

[5] Boggs S. Computer-Assisted Personalized Sedation—The Beginning or the End of the Anesthesia Provider? In: Anesthesia Business Consultants [Internet]. [cited 19 Dec 2019]. Available: https://www.anesthesiallc.com/publications/blog/entry/computer-assisted-personalized-sedation-the-beginning-or-the-end-of-the-anesthesia-provider

[6] Hatib F, Jian Z, Buddi S, Lee C, Settels J, Sibert K, et al. Machine-learning Algorithm to Predict Hypotension Based on High-fidelity Arterial Pressure Waveform Analysis. *Anesthesiology.* 2018;129: 663–674. doi:10.1097/ALN.0000000000002300

[7] Kendale S, Kulkarni P, Rosenberg AD, Wang J. Supervised Machine-learning Predictive Analytics for Prediction of Postinduction Hypotension. *Anesthesiol J Am Soc Anesthesiol.* 2018;129: 675–688. doi:10.1097/ALN.0000000000002374

[8] Lundberg SM, Nair B, Vavilala MS, Horibe M, Eisses MJ, Adams T, et al. Explainable machine-learning predictions for the prevention of hypoxaemia during surgery. *Nat Biomed Eng.* 2018;2: 749–760. doi:10.1038/s41551-018-0304-0

[9] Saadeh W, Khan FH, Altaf MAB. Design and Implementation of a Machine Learning Based EEG Processor for Accurate Estimation of Depth of Anesthesia. *IEEE Trans Biomed Circuits Syst.* 2019;13: 658–669. doi:10.1109/TBCAS.2019.2921875

[10] Lee CK, Hofer I, Gabel E, Baldi P, Cannesson M. Development and Validation of a Deep Neural Network Model for Prediction of Postoperative In-Hospital Mortality. *Anesthesiology.* 2018;129: 649–662. doi:10.1097/ALN.0000000000002186

[11] Novak R. Robot Anesthesia. In: The anesthesia consultant [Internet]. 27 Nov 2012 [cited 19 Dec 2019]. Available: https://theanesthesiaconsultant.com/2012/11/27/robot-anesthesia/

CHAPTER 2

Dermatological Machine Learning Clinical Decision Support System

Pushkar Aggarwal

University of Cincinnati College of Medicine
Cincinnati, Ohio

CONTENTS

2.1 BACKGROUND

Dermatology is a subject that relies on morphological features and the majority of diagnoses are based on visual pattern recognition. At present, the skin imaging technology is represented by dermoscopy, very high-frequency ultrasound, and reflectance confocal microscopy. Each method of skin imaging equipment has its own advantages and limitations. Dermatologists need to choose different imaging methods according to different conditions of skin lesions. The skin imaging technology has become a vitally important tool for clinical diagnosis of skin diseases and is widely accepted and applied worldwide [1]. As such, dermatology is exceedingly suitable for applying artificial intelligence (AI) image recognition capabilities for assisted diagnosis.

In 2013, one out of every four Americans saw a physician regarding a skin disease [2]. The overall prevalence of skin disease in the U.S. is estimated to be around 27%. In those who are 65 years or older, the prevalence increases to around 49%, and the average number of skin diseases per person increases from 1.6 to 2.2. Furthermore, of the total number of deaths in 2013, skin disease accounted for almost 1 out of every 100. Assuming a potential life expectancy of 75 years, it was found that fatal skin disease resulted in almost 11 years of potential life loss [2]. Melanoma is the most deadly skin cancer, accounting for 75% of all skin cancer-related death, and is responsible for over 10,000 deaths annually in the U.S. [3]. Melanoma is the leading cause of cancer death in 25–30 years old women and the second most commonly diagnosed cancer in those who are 15–29 years of age [4]. The incidence of melanoma doubled from 11.2 per 100,000 people in 1982 to 22.7 per 100,000 people in 2011. Other skin conditions while not being as deadly as melanoma can still have a significant impact on a person. Acne affects about 50 million Americans annually and is the most common skin condition in the U.S. [5]. Rosacea and psoriasis affect about 15 million people and 8 million people in the U.S., respectively [6,7]. Non-melanoma skin cancer and melanoma combine for about $6 billion in medical costs each year. Other skin conditions such as acne, psoriasis, seborrheic dermatitis, and atopic dermatitis account for $846, $737, $339, and $314 million each year, respectively [2]. Therefore, AI implementation in dermatology has the potential to significantly benefit the health and finances of a large part of the population.

AI applies automated learning and provides output based upon large data. Previously, large data were not available or were not assimilated together in a standardized form. The advent and extensive use of computers have helped in assimilating large data sets in many medical fields, including dermatology. AI tries to mimic the human brain in reproducing human cognition and can be an asset in dermatology clinical evaluations.

2.2 MELANOMA

Much of the machine learning implementation in the field of dermatology encompasses the binary classification of malignant melanoma versus benign nevi. One criterion that is often used in the clinical diagnosis of melanoma is the ABCDE criteria – asymmetry, border (irregular), color (two or more colors), diameter greater than 6 mm, and enlargement or evolution in size [8]. The first four criteria are potential criteria that a machine learning algorithm can use during its assessment of the lesion.

One of the major studies in the field of machine learning in melanoma diagnosis involved training a convolutional neural network (CNN) with about 130,000 images that encompassed more than 2,000 different diseases [9]. This CNN was then used to classify melanocytic lesions as either benign or malignant. The analysis was performed separately on photographic images and on dermoscopic images. On photographic images, the CNN has an area under the curve (AUC) of 0.96 when tested on 225 images, and on dermoscopic images, the CNN has an AUC of 0.94 when tested on 1,010 images. In this study, dermatologists were also shown the same test images that were inputted into the CNN, and the dermatologists were asked to classify each image as benign or malignant. For both the photographic and dermoscopic images, the CNN outperformed the average dermatologist in this classification.

A similar study was performed to assess the performance of machine learning in differentiating between malignant melanoma and benign melanocytic as compared to the ability of dermatologists to do the same [10]. In this study, dermatologists were first given the image and asked whether the lesion was benign or malignant. Next, they were provided clinical information and supplemental close-up images and asked to perform the same differentiation. At the dermatologists' mean sensitivity, the CNN had a statistically significant higher specificity than the dermatologists' specificity. The statistically significant higher specificity of the CNN occurred in the stage in which dermatologists were not given clinical information and supplemental close-up images and in the stage in which they were given that information. Furthermore, the mean AUC of the CNN was higher than the mean receiver operating curve area of dermatologists in both stages. This study shows that even with a lack of clinical information, the machine learning neural network was able to outperform dermatologists. Overall, machine learning has been shown to provide very good results in differentiating malignant melanoma from benign nevi.

2.3 NON-MELANOMA MACHINE LEARNING

Machine learning has been implemented in the dermatological field beyond just binary classification of malignant melanoma. Some examples include classification of acne, rosacea, impetigo, psoriasis, atopic dermatitis, seborrheic dermatitis, lichen planus, and pityriasis rosea, among many more [11,12]. Some of these neural networks were tasked with classifying multiple different diseases as compared to a binary classification. This not only presents a significant challenge for the neural network, but also simulates real-world conditions better.

One study examined the ability of a CNN as a binary classification for onychomycosis. The CNN was trained with over 49,000 images and was found to have a higher diagnostic accuracy than dermatologists who were given the same test images [13]. Another study used machine learning to classify ten types of lesions – actinic keratosis, basal cell carcinoma, melanocytic nevus/mole, squamous cell carcinoma, seborrhoeic keratosis, intraepithelial carcinoma, pyogenic granuloma, hemangioma, dermatofibroma, and malignant melanoma [14]. As one would expect, the more the classifying categories that the model is expected to differentiate, the lower the accuracy. Part of this is due to the limited number of images that are often available for some of the categories. Also, the chances of the model guessing and getting the correct answer have decreased fivefold from a binary classifier to a ten-category classifier. In the study, the ten-category classifier model had an accuracy of 81.8% while another run was performed with the model being only a five-category classifier (the first five of the ten types of lesions are listed above) and this model had an accuracy of 85.8%. Both of these models still showed good accuracy but also demonstrated the effect of increasing the number of categories. In order to keep the accuracy high as the number of categories for the model to classify increases, it will be imperative to input clinical information such as age, gender, race, time of onset, duration, location, irritation, itching, stinging, type of discharge, evolution, and family history among others to the neural network. This is likely the next step in the field of machine learning in dermatology.

2.4 NON-SKIN IMAGE RECOGNITION MACHINE LEARNING

The primary thought that comes to mind when thinking of the applicability of machine learning in the field of dermatology is the use of skin images to classify diseases. However, machine learning encompasses far more as it can use all types of data (pixilated or non-pixilated).

Apart from image recognition, machine learning has to been used to predict the severity of epidermolysis bullosa simplex [15]. In this study, the neural network was provided the position and type of mutation in the genome and tasked with predicting the severity of the disease. The model had a 78% accuracy rate, although the training and testing data were limited. However, this provides an example of the non-image recognition application of machine learning in dermatology. Another study used near-infrared Fourier transform Raman spectra to assess the ability of a neural network in the diagnosis of melanoma [16]. As opposed to feeding the neural network skin images of the lesion, punch biopsies were performed, and then an interferometer was used for obtaining the Raman spectra. The neural network had a sensitivity of 85% and a sensitivity of 99% for the diagnosis of melanoma. This is another example of how information other than skin images can be used by neural networks in aiding the clinician's diagnosis.

2.5 DATA AUGMENTATION

In the last few years, there has been a major push to develop methods to improve the accuracy of neural networks. One such method is through the use of data/image augmentation. This technique involves the use of various techniques such as cropping, altering brightness, and altering shear among others in order to simulate the real-world variability of images and to provide the neural network with multiple images from just one image. The latter is especially important as there is a paucity of high-quality dermatological images with an associated accurate and verified diagnosis. In addition, the data augmentation can help to decrease the likelihood of overfitting of the model. Data augmentation has been implemented in dermatological machine learning with good results.

For example, a deep learning model that was used to classify acne, atopic dermatitis, rosacea, psoriasis, and impetigo was re-run with data augmentation in order to assess its impact on the model [11]. Data augmentation techniques used in this analysis included rotation, zoom, shear, and horizontal and vertical flipping. These techniques helped to provide the model with some of the variability that can exist in the location and size of the lesion and also the angle at which the image is taken. Addition of these data augmentation techniques resulted in an average Matthews correlation coefficient increase of 7.7%. Furthermore, the AUC for each of the dermatological conditions being classified increased. The mean AUC increase was 13.2% with a standard deviation of 0.033. These results highlight the significant improvement that data augmentation can have on the accuracy of the deep learning models in classifying dermatological lesions. Furthermore, it can be especially useful when the deep learning model is classifying multiple conditions/diseases as opposed to being a binary classifier.

In another example, in the classification of melanoma using a deep learning model, eight augmentation techniques and a combination (mix and match) of these eight were implemented and assessed for their improvement/decrement in the accuracy of the model [17]. The augmentation techniques included saturation, contrast, and brightness; saturation, contrast, brightness, and hue; affine (rotate, shear, scaling, and adding pixels symmetrically at the edge); flipping; cropping; random replacement of image with noise; warping; and mixing two lesions into one image. These changes can help to account for the variability in images taken by different cameras, by different picture takers and account for the variability in the setting/background among others. Another feature of this study was that three different CNNs were run in parallel to account for the variability among the CNNs. The study found that geometric augmentation (affine, cropping, and warping) had a more consistent improvement in all three CNNs than did color augmentation (saturation, contrast, brightness, and hue). Some augmentation techniques such as random erasing resulted in worse performance or only slight improvements in the model. Cropping was shown to significantly improve the accuracy of the model. The highest AUC in this study was found with the following combined augmentation techniques: random cropping, affine, flipping, and saturation and contrast, brightness, and hue. Overall, data augmentation has proven to be a very useful method by which the accuracy of a neural network can be improved. More complex data augmentation techniques such as Gaussian blur are likely to be implemented in the future to dermatological image analysis to assess their impact on the model.

2.6 LIMITATIONS

Some of the issues/limitations with the adaptation of AI at present are enumerated below:

a. Ethical issues and data privacy in sharing of patient data and images

b. Quality of images taken by patients or under sub-optimal lighting conditions

c. Lack of standardization of training images

d. Transportability/sharing of images

e. Quality and capability of image recognition programs

f. Reliability – sensitivity and specificity of output

g. Lack of integration of clinical symptoms, patient characteristics, other disease status, etc.

h. Lack of clinical expertise and clinical experience of health professionals in the programs

i. Lack of integration of genetic characteristics

j. Software programmers and physicians – experts in their own fields – are less likely to integrate their thoughts/expertise

k. Complex and multitude of dermatology manifestations

l. Deciphering the root cause of the dermatological manifestation

m. Legal issues

n. Regulatory issues and commercialization

o. Lack of humanity and care of physicians/communication with patients

p. Integration of cognitive recognition/computing

q. Differentiating similar dermatological manifestations due to underlying different clinical conditions.

2.7 FUTURE DIRECTIONS

The future of AI in dermatology will be the integration of various AI applications in medicine and not just solely dermatological image recognition. The following AI applications may be integrated.

a. Lab and diagnostic test results interpretation using AI

b. Personal characteristics (sex, race, age, etc.) disposition to some diseases using AI

c. Clinical symptoms processing using AI

d. Cognitive computing

e. Genetic dispositions and changes in genetic markers

f. Latest research and guidelines for diagnosis as well as probable treatments

g. Changes in images during the treatment phase

h. Adverse event analysis from various probable treatments

The output of the AI model would be the probable diagnosis aid as well as the probable treatment direction for consideration by the dermatologist. The clinical decision support system would aid the dermatologist not only in accurate diagnosis and treatment therapies, but also in monitoring the progress/remission of the disease.

2.8 CONCLUSION

Machine learning has been used in various aspects in the field of dermatology. A large part of the already conducted research has been on the diagnosis of melanoma using machine learning. However, other skin diseases such as psoriasis and atopic dermatitis are also being integrated. In addition, non-image machine learning for both diagnosing and for prognosis/severity of dermatological conditions has also been developed. Future research will likely consist of developing ways to improve the accuracy of the model, for example, by addition of new data augmentation techniques or improvement/fine-tuning of old data augmentation techniques and by the addition of clinical information such as age, gender, race, time of onset, location, evolution, and family history to the dermatological image being used to train the neural network. In the coming years, AI has the potential to provide a second opinion and ultimately expert opinion to the dermatologists and act as a clinical decision system with high sensitivity and specificity.

REFERENCES

1. Li C-X, Shen C-B, Xue K, Shen X, Jing Y, Wang Z-Y, et al. Artificial intelligence in dermatology: past, present, and future. *Chin Med J (Engl).* 2019;132: 2017–2020. doi:10.1097/CM9.0000000000000372
2. Lim HW, Collins SAB, Resneck JS, Bolognia JL, Hodge JA, Rohrer TA, et al. The burden of skin disease in the United States. *J Am Acad Dermatol.* 2017;76: 958-972.e2. doi:10.1016/j.jaad.2016.12.043
3. Esteva A, Kuprel B, Novoa RA, Ko J, Swetter SM, Blau HM, et al. Dermatologist-level classification of skin cancer with deep neural networks. *Nature.* 2017;542: 115–118. doi:10.1038/nature21056
4. Mealnoma Fact Sheet. Melanoma Research Foundation; Available: https://melanoma.org/sites/default/files/2017MelanomaFactSheet.pdf
5. Skin conditions by the numbers. In: American Academy of Dermatolgoy [Internet]. Available: https://www.aad.org/media/stats-numbers

6. Okhovat J-P, Armstrong AW. Updates in Rosacea: Epidemiology, Risk Factors, and Management Strategies. *Curr Dermatol Rep.* 2014;3: 23–28. doi:10.1007/s13671-014-0070-5
7. Psoriasis Statistics. In: National Psoriasis Foundation [Internet]. Available: https://www.psoriasis.org/content/statistics
8. Clinical Diagnosis of Melanoma. *Am Fam Physician.* 2008;78: 1205.
9. Esteva A, Kuprel B, Novoa RA, Ko J, Swetter SM, Blau HM, et al. Dermatologist-level classification of skin cancer with deep neural networks. *Nature.* 2017;542: 115–118. doi:10.1038/nature21056
10. Haenssle HA, Fink C, Schneiderbauer R, Toberer F, Buhl T, Blum A, et al. Man against machine: diagnostic performance of a deep learning convolutional neural network for dermoscopic melanoma recognition in comparison to 58 dermatologists. *Ann Oncol Off J Eur Soc Med Oncol.* 2018;29: 1836–1842. doi:10.1093/annonc/mdy166
11. Aggarwal SLP. Data augmentation in dermatology image recognition using machine learning. *Skin Res Technol Off J Int Soc Bioeng Skin ISBS Int Soc Digit Imaging Skin ISDIS Int Soc Skin Imaging ISSI.* 2019;25: 815–820. doi:10.1111/srt.12726
12. Bobrova M, Taranik M, Kopanitsa G. Using Neural Networks for Diagnosing in Dermatology. *Stud Health Technol Inform.* 2019;261: 211–216.
13. Han SS, Park GH, Lim W, Kim MS, Na JI, Park I, et al. Deep neural networks show an equivalent and often superior performance to dermatologists in onychomycosis diagnosis: Automatic construction of onychomycosis datasets by region-based convolutional deep neural network. *PloS One.* 2018;13: e0191493. doi:10.1371/journal.pone.0191493
14. Kawahara J, BenTaieb A, Hamarneh G. Deep features to classify skin lesions. 2016 IEEE 13th International Symposium on Biomedical Imaging (ISBI). 2016. pp. 1397–1400. doi:10.1109/ISBI.2016.7493528
15. Eapen BR. "Neural network" algorithm to predict severity in epidermolysis bullosa simplex. *Indian J Dermatol Venereol Leprol.* 2005;71: 106–108. doi:10.4103/0378-6323.13995
16. Gniadecka M, Philipsen PA, Wessel S, Gniadecki R, Wulf HC, Sigurdsson S, et al. Melanoma Diagnosis by Raman Spectroscopy and Neural Networks: Structure Alterations in Proteins and Lipids in Intact Cancer Tissue. *J Invest Dermatol.* 2004;122: 443–449. doi:10.1046/j.0022-202X.2004.22208.x
17. Perez F, Vasconcelos C, Avila S, Valle E. Data Augmentation for Skin Lesion Analysis. ISIC Skin Image Anal Workshop. 2018. Available: https://arxiv.org/pdf/1809.01442.pdf

CHAPTER 3

Vision and AI

Mohini Bindal

Baylor College of Medicine
Houston, Texas

Pushkar Aggarwal

University of Cincinnati College of Medicine
Cincinnati, Ohio

CONTENTS

3.1 INTRODUCTION

The current world population is 7.7 billion, of which at least 2.2 billion (28.6%) has visual impairment [1]. In 2015, it was estimated that 36 million people were blind [2]. Early diagnosis and treatment of ophthalmological diseases are crucial in order to decrease this prevalence and to improve the quality of life of those affected. In the last few years, machine learning has made significant strides in various aspects of healthcare, including ophthalmology. In ophthalmology, a majority of research on the integration of machine learning has focused on the diagnosis of diabetic retinopathy and age-related macular degeneration (AMD). In the last few years, researchers have been investigating the application of machine learning to other diseases, such as glaucoma.

3.2 DIABETIC RETINOPATHY

In 2010, it was estimated that 126.6 million people have diabetic retinopathy, of which 37.3 million have vision-threatening diabetic retinopathy. It was also predicted that by 2030, these numbers would increase to 191.0 million and 56.3 million, respectively [3]. Globally, diabetic retinopathy is the leading cause of vision loss in those between 20 and 74 years of age. However, only 33% of those with diabetes mellitus have characteristic symptoms [4]. Machine learning presents an opportunity by which early detection and correct diagnosis of diabetic retinopathy can be performed.

Gulshan et al. at Google trained a convolutional neural network (CNN) on over 120,000 retinal images [5]. These retinal images were first graded by ophthalmologists for image quality and for the presence of diabetic retinopathy or diabetic macular edema. In addition to labeling the images, ophthalmologists assessed the severity of the images identified as diabetic retinopathy on the scale of none, mild, moderate, severe, or proliferative. Next, the images were presented to the CNN for training. Two sets of testing were performed and the CNN achieved an area under the curve (AUC) of 0.991 (95% confidence interval (CI), 0.988–0.993) on the first testing data set and 0.990 (95% CI, 0.986–0.995) on the second testing data set. Given that the highest AUC possible is 1.0, the above model performed exceptionally well.

One of the limitations of machine learning in healthcare is that most often the images that the CNN is trained and validated on are images of one or only a few ethnicities. The model is never exposed to the inter-ethnicity differences and as such its performance would be expected to drop significantly if it was to be used for a different population. Ting et al. tried to account for this variability [6]. Their CNN was trained primarily on retinal images from people of Chinese, Malay, and Indian ethnicity. However, during validation, the CNN was provided images from people of the following races/ethnicities: Chinese, Malay, Indian, African American, White, and Hispanic. For detection of diabetic retinopathy, 76,370 images were used during training, and 112,648 images were used during testing. The model had an AUC of 0.936 (95% CI, 0.925–0.943), a sensitivity of 90.5% (95% CI, 87.3%–93.0%), and a specificity of 91.6% (95% CI, 91.0%–92.2%). The inclusion of multiple ethnicities is expected to lower the accuracy of the model but achieving an AUC higher than 0.93 indicates that machine learning has the potential to tease out inter-ethnicity differences when analyzing retinal images.

In late 2018, Abràmoff et al. conducted a groundbreaking study in the use of artificial intelligence in the detection of diabetic retinopathy [7]. In this study, 900 people with a history of diabetes but no history of diabetic retinopathy were enrolled. The study population consisted of mostly Caucasians and African Americans but also included Asians (1.5%), American Indians or Alaskan Natives (0.4%), and Hispanics (~0.2%). During testing, the model had a sensitivity of 87.2% (95% CI, 81.8%–91.2%) and a specificity of 90.7% (95% CI, 88.3%–92.7%). For reference, the British Diabetic Association proposed that screening methods for diabetic retinopathy should have at least 80% sensitivity and specificity [8]. Based on the results of the study of Abràmoff et al., the Food and Drug Administration (FDA) authorized the use of their system by healthcare providers in the detection of "more than mild diabetic retinopathy in adults (22 years of age or older) diagnosed with diabetes who have not been previously diagnosed with diabetic retinopathy" [9]. As such, this became the first autonomous diagnostic artificial intelligence system to be authorized by the FDA in medicine.

3.3 AGE-RELATED MACULAR DEGENERATION

Aside from diabetic retinopathy, machine learning in ophthalmology has been studied extensively on the diagnosis of age-related macular degeneration (AMD). AMD is the leading cause of severe central visual acuity loss in those over 50 years of age. It has been estimated that 15 million people in North America suffer from AMD [10]. Direct healthcare cost of visual impairment due to AMD is estimated to be $255 billion globally [11].

In the implementation of machine learning in diagnosing AMD, one study examined the use of a binary classifier of normal versus AMD in optical coherence tomography (OCT) images, the most common imaging modality in ophthalmology [12]. About 50,000 normal macular OCT images and about 50,000 AMD images were used for training and validation of the deep neural network. Three analyses of the performance of the neural network were completed. On each image, the CNN had an AUC of 0.9277. When the images from the same OCT scan were grouped together and the probabilities from each image were averaged, the AUC improved to 0.9382. Finally, the probabilities from all the images from one patient were averaged together, and the AUC improved to 0.9746. Similar to the use of machine learning in diagnosing diabetic retinopathy, its use in diagnosing AMD looks promising.

Grassman et al. performed a similar analysis on the use of CNN in the diagnosis of AMD [13]. However, color fundus images were used as opposed to OCT images and six different neural net architectures were included in the study. The latter was especially important because various neural net architectures exist (Inception, Resnet, VGG, AlexNet, and GoogLeNet among others). While the six neural network architectures performed relatively similarly in the study, with the use of random forests, a model ensemble was created that combined the six neural networks. This ensemble outperformed each of the neural networks in the seven metrics that were measured. Researchers are looking for methods by which the accuracy of the CNN can be further increased beyond the baseline, and the mixing of the various neural networks into a model ensemble is an intriguing way to accomplish this.

3.4 GLAUCOMA

Compared to diabetic retinopathy and AMD, there has been significantly less research on the use of machine learning in diagnosing glaucoma. In 2013, the global prevalence of glaucoma in those aged 40–80 years was estimated to be 64.3 million and predicted to increase to 111.8 million in 2040 [14].

Deep learning for the detection of glaucomatous optic neuropathy has been performed by Li et al. [15]. One of the difficulties in assessing for glaucoma is that no cup-to-disc ratio has been established that defines pathological cupping because of the wide range of cup-to-disc ratio values in the normal population [16]. Li et al. defined referable glaucomatous optic neuropathy with a vertical cup-to-disc ratio of 0.7 or higher. In this study, a total of 31,745 fundus photographs were included in the training of the neural network, and 8,000 were included for the validation. The neural network achieved an AUC of 0.986 (95% CI, 0.984–0.988) and had a sensitivity and specificity of 95.6% and 92.0%, respectively. In addition, the most common reason for a false negative from the model was due to a coexisting eye condition such as myopia, diabetic retinopathy, and AMD. Coexisting conditions are often present during testing and are one of the areas in which deep learning has room to improve. As more diseases are presented to a neural network, it is expected that there will be a decrease in the accuracy of the neural network; however, if enough high-quality images are shown, the model may be able to return to higher accuracy levels. The primary reason for a false positive from the model was due to physiologic cupping. This represents one of the major barriers in using machine learning for glaucoma as cupping does not always indicate the presence of glaucoma. Information such as the previous cup-to-disc ratio, clinical presentation, and inner eye pressure among others would need to be provided to overcome this challenge.

3.5 MULTI-CLASSIFIER AND IMPROVING PERFORMANCE

As described above, one of the major challenges in machine learning is going from a binary classifier to a multi-classifier of disease processes while at the same time maintaining or improving the sensitivity and specificity of the model. De Fauw et al. [17] tried to tackle this and also used three-dimensional optical coherence tomography scans as opposed to the two-dimensional photographs that are often used in assessing the performance of machine learning in healthcare. The model first contained a segmentation network that analyzed the OCT image and labeled the segments of the image in one of the 15 possible classes. Some of the possible labels included neurosensory retina, intraretinal fluid, retinal pigment epithelium, and artifact such as from blinking. Next, the model contained a classification network that identified the image as urgent, semi-urgent, routine, or observation. The classification network also categorized the image among ten different OCT pathologies. Overall, the neural network achieved an AUC over 0.99 for most pathologies with the lowest being 0.9663. These results were on par with the performance of experts in the ophthalmology field when they were provided the OCT images. The results of this study show that machine learning can continue to provide high accuracy even when it is expected to diagnose among multiple pathologies.

Data augmentation has been studied extensively in the last few years in order to further improve the capabilities of machine learning. Data augmentation includes changing aspects of one image so that the neural network is exposed to variability that is often present in the real world. In ophthalmology, one study looked specifically at the impact of data augmentation in the performance of the neural network [18]. OCT images were inputted into the neural network and the model was expected to differentiate between five different OCT conditions: – acute macular degeneration, central serous retinopathy, diabetic retinopathy, macular hole, and normal. The specific data augmentation techniques used in this analysis included rotation, width and height shear, horizontal flip, and Gaussian noise. In Gaussian noise data augmentation, noise is added to the image based on the Gaussian distribution resulting in distortion of the high-frequency features of the model. The addition of these data augmentation techniques led to a 6% improvement in AUC (from 0.91 to 0.97) and the average sensitivity, specificity, positive predictive value (PPV), and negative predictive value (NPV) all increased. Data augmentation is a powerful tool in improving the capabilities of the CNN and future research will likely consist of fine-tuning these techniques in order to identify which ones have the most beneficial effect on performance and which combination of these techniques leads to the best overall performance.

3.6 MACHINE LEARNING FOR PREDICTING SURVIVAL/PROGNOSIS

Although most of the integration of machine learning in the field of ophthalmology has focused on image analysis, there has been some research on other applications of machine learning. For example, Damato et al. investigated the use of an artificial neural network on estimating the survival probability in patients after treatment of choroidal melanoma [19]. Patient characteristics such as age, sex, largest basal tumor diameter, ciliary body involvement, extraocular extension, tumor cell type, closed loops, mitotic rate, and the presence of monosomy chromosome 3 were used by the neural network to generate survival curves. The characteristics and risk factors were analyzed both individually and in combination. From the study, it was found that the most predictive factor in tumors of high-grade malignancy was the basal tumor diameter. In addition, combination analysis showed that the addition of cytogenetic and histological data in the model led to a decreased importance in certain factors including the ciliary body involvement and extraocular extension. Finding such interactions among several risk factors in order to predict survival is one of the advantages of the use of machine learning in healthcare.

3.7 CONCLUSION

Machine learning has made significant progress in diagnosing diabetic retinopathy and AMD. In the last few years, it has also been used for other ophthalmological conditions, including glaucoma, cataracts, and retinopathy of prematurity among others. Based on statistical measures such as AUC, sensitivity, and specificity, the neural networks indicate excellent performance in detecting many of these disease processes. The next stage of machine learning in ophthalmology will likely consist of the addition of fundus and OCT images from several ethnicities/races to better account for inter-ethnic variability. In addition, because of the success of machine learning in binary classification, further research will likely focus on using neural networks to make predictions among several disease processes.

In 2018, the FDA approved the use of artificial intelligence in the detection of diabetic retinopathy, and it is expected that as the deep learning models continue to improve, their adoption into the real-world healthcare setting will continue to grow. Finally, outside of image detection, machine learning has been shown to be useful in identifying risk factors for predicting the severity of ophthalmological diseases.

REFERENCES

[1] Vision impairment and blindness. In: World Health Organization [Internet]. [cited 19 Dec 2019]. Available: https://www.who.int/news-room/fact-sheets/detail/blindness-and-visual-impairment

[2] Bourne RRA, Flaxman SR, Braithwaite T, Cicinelli MV, Das A, Jonas JB, et al. Magnitude, temporal trends, and projections of the global prevalence of blindness and distance and near vision impairment: a systematic review and meta-analysis. *Lancet Glob Health.* 2017;5: e888–e897. doi:10.1016/S2214-109X(17)30293-0

[3] Zheng Y, He M, Congdon N. The worldwide epidemic of diabetic retinopathy. *Indian J Ophthalmol.* 2012;60: 428–431. doi:10.4103/0301-4738.100542

[4] Lee R, Wong TY, Sabanayagam C. Epidemiology of diabetic retinopathy, diabetic macular edema and related vision loss. *Eye Vis.* 2015;2. doi:10.1186/s40662-015-0026-2

[5] Gulshan V, Peng L, Coram M, Stumpe MC, Wu D, Narayanaswamy A, et al. Development and Validation of a Deep Learning Algorithm for Detection of Diabetic Retinopathy in Retinal Fundus Photographs. *JAMA.* 2016;316: 2402–2410. doi:10.1001/jama.2016.17216

[6] Ting DSW, Cheung CY-L, Lim G, Tan GSW, Quang ND, Gan A, et al. Development and Validation of a Deep Learning System for Diabetic Retinopathy and Related Eye Diseases Using Retinal Images From Multiethnic Populations With Diabetes. *JAMA.* 2017;318: 2211–2223. doi:10.1001/jama.2017.18152

[7] Abràmoff MD, Lavin PT, Birch M, Shah N, Folk JC. Pivotal trial of an autonomous AI-based diagnostic system for detection of diabetic retinopathy in primary care offices. *NPJ Digit Med.* 2018;1. doi:10.1038/s41746-018-0040-6

[8] Squirrell DM, Talbot JF. Screening for diabetic retinopathy. *J R Soc Med.* 2003;96: 273–276.

[9] Abràmoff MD, Lavin PT, Birch M, Shah N, Folk JC. Pivotal trial of an autonomous AI-based diagnostic system for detection of diabetic retinopathy in primary care offices. *NPJ Digit Med.* 2018;1. doi:10.1038/s41746-018-0040-6

[10] Age-Related Macular Degeneration. In: American Academy of Ophthalmology [Internet]. [cited 19 Dec 2019]. Available: https://www.aao.org/bcscsnippetdetail.aspx?id=9711f063-ed7b-452b-8708-c4dad0d893e8

[11] Age-Related Macular Degeneration: Facts & Figures. In: BrightFocus Foundation [Internet]. 4 Jul 2015 [cited 19 Dec 2019]. Available: https://www.brightfocus.org/macular/article/age-related-macular-facts-figures

[12] Lee CS, Baughman DM, Lee AY. Deep Learning Is Effective for Classifying Normal versus Age-Related Macular Degeneration OCT Images. *Ophthalmol Retina*. 2017;1: 322–327. doi:10.1016/j.oret.2016.12.009

[13] Grassmann F, Mengelkamp J, Brandl C, Harsch S, Zimmermann ME, Linkohr B, et al. A Deep Learning Algorithm for Prediction of Age-Related Eye Disease Study Severity Scale for Age-Related Macular Degeneration from Color Fundus Photography. *Ophthalmology*. 2018;125: 1410–1420. doi:10.1016/j.ophtha.2018.02.037

[14] Tham Y-C, Li X, Wong TY, Quigley HA, Aung T, Cheng C-Y. Global prevalence of glaucoma and projections of glaucoma burden through 2040: a systematic review and meta-analysis. *Ophthalmology*. 2014;121: 2081–2090. doi:10.1016/j.ophtha.2014.05.013

[15] Li Z, He Y, Keel S, Meng W, Chang RT, He M. Efficacy of a Deep Learning System for Detecting Glaucomatous Optic Neuropathy Based on Color Fundus Photographs. *Ophthalmology*. 2018;125: 1199–1206. doi:10.1016/j.ophtha.2018.01.023

[16] Ting DSW, Pasquale LR, Peng L, Campbell JP, Lee AY, Raman R, et al. Artificial intelligence and deep learning in ophthalmology. *Br J Ophthalmol*. 2019;103: 167–175. doi:10.1136/bjophthalmol-2018-313173

[17] Fauw JD, Ledsam JR, Romera-Paredes B, Nikolov S, Tomasev N, Blackwell S, et al. Clinically applicable deep learning for diagnosis and referral in retinal disease. *Nat Med*. 2018;24: 1342–1350. doi:10.1038/s41591-018-0107-6

[18] Aggarwal P. Machine learning of retinal pathology in optical coherence tomography images. *J Med Artif Intell*. 2019;2. doi:10.21037/jmai.2019.08.01

[19] Damato B, Eleuteri A, Fisher AC, Coupland SE, Taktak AFG. Artificial Neural Networks Estimating Survival Probability after Treatment of Choroidal Melanoma. *Ophthalmology*. 2008;115: 1598–1607. doi:10.1016/j.ophtha.2008.01.032

CHAPTER 4

Thermal Dose Modeling for Thermal Ablative Cancer Treatments by Cellular Neural Networks

Jinao Zhang and Sunita Chauhan

Monash University
Clayton, Australia

Wa Cheung and Stuart K. Roberts

The Alfred Hospital
Melbourne, Australia

CONTENTS

4.1 INTRODUCTION

Thermal ablative therapy is a type of cancer treatment in which cancer cells are killed *in situ* by inducing temperature alteration to cause cellular coagulation necrosis. The commonly deployed thermal ablative methods include hyperthermia (e.g., ablation using radiofrequency (RFA), microwave (MWA), laser and high-intensity focused ultrasound (HIFU)) and hypothermia (cryoablation), among which RFA is currently the most recommended first-line ablation technique [1]. In the treatment of hepatic cancers, thermal ablative therapy allows the treatment of primary (mainly hepatocellular carcinoma (HCC)) and secondary liver tumours without surgery and provides an alternative for patients who are not suitable for surgery or who do not wish to have surgery. Thermal ablation of small (<3 cm) liver tumours is very effective, achieved complete tumour necrosis in nearly all patients and provided similar survival outcomes to those undergoing liver resection [2]. It can achieve excellent long-term overall and tumour-specific survivals as a first-line stand-alone or bridge therapy to liver transplantation [3]. Moreover, the deployed methods in thermal ablative therapy are typically minimally invasive (such as percutaneous RFA) or non-invasive (such as HIFU), which are associated with benefits of less morbidity and mortality than those undergoing surgery.

To assist the operator of thermal ablation with better patient safety and greater ablation accuracy, computer-assisted treatment planning and analysis are becoming increasingly important to provide *in silico* analysis and estimation of tissue temperature and thermal damage [4]. To enable the operator of ablation to visualise the simulated results immediately to aid the treatment procedures, the numerical computation demands real-time solutions. It was reported that real-time computation and analysis of soft tissue temperature and associated thermal doses could help to improve the safety and effectiveness of the treatment [5] by precise management of the thermal energy to produce desired thermal damage to the tumour while avoiding thermally hot-spots and unintended thermal injuries in the surrounding healthy tissues. Not only can it lead to technological advancement in clinical procedures but also practical improvement in patient outcomes.

However, most of the conventional numerical methods [6–8] were developed for accurate approximation of the characteristics of bio-heat transfer in soft tissues without considering the need for fast computation. For instance, it was reported that using conventional methods to simulate a process of thermal ablation consumed calculation time ranging from several minutes to a few hours [9], which was primarily attributed to solving the non-linear bio-heat transfer at each time step during the simulation. Based on the finite difference method (FDM) [10], Schwenke et al. [11] and Kalantzis et al. [12] studied graphics processing unit (GPU)-based techniques for fast simulation of focused ultrasound treatments. Zhang et al. [13,14] and Mariappan et al. [15] presented GPU-accelerated finite element methodologies for high-speed solutions of bio-heat transfer for thermal ablation. He and Liu [16] devised an alternating direction explicit method, and Carluccio et al. [17] developed a methodology based on spatial filters to reduce computation time. Other methods such as fast explicit dynamics finite element algorithms [18,19], fast Fourier transform-based FDM algorithm [20], model order reduction method [21], finite volume-based multigrid methods [22,23] and meshless point collocation-based dynamic mode decomposition method [24] were also studied for fast bio-heat transfer analysis.

Recently, cellular neural networks (CNNs) have gained attention to be used in the biomechanics area [25–28] for fast numerical computation [29] due to the collective and simultaneous computing activity of cells. CNN was developed by Chua and Yang [30], which was primarily used for image processing such as noise removal, pattern recognition and feature extraction [31] (see the review paper [32] and book [33]). It was evident that CNN solutions could achieve excellent approximations to many non-linear partial differential equations including the reaction-diffusion equation, Burgers' equation, Navier–Stokes equation and heat equation [34,35], and therefore various non-linear dynamic systems including the mechanical vibrating systems [36], pattern formation and wave propagation [37], differential equations [29], deformable models [38,39] and bio-heat transfer problems [40,41] were modelled by CNN for efficient and effective solutions. In this work, given the computational characteristics, CNN is employed to efficiently solve the bio-heat transfer equation for thermal dose Modeling in biological soft tissues to provide computer-assisted planning and analysis for thermal ablative cancer treatments. It presents CNN formulations of the bio-heat transfer equation on 2D and 3D regular and irregular grids of the computational domain, and it employs the presented CNN models to predict soft tissue temperature distributions and to estimate the associated thermal doses, which are demonstrated using a clinically relevant scenario of local thermal ablation of liver tumours.

The remainder of this work is structured as follows: Section 4.2 introduces the fundamental governing equations for soft tissue thermal dose modeling, followed by introducing CNN architectures and CNN formulations on 2D and 3D regular and irregular grids in Section 4.3. Section 4.4 presents *in silico* results of a patient-specific thermal dose estimation and an application to HIFU ablation of hepatic tumours. Discussions are presented in Section 4.5, and Section 4.6 concludes the present work.

4.2 SOFT TISSUE THERMAL DOSE MODELING

The irreversible cellular protein denaturation and coagulation necrosis occur when soft biological tissues are attained with a certain temperature for a duration of time. Although some studies [42,43] assumed a regular shape such as a sphere or an ellipsoid for the approximation of the coagulation necrosis zone (lesion), it was shown that the extent of a lesion was related to the thermal dose attained in the tissue, which was a measure of tissue heat exposure history. An empirical measure of thermal dose, CEM_{43}, which relates the extent of a lesion to the cumulative equivalent minutes (CEM) of heat exposure at a tissue temperature of 43°C [44] is used in the present work, and it is considered that tumour necrosis occurs for 240 CEM_{43} [45]. Mathematically, CEM_{43} is computed by [44]

$$\mathrm{CEM}_{43} = \int^{t} R^{(43-T(t))} dt \tag{4.1}$$

where t is the duration of heat exposure, $T(t)$ is the local tissue temperature, and R is the constant, which is given by

$$R = \begin{cases} 0.25, & (T(t) < 43°\mathrm{C}) \\ 0.5, & (T(t) \geq 43°\mathrm{C}) \end{cases} \tag{4.2}$$

To determine the amount of CEM_{43}, the time evolution of the soft tissue temperature field (temperature-history) must be computed and recorded. The behaviour of heat transfer in biological soft tissues is modelled by the

Pennes bio-heat transfer equation [46], which accounts for the effects of heating and cooling of heat conduction, blood perfusion, metabolic heat generation, and external heat sources. It was validated against experiments [47,48] that the Pennes bio-heat model can offer reliable tissue temperature predictions, and it was widely used to model tumour management by hyperthermia and thermal ablative treatments [49–52]. For soft tissues of mass density ρ, specific heat capacity C, thermal conductivity k, blood perfusion rate w_b, blood specific heat capacity C_b, arterial blood temperature T_a, metabolic heat generation rate Q, and subject to an external heat source H, the Pennes bio-heat transfer equation is given by [46]

$$\rho C \frac{\partial T(t)}{\partial t} = \nabla \cdot \left(k \nabla T(t)\right) - w_b C_b \left(T(t) - T_a\right) + Q + H \tag{4.3}$$

where $\nabla \cdot$ represents the divergence operator, and ∇ represents the gradient operator.

4.3 CELLULAR NEURAL NETWORKS

4.3.1 Architecture

A CNN is a dynamic information-processing system that processes signals in real-time in a large-scale non-linear analogue circuit; the fundamental unit of a circuit in CNN is called a cell, and every cell is a time-continuous non-linear dynamic signal processing unit made of capacitors, resistors, and voltage-controlled current sources of linear and non-linear types [30]. Cells are interconnected and communicate with their adjacent neighbours [53]; as a result, it leads to a global propagation that cells not directly connected influence each other implicitly [54]. An example of a 2D CNN is shown in Figure 4.1. Owing to the behaviours of non-linear cell dynamics, local cell interaction, global cell propagation and simultaneous cell activity, CNNs are well suited for high-speed parallel signal processing such as

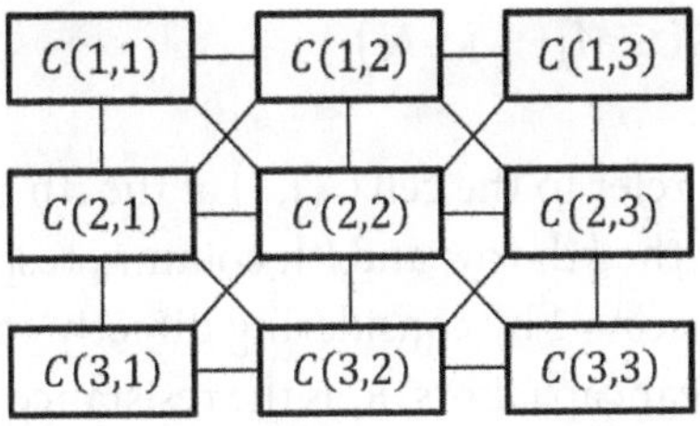

FIGURE 4.1 A 2D CNN of grid size 3×3: the rectangles are the cells, and the connections between cells denote local cell interactions.

fast computation of non-linear partial differential equations [29]. Hence, in analogy to the heat transfer equation with a given input of heat source that governs the non-linear bio-heat transfer behaviour in biological soft tissues, the presented CNN is formulated as the global propagation of a given current source (analogy to the heat source) through the locally interconnected activity of non-linear cell dynamics.

Consider a 2D CNN made of a rectangular computing array of $M \times N$ cells in M rows and N columns, the dynamics of CNN are given by [30]:

i. Cell state $v_{xij}(t)$

$$C_x \frac{dv_{xij}(t)}{dt} = -\frac{1}{R_x} v_{xij}(t) + \sum_{C(k,l)\in N_r(i,j)} A(i,j;k,l) v_{ykl}(t) + \sum_{C(k,l)\in N_r(i,j)} B(i,j;k,l) v_{ukl}(t) + I_{ij} \tag{4.4}$$

ii. Cell output $v_{yij}(t)$

$$v_{yij}(t) = \frac{1}{2}\left(\left|v_{xij}(t)+K\right| - \left|v_{xij}(t)-K\right|\right),\ K \geq 1 \tag{4.5}$$

iii. Constraint conditions

$$\left|v_{xij}(0)\right| \leq K;\ \left|v_{uij}\right| \leq K \tag{4.6}$$

iv. r-neighbourhood

$$N_r(i,j) = \left\{C(k,l) \mid \max\left\{|k-i|, |l-j|\right\} \leq r, 1 \leq k \leq M; 1 \leq l \leq N\right\} \quad (1 \leq i \leq M; 1 \leq j \leq N) \tag{4.7}$$

where (i,j) and (k,l) refer to the cell $C(i,j)$ at the ith row and jth column and the cell $C(k,l)$ at the kth row and lth column, respectively; r is a positive integer (in our case $r=1$ by considering directly connected cells); C_x is the capacitance of linear capacitors, R_x is the resistance of linear resistors, I_{ij} is the current of current sources, $A(i,j;k,l)$ is the output feedback operator

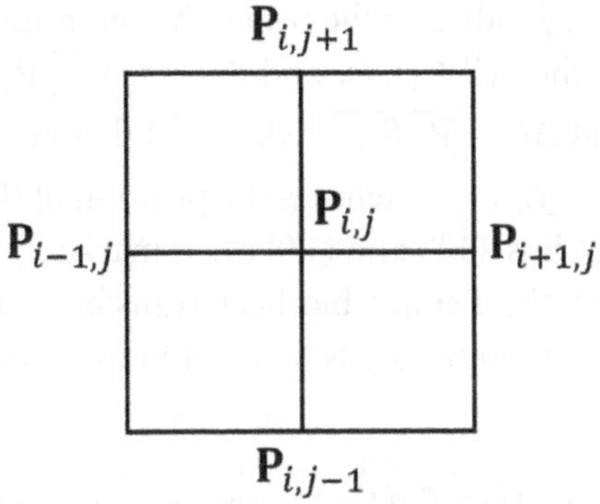

FIGURE 4.2 Bio-heat conduction on a 2D rectangular grid.

defining cell interactions with its adjacent neighbours and $B(i,j;k,l)$ is the input control operator defining the impact of input on the cell state; $v_{uij}(t)$, $v_{xij}(t)$ and $v_{yij}(t)$ are the input, state, and output of cell $C(i,j)$ at time t.

When there is no cell input, Eq. (4.4) can be written as

$$C_x \frac{dv_{xij}(t)}{dt} = -\frac{1}{R_x} v_{xij}(t) + \sum_{C(k,l)\in N_r(i,j)} A(i,j;k,l) v_{ykl}(t) + I_{ij} \tag{4.8}$$

which becomes an autonomous CNN [37].

4.3.2 CNN Formulation of Bio-Heat Transfer on 2D Grids

4.3.2.1 2D Regular Grids

As illustrated in Figure 4.2, the CNN formulation of bio-heat transfer on a 2D rectangular grid is achieved by using FDM to discretise the Pennes bio-heat transfer equation in the spatial domain, yielding:

$$\begin{aligned}\rho_{i,j}C_{i,j}\frac{\partial T_{i,j}(t)}{\partial t} &= -\left(\frac{2k_{i,j}}{\Delta u_{i-1}\Delta u_i} + \frac{2k_{i,j}}{\Delta v_{j-1}\Delta v_j} + w_{b,i,j}C_{b,i,j}\right)T_{i,j}(t)\\ &+ \frac{2k_{i+1,j}T_{i+1,j}(t)}{\Delta u_i(\Delta u_{i-1}+\Delta u_i)} + \frac{2k_{i-1,j}T_{i-1,j}(t)}{\Delta u_{i-1}(\Delta u_{i-1}+\Delta u_i)} + \frac{2k_{i,j+1}T_{i,j+1}(t)}{\Delta v_j(\Delta v_{j-1}+\Delta v_j)}\\ &+ \frac{2k_{i,j-1}T_{i,j-1}(t)}{\Delta v_{j-1}(\Delta v_{j-1}+\Delta v_j)} + w_{b,i,j}C_{b,i,j}T_{a,i,j} + Q_{i,j} + H_{i,j}\end{aligned} \tag{4.9}$$

where the subscript i, j indicates the respective quantities at the grid point i,j associated with the cell $C(i,j)$, and $\Delta u_{i-1} = \left\|\overrightarrow{\mathbf{P}_{i-1,j}\mathbf{P}_{i,j}}\right\|$, $\Delta u_i = \left\|\overrightarrow{\mathbf{P}_{i,j}\mathbf{P}_{i+1,j}}\right\|$, $\Delta v_{j-1} = \left\|\overrightarrow{\mathbf{P}_{i,j-1}\mathbf{P}_{i,j}}\right\|$ and $\Delta v_j = \left\|\overrightarrow{\mathbf{P}_{i,j}\mathbf{P}_{i,j+1}}\right\|$ where $\|\vec{\cdot}\|$ denotes the magnitude of a vector, and $\mathbf{P}_{i,j}\left(x_{i,j}, y_{i,j}, z_{i,j}\right)$ denotes the position of the grid point i,j.

It can be seen that Eqs. (4.8) and (4.9) are remarkably similar; therefore, the discrete form of the Pennes bio-heat transfer equation (Eq. 4.9) is embedded into the autonomous CNN (Eq. 4.8) by associating the following parameters:

$$C_x = \rho_{i,j}C_{i,j}; v_{xij}(t) = T_{i,j}(t);\ I_{ij} = w_{b,i,j}C_{b,i,j}T_{a,i,j} + Q_{i,j} + H_{i,j}$$

$$A = \begin{pmatrix} 0 & \dfrac{2k_{i,j+1}}{\Delta v_j\left(\Delta v_{j-1}+\Delta v_j\right)} & 0 \\ \dfrac{2k_{i-1,j}}{\Delta u_{i-1}\left(\Delta u_{i-1}+\Delta u_i\right)} & -\left(\dfrac{2k_{i,j}}{\Delta u_{i-1}\Delta u_i}+\dfrac{2k_{i,j}}{\Delta v_{j-1}\Delta v_j}+w_{b,i,j}C_{b,i,j}\right)+\dfrac{1}{R_x} & \dfrac{2k_{i+1,j}}{\Delta u_i\left(\Delta u_{i-1}+\Delta u_i\right)} \\ 0 & \dfrac{2k_{i,j-1}}{\Delta v_{j-1}\left(\Delta v_{j-1}+\Delta v_j\right)} & 0 \end{pmatrix} \tag{4.10}$$

4.3.2.2 2D Irregular Grids

To establish CNN on 2D irregular grids such as a triangular grid, the original definition of "*r*-neighbourhood" is generalised from the rectangular grid to handle arbitrary grids, in which the grid points are positioned arbitrarily and linked to their neighbouring points. The *r*-neighbourhood of the cell $C(i)$ associated with the grid point i is defined by

$$N_r(i) = \left\{C(j) \mid \text{links}\left(C(i), C(j)\right) \le r\right\} \tag{4.11}$$

The state of a cell in the autonomous CNN is expressed by the following equation:

$$C_x \frac{dv_{xi}(t)}{dt} = -\frac{1}{R_x}v_{xi}(t) + \sum_{c(j)\in N_r(i)} A(i;j)v_{yj}(t) + I_i \tag{4.12}$$

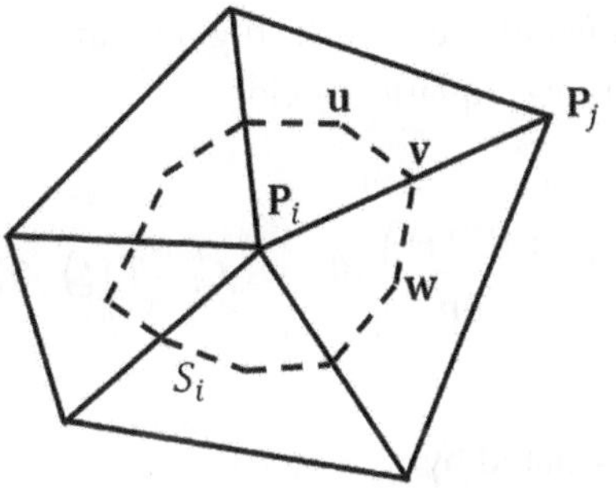

FIGURE 4.3 Bio-heat conduction on a 2D triangular grid. The control area S_i (surrounded by the dashed lines) of the point i is formed by connecting each centroid (such as $\mathbf{u}$ and $\mathbf{w}$) of the adjacent triangles and the mid-points (such as $\mathbf{v}$) of the adjacent edges connecting $\mathbf{P}_i$ and $\mathbf{P}_j$.

where the subscripts i and j denote the respective quantities at the grid points i and j associated with the cells $C(i)$ and $C(j)$.

To discretise the Pennes bio-heat transfer equation on the 2D irregular grids, the CNN formulation is achieved with the assistance of the concept of control area [55]. The problem domain is divided into a finite number of non-overlapping control areas with computation (grid) points located at centres, over which the conservation of energy is enforced in a discrete manner. An example of a control area of the point i is illustrated in Figure 4.3, and it is formed by connecting each centroid of the triangles and the mid-points of the edges adjacent to P_i.

For the point i enclosed by the control area S_i, the discrete form of the Pennes bio-heat transfer equation can be expressed as

$$\int_{S_i}\left(\rho_i C_i \frac{\partial T_i(t)}{\partial t} + w_{b,i}C_{b,i}\left(T_i(t) - T_{a,i}\right) - Q_i - H_i\right)dS = \int_{S_i}\nabla\cdot\left(k_i \nabla T_i(t)\right)dS \quad (4.13)$$

Applying Gauss's divergence theorem yields

$$\int_{S_i}\left(\rho_i C_i \frac{\partial T_i(t)}{\partial t} + w_{b,i}C_{b,i}\left(T_i(t) - T_{a,i}\right) - Q_i - H_i\right)dS$$

$$= \int_{\partial S_i} k_i \nabla T_i(t)\cdot\mathbf{n}\,dl = \int_{\partial S_i} k_i\left(\frac{\partial T(t)}{\partial \mathbf{n}}\right)_i dl \quad (4.14)$$

where **n** is the unit normal vector pointing outwards at the boundary of S_i.

Rearranging the above equation yields

$$\rho_i C_i \frac{\partial T_i(t)}{\partial t} = \frac{1}{S_i} \int_{\partial S_i} k_i \left(\frac{\partial T(t)}{\partial \mathbf{n}} \right)_i dl - w_{b,i} C_{b,i} \left(T_i(t) - T_{a,i} \right) + Q_i + H_i \quad (4.15)$$

which can be approximated by

$$\begin{aligned} \rho_i C_i \frac{\partial T_i(t)}{\partial t} = \frac{1}{S_i} \sum_{j \in N_r(i)} \frac{\left(k_j T_j(t) - k_i T_i(t) \right)}{l_{ij}} (l_{uv} + l_{vw}) \\ - w_{b,i} C_{b,i} \left(T_i(t) - T_{a,i} \right) + Q_i + H_i \end{aligned} \quad (4.16)$$

where $l_{ij} = \left\| \overrightarrow{\mathbf{P}_i \mathbf{P}_j} \right\|$, $l_{uv} = \left\| \overrightarrow{\mathbf{uv}} \right\|$ and $l_{vw} = \left\| \overrightarrow{\mathbf{vw}} \right\|$.

Rearranging the above equation leads to

$$\begin{aligned} \rho_i C_i \frac{\partial T_i(t)}{\partial t} = -\left(\frac{1}{S_i} \sum_{j \in N_r(i)} \frac{k_i (l_{uv} + l_{vw})}{l_{ij}} + w_{b,i} C_{b,i} \right) T_i(t) \\ + \frac{1}{S_i} \sum_{j \in N_r(i)} \frac{k_j (l_{uv} + l_{vw})}{l_{ij}} T_j(t) + w_{b,i} C_{b,i} T_{a,i} + Q_i + H_i \end{aligned} \quad (4.17)$$

It can be seen that Eqs. (4.12) and (4.17) are remarkably similar; therefore, the discrete form of the Pennes bio-heat transfer equation (Eq. 4.17) is embedded into the autonomous CNN (Eq. 4.12) by associating the following parameters:

$$C_x = \rho_i C_i;\ v_{xi}(t) = T_i(t);\ v_{yj}(t) = T_j(t);\ I_i = w_{b,i} C_{b,i} T_{a,i} + Q_i + H_i$$

$$A(i;i) = -\left(\frac{1}{S_i} \sum_{j \in N_r(i)} \frac{k_i (l_{uv} + l_{vw})}{l_{ij}} + w_{b,i} C_{b,i} \right) + \frac{1}{R_x} \quad (4.18)$$

$$A(i;j) = \frac{1}{S_i} \frac{k_j (l_{uv} + l_{vw})}{l_{ij}}$$

4.3.3 CNN Formulation of Bio-Heat Transfer on 3D Grids

4.3.3.1 3D Regular Grids

The CNN formulation on 3-D regular grids can be expressed using a generalisation of 2D CNN to higher dimension cases, by a 3D rectangular array of cells. Define a grid point i, j, k associated with the cell $C(i, j, k)$, and $\Delta w_{k-1} = \left\|\overrightarrow{\mathbf{P}_{i,j,k-1}\mathbf{P}_{i,j,k}}\right\|$ and $\Delta w_k = \left\|\overrightarrow{\mathbf{P}_{i,j,k}\mathbf{P}_{i,j,k+1}}\right\|$ where $\mathbf{P}_{i,j,k}$ is the position of the grid point i, j, k. In analogy to the 2D regular grid case using FDM, the discrete form of the Pennes bio-heat transfer equation on a 3D regular grid can be expressed as

$$\begin{aligned}\rho_{i,j,k}C_{i,j,k}\frac{\partial T_{i,j,k}(t)}{\partial t} = &-\left(\frac{2k_{i,j,k}}{\Delta u_{i-1}\Delta u_i}+\frac{2k_{i,j,k}}{\Delta v_{j-1}\Delta v_j}+\frac{2k_{i,j,k}}{\Delta w_{k-1}\Delta w_k}+w_{b,i,j,k}C_{b,i,j,k}\right)T_{i,j,k}(t)\\&+\frac{2k_{i+1,j,k}T_{i+1,j,k}(t)}{\Delta u_i(\Delta u_{i-1}+\Delta u_i)}+\frac{2k_{i-1,j,k}T_{i-1,j,k}(t)}{\Delta u_{i-1}(\Delta u_{i-1}+\Delta u_i)}\\&+\frac{2k_{i,j+1,k}T_{i,j+1,k}(t)}{\Delta v_j(\Delta v_{j-1}+\Delta v_j)}+\frac{2k_{i,j-1,k}T_{i,j-1,k}(t)}{\Delta v_{j-1}(\Delta v_{j-1}+\Delta v_j)}\\&+\frac{2k_{i,j,k+1}T_{i,j,k+1}(t)}{\Delta w_k(\Delta w_{k-1}+\Delta w_k)}+\frac{2k_{i,j,k-1}T_{i,j,k-1}(t)}{\Delta w_{k-1}(\Delta w_{k-1}+\Delta w_k)}\\&+w_{b,i,j,k}C_{b,i,j,k}T_{a,i,j,k}+Q_{i,j,k}+H_{i,j,k}\end{aligned} \tag{4.19}$$

The parameters of the autonomous CNN are associated with the parameters of the discrete Pennes bio-heat transfer equation, leading to:

$$C_x = \rho_{i,j,k}C_{i,j,k};\, v_{xijk}(t) = T_{i,j,k}(t);\; I_{ijk} = w_{b,i,j,k}C_{b,i,j,k}T_{a,i,j,k}+Q_{i,j,k}+H_{i,j,k}$$

$$A(i,j,k;i,j,k) = -\left(\frac{2k_{i,j,k}}{\Delta u_{i-1}\Delta u_i}+\frac{2k_{i,j,k}}{\Delta v_{j-1}\Delta v_j}+\frac{2k_{i,j,k}}{\Delta w_{k-1}\Delta w_k}+w_{b,i,j,k}C_{b,i,j,k}\right)+\frac{1}{R_x}$$

$$A(i,j,k;i+1,j,k) = \frac{2k_{i+1,j,k}}{\Delta u_i(\Delta u_{i-1}+\Delta u_i)};\; A(i,j,k;i-1,j,k) = \frac{2k_{i-1,j,k}}{\Delta u_{i-1}(\Delta u_{i-1}+\Delta u_i)}$$

$$A(i,j,k;i,j+1,k) = \frac{2k_{i,j+1,k}}{\Delta v_j(\Delta v_{j-1}+\Delta v_j)};\; A(i,j,k;i,j-1,k) = \frac{2k_{i,j-1,k}}{\Delta v_{j-1}(\Delta v_{j-1}+\Delta v_j)}$$

$$A(i,\, j,\, k;i,\, j,\, k+1) = \frac{2k_{i,\,j,\,k+1}}{\Delta w_k(\Delta w_{k-1} + \Delta w_k)};\; A(i,\, j,\, k;i,\, j,\, k-1)$$

$$= \frac{2k_{i,\,j,\,k-1}}{\Delta w_{k-1}(\Delta w_{k-1} + \Delta w_k)} \tag{4.20}$$

4.3.3.2 3D Irregular Grids

On 3D irregular grids, the CNN formulation of bio-heat transfer is achieved with an extension of the control areas in 2D to control volumes in 3-D [56]. In analogy to a control area in 2D triangular grids, a control volume in 3D tetrahedral grids is established by a dual mesh joining at the edge-midpoints, face-centroids and centroids of tetrahedrons adjacent to a computation point. Similar to the 2D irregular case, for the point i enclosed by the control volume Ω_i, the discrete form of the Pennes bio-heat transfer equation can be expressed as

$$\rho_i C_i \frac{\partial T_i(t)}{\partial t} = -\left(\frac{1}{\Omega_i} \sum_{j \in N_r(i)} \frac{k_i \sum^n S_{ij,n}}{l_{ij}} + w_{b,i} C_{b,i} \right) T_i(t)$$

$$+ \frac{1}{\Omega_i} \sum_{j \in N_r(i)} \frac{k_j \sum^n S_{ij,n}}{l_{ij}} T_j(t) + w_{b,i} C_{b,i} T_{a,i} + Q_i + H_i \tag{4.21}$$

where $\sum^n S_{ij,n}$ denotes the sum of boundary surfaces [57] that are attached to the edge connecting $\mathbf{P}_i$ and $\mathbf{P}_j$.

The parameters of the autonomous CNN are associated with the parameters of the discrete Pennes bio-heat transfer equation, resulting in:

$$C_x = \rho_i C_i; v_{xi}(t) = T_i(t); v_{yj}(t) = T_j(t); I_i = w_{b,i} C_{b,i} T_{a,i} + Q_i + H_i$$

$$A(i;i) = -\left(\frac{1}{\Omega_i} \sum_{j \in N_r(i)} \frac{k_i \sum^n S_{ij,n}}{l_{ij}} + w_{b,i} C_{b,i} \right) + \frac{1}{R_x}$$

$$A(i;j) = \frac{1}{\Omega_i} \frac{k_j \sum^n S_{ij,n}}{l_{ij}} \tag{4.22}$$

4.3.4 Initial and Boundary Conditions

The initial and boundary conditions must be specified in order to fully describe the CNN models. The initial condition is achieved by assigning the initial state of the cell with the initial temperature of the tissue, i.e.,

$$v_x(0) = T(0) \tag{4.23}$$

The boundary condition of the Dirichlet type is enforced by assigning the fixed-state cells with a prescribed constant temperature, i.e.,

$$v_{x,b}(t) = T \tag{4.24}$$

where $v_{x,b}(t)$ represents the state of the cell at the specified domain boundary at time t.

The time evolution of CNN directly provides the soft tissue temperature field governed by the Pennes bio-heat transfer equation, which is subsequently used for thermal dose computation.

4.4 NUMERICAL EXAMPLES

4.4.1 Patient-Specific Thermal Dose Computation

A set of patient-specific virtual digital models of heterogenous tissues is employed to analyse thermal doses in a personalised thermal ablative treatment of hepatic tumours. As illustrated in Figure 4.4, the patient-specific anatomical models were constructed from a computed tomography (CT) medical image dataset of an anonymised patient (the dataset is available at https://www.ircad.fr/research/3dircadb/), which was segmented and reconstructed into the liver and the bone. The thermal dose CEM_{43} was computed from the tissue heat exposure history (Eq. 4.1) where the tissue temperature was calculated by the bio-heat transfer-embedded CNN whose performance was previously evaluated in Ref. [41]. The heterogeneity of tissues was modelled by setting parameters of cells to different values based on the tissue/tumour material properties at different regions.

As illustrated in Figure 4.5, a volumetric heat source of a Gaussian distribution type was used as the externally applied heat source. The simulated heat source was employed to demonstrate the applicability of the CNN methodology in estimating tissue temperature and thermal doses, and they can be substituted by different heat sources of various sizes and shapes such as those induced by the different thermal ablative modalities.

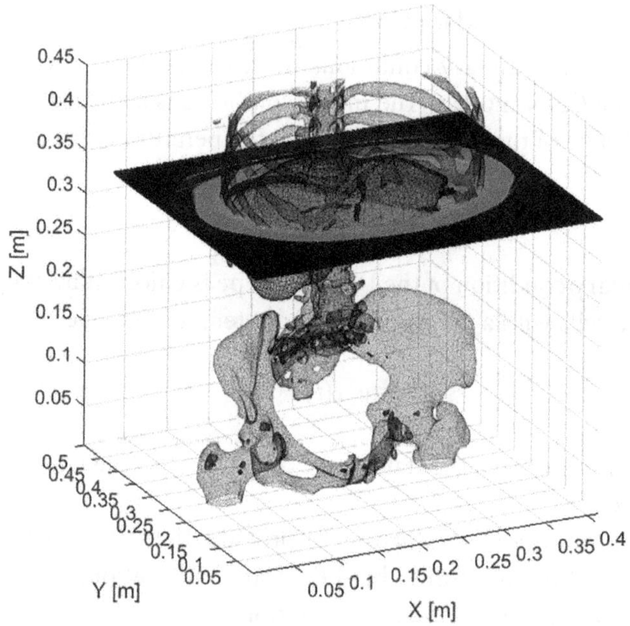

FIGURE 4.4 Mesh of the patient-specific anatomical models for simulation: the models are constructed from a CT image dataset (a DICOM slice is shown), which is segmented and reconstructed into the liver and the bone.

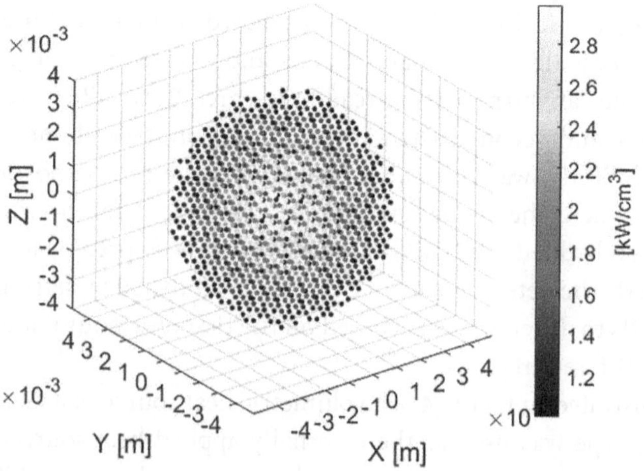

FIGURE 4.5 A simulated volumetric heat source of a Gaussian distribution type is used as the heat source to be fed into the Pennes bio-heat transfer equation for thermal dose computation.

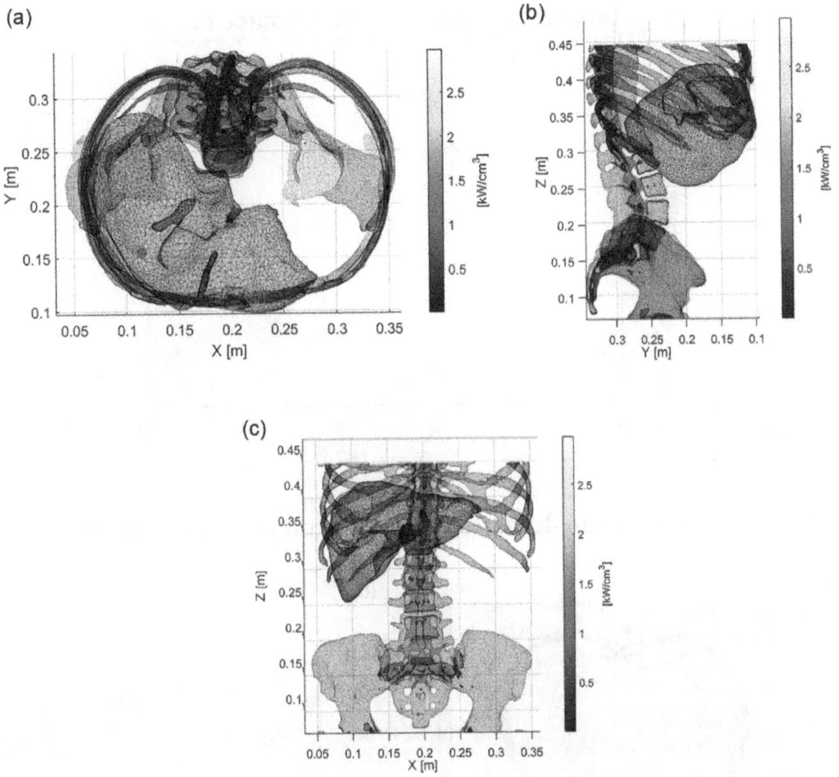

FIGURE 4.6 Geometric placement of the volumetric heat source in the liver from different viewing angles (a), (b) and (c).

Figure 4.6 presents the geometric placement of the simulated volumetric heat source in the liver relative to the patient-specific anatomical models.

A thermal simulation was applied for 5 seconds with the heat source on and for 5 seconds with the heat source off. The thermal material properties used for the liver were $\rho = 1{,}060$ [kg/m³], $k = 0.518\left[\mathrm{W}/(\mathrm{m}\cdot\mathrm{K})\right]$ and $C = 3{,}700\left[\mathrm{J}/(\mathrm{kg}\cdot\mathrm{K})\right]$. The initial tissue temperature was set to $T(0) = 37°\mathrm{C}$. During the simulation, the temperature history of the tissue at the heat source centre was recorded and is presented in Figure 4.7. The thermal dose 240 CEM_{43} to cause tissue thermal damage at the completion of the simulation is shown in Figure 4.8.

4.4.2 Application to Hepatic Tumour Ablation Using HIFU

As mentioned previously, the thermal ablative management of hepatic tumours can be achieved with various modalities, such as RFA, MWA,

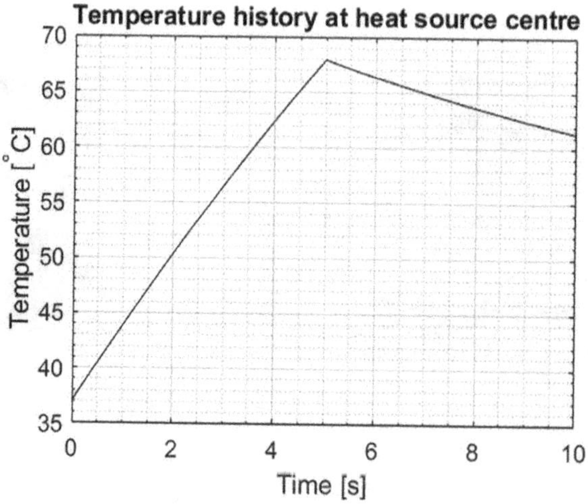

FIGURE 4.7 Temperature-history of the tissue at the heat source centre.

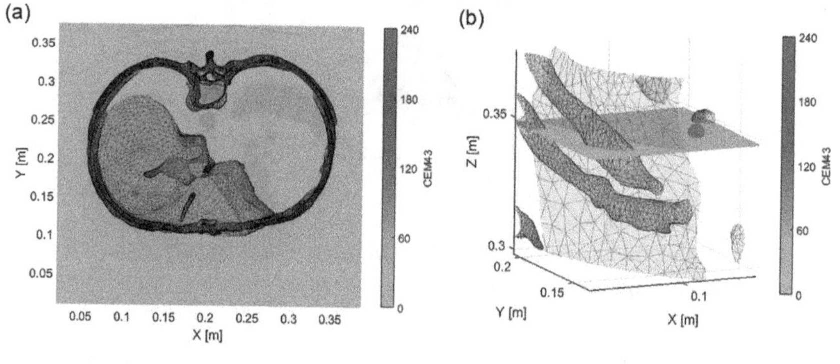

FIGURE 4.8 240 CEM_{43} to cause tissue thermal damage at the completion (10 seconds) of the simulation: (a) the induced lesion in the liver and (b) the 3D volumetric lesion in the liver; the colourmap is applied to the heat source region only and does not apply to the CT slice.

laser and HIFU, to induce heat to produce cellular thermal damage for cancer treatment. Compared to RFA, MWA and laser, HIFU has an inherent advantage in that it does not require the introduction of an applicator to achieve the ablative effect and is the only non-invasive option. As illustrated in Figure 4.9, HIFU treatment uses a HIFU transducer to induce ultrasound of high-intensity to focus at the tumour region where the mechanical vibration energy is absorbed by tissues in the form of heat, acting as heat sources to increase local tissue temperature to cause tumour coagulative necrosis via the intact skin.

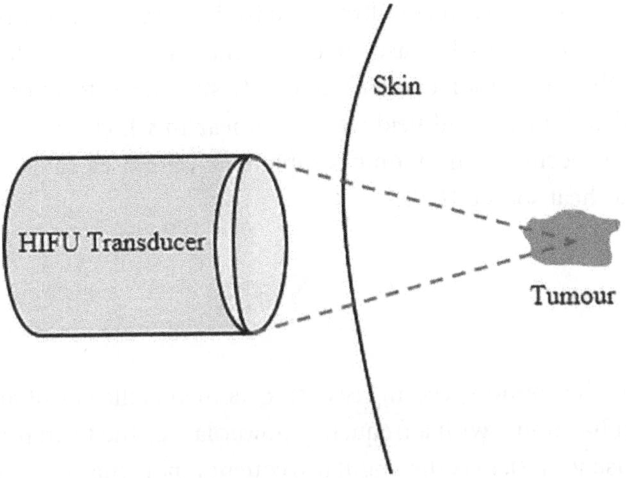

FIGURE 4.9 Diagram of the principle of HIFU ablation: a HIFU transducer is placed outside the patient skin to induce ultrasound of high intensity to focus on the target tumour to cause cellular coagulative necrosis.

An *in silico* simulation of a patient-specific HIFU treatment of liver tumours was conducted using CNN. In addition to the liver and the bone, the CT images were further segmented into the skin, fat and muscle; the HIFU transducer was positioned outside the patient skin where the medium was segmented as water. The ultrasound wave was propagated through water, skin, fat and muscle and focused on the liver tumour. The propagation of ultrasound was simulated by the non-linear full-wave Westervelt equation [58] on a uniform $208 \times 112 \times 112$ mesh-grid occupying a computational domain of $121.3 \times 65.3 \times 65.3$ mm. A HIFU transducer of diameter $D = 60$ mm and radius of curvature $R = 75$ mm operated at the frequency $f = 1$ MHz with a surface pressure of 0.3 MPa was used for simulation. The typical acoustic property values of each type of tissues are presented in Table 4.1.

TABLE 4.1 Acoustic Properties of the Heterogeneous Tissues

	Density [kg/m³]	Sound Speed [m/s]	Attenuation [dB/MHz/cm]	B/A
Water	998	1,482	0.00217	5.2
Skin	1,090	1,615	0.35	7.9
Fat	985	1,465	0.40	8.5
Muscle	1,055	1,575	0.60	7.0
Liver	1,060	1,595	0.50	6.6

Due to the propagation of ultrasound in the tissue, an acoustic pressure field is developed, which is used to obtain the HIFU-induced heat sources owing to the attenuation of ultrasound in tissues in the form of heat. Since the simulated ultrasound field was non-linear in which higher harmonic frequencies occur, the harmonic components were used to determine the non-linear heat source H, i.e.,

$$H = \frac{1}{\rho c} \sum_{k=1}^{K} \alpha_k p_k^2 \tag{4.25}$$

where c is the sound speed in tissues, α_k is the coefficient of attenuation of the kth harmonic with a frequency power law of the form $\alpha = \alpha_0 \omega^y$ [59] (in our case $y = 1.3$), ω is the angular frequency, p_k is the acoustic pressure of the kth harmonic component and K is the number of harmonics (in our case $K = 3$ for a balance between numerical accuracy and computational resources). The calculated heat source H is substituted into Eq. (4.3) for computation of the temperature field in the liver tissues.

Figure 4.10 illustrates the geometric placement of the HIFU transducer and the induced heat source calculated from the ultrasound pressure field. The thermal energy was induced in the target region by placing the focused ultrasound transducer such that the geometrical focal point was located inside the target region while avoiding the ribs where the bone

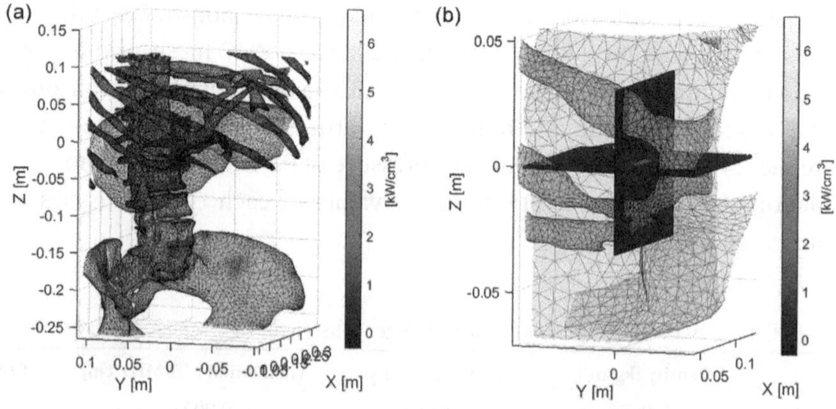

FIGURE 4.10 (a) Heat deposition is induced in the target region by placing the focused ultrasound transducer in such a way that the geometrical focal point is located inside the target region and the ultrasound can pass through the intercostal windows (the gaps between the ribs) and (b) a close-up look of (a).

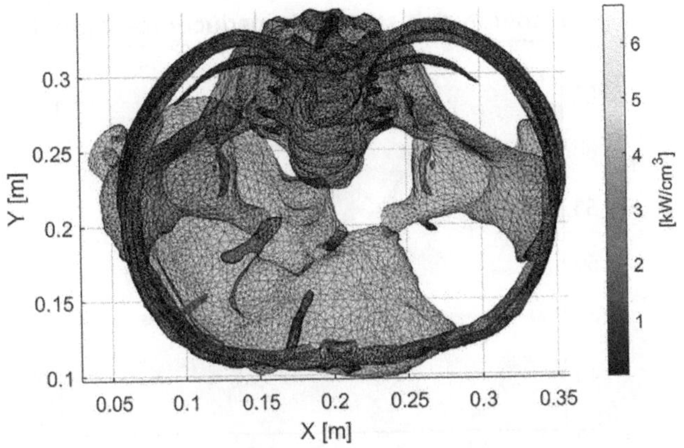

FIGURE 4.11 HIFU-induced volumetric heat source at the target liver region.

tissues and gas/air trapped cavities can interfere with the HIFU modality and affect the dose delivery, so it is imperative to plan the treatment accordingly. It is also worth mentioning that owing to the positioning of the HIFU transducer between the ribs (intercostal window), it may limit the reachability of the desired HIFU dose in the liver and may call for using multiple HIFU probes to work in conjunction through multiple routes [60,61]. The volumetric heat source is induced in the target liver region as shown in Figure 4.11.

A thermal simulation was applied for 3.5 seconds with the heat source on and for 11.5 seconds with the heat source off. The thermal material properties of the liver were the same as those mentioned in Section 4.4.1. The initial tissue temperature was set to $T(0) = 37°C$. During the simulation, the temperature history of the tissue at the transducer focal point was recorded and is presented in Figure 4.12. The thermal dose 240 CEM_{43} to cause tissue thermal damage at the completion of the simulation is shown in Figure 4.13.

4.5 DISCUSSIONS

Compared to conventional numerical methods, CNN provides a fast means for solving the bio-heat transfer equation for thermal dose modeling owing to the collective and simultaneous computing activity of cells. The non-linear bio-heat transfer dynamics is modelled by the non-linear cell dynamics to evolve in time in the manner of local interaction and global propagation of cells. Soft tissue thermal heterogeneity is accommodated by setting parameters of cells to different values based on tissue/

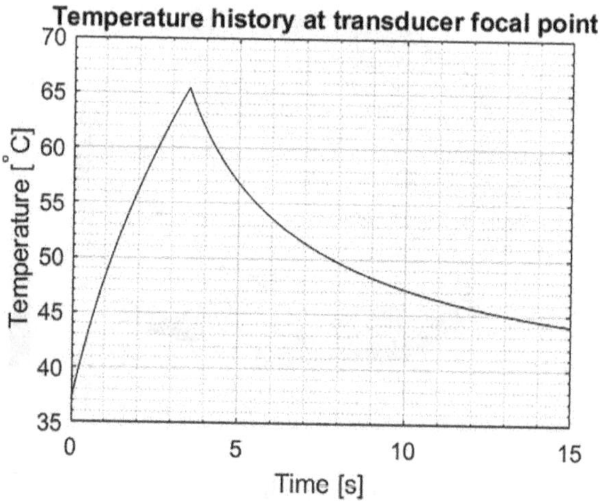

FIGURE 4.12 Temperature-history of the tissue at the transducer focal point.

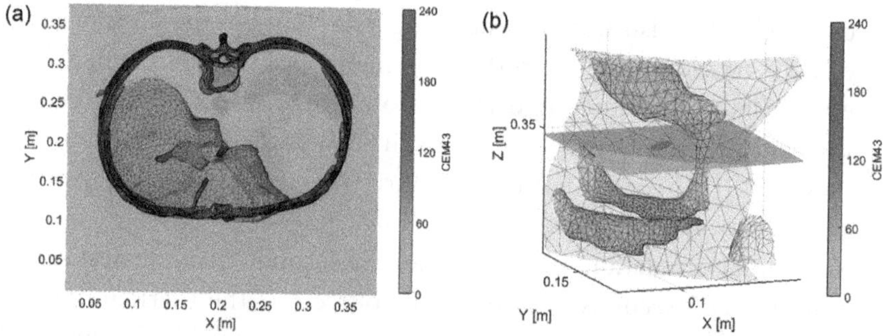

FIGURE 4.13 240 CEM_{43} to cause tissue thermal damage at the completion (15 seconds) of the simulation: (a) the induced lesion in the liver and (b) the 3D volumetric lesion in the liver; the colourmap is applied to the heat source region only and does not apply to the CT slice.

tumour material properties at different regions. Compared to the conventional area of applications of CNN, which is primarily used for image processing, the presented CNNs are formulated to incorporate the mechanism of bio-heat transfer for efficient and effective computation of the soft tissue temperature field and for computer-assisted thermal ablative cancer treatments.

The computation for thermal doses (Eq. 4.1) indicates that the quantity of thermal doses is affected by the tissue heat exposure history, which is associated with the tissue temperature and heating duration. As the variation of tissue temperature is governed by the bio-heat transfer equation in which the exciting input is the heat source that is induced by the various thermal modalities, the thermal doses can be controlled by the operator of ablation via the instrument power and heating time. The same amount of thermal doses at a material point in tissues may be achieved by (1) a high power input with a short heating duration or (2) a low power input with a long heating duration; however, the thermal dose distributions (such as those in Figures 4.8 and 4.13) may work out differently for (1) and (2) as the variation of thermal doses will be more prone to the effects of heat diffusion and blood perfusion during a long heating period, whereas these effects are less pronounced when the heating time is short. In addition, it is worth noting that tissue heating is a dynamic process accompanied by a dynamic change of tissue material properties and physical tissue geometries due to the temperature-dependent material properties [62] and tissue deformations (such as organ movements [63] and the effects of thermal expansion and contraction), compensating both may lead to more precise thermal dose computation.

Whilst minimally invasive thermal modalities such as RFA and MWA are effective in treating hepatic tumours and providing a safer option than liver resection, they exhibit some limitations. For instance, RFA is associated with a major complication rate of ≈4% and a low mortality rate of ≤1% [64]. Most complications, such as bowel perforation or bile duct injury, are due to thermal injuries to organ tissues adjacent to the liver, particularly for subcapsular tumours and tumours near the porta hepatis and gallbladder [65]. Intraoperative RFA has been employed to avoid these complications, but this approach is more invasive, which may lead to further complications and side effects. Moreover, tumours in the neighbourhood of large blood vessels can be difficult to ablate completely because of a heat sink effect due to blood perfusion that limits the ability to achieve the high temperature required for thermal ablation. Experimental studies [66,67] indicate that this problem is less pronounced if heat sources are induced with high energy intensity and a short heating duration (≤ 2 seconds), since the heating would be rapid and less affected by the heat diffusion and blood perfusion effects.

As mentioned in Section 4.4.2, compared to RFA and MWA, the HIFU tumour ablation represents the advantage of being a non-invasive means for hepatic cancer treatment; however, on the other hand, it demands precise tracking of organ movements in order to synchronise the focal region of the HIFU transducer with the target tumours to accurately induce the desired level of thermal injury [68]. Due to the physiological motion of the liver, which is primarily caused by the respiratory cycle [69] and, to a lesser extent, by cardiac motion and bowel movements, the target tumour moves and deforms continuously that complicates both precise and effective HIFU energy deposition. Consequently, more recent approaches were focused on continuous target-tracking techniques, which can lock the ultrasound beam to the target during the motion cycle and thus allow continuous energy deposition. Both real-time magnetic resonance imaging (MRI) and diagnostic ultrasound have been demonstrated as viable tracking modalities [70,71]. In addition, due to organ movements, soft tissue deformations [72,73] must be considered when calculating thermal doses, the soft tissue temperature field must be computed based on the deformed state of tissues for accurate computation of thermal doses under tissue deformations [74].

4.6 CONCLUSION

This work presents a CNN-based methodology for fast computation and analysis of soft tissue temperature and thermal doses for the management of hepatic tumours in thermal ablative treatments. To avoid the complex and expensive numerical non-linear solution procedures, CNN models are developed by formulating the non-linear bio-heat transfer equation as the non-linear collective and simultaneous local and global cell activities of CNN, leading to neural network models on 2D and 3D regular and irregular grids with the mechanism of bio-heat transfer embedded for fast temperature computation for computer-assisted thermal ablative treatments. The application of the CNN models is demonstrated using a clinically relevant scenario of thermal dose modeling in a patient-specific HIFU treatment of liver cancers for tumour management.

ACKNOWLEDGEMENT

The funding from the National Health and Medical Research Council (NHMRC), Australia, Project Grant APP1093314 is gratefully acknowledged.

REFERENCES

1. D. J. Breen, and R. Lencioni, "Image-guided ablation of primary liver and renal tumours," *Nat Rev Clin Oncol*, vol. 12, no. 3, pp. 175–86, 2015.
2. Y. Fang, W. Chen, X. Liang, D. Li, H. Lou, R. Chen, K. Wang, and H. Pan, "Comparison of long-term effectiveness and complications of radiofrequency ablation with hepatectomy for small hepatocellular carcinoma," *J Gastroenterol Hepatol*, vol. 29, no. 1, pp. 193–200, 2014.

3. M. W. Lee, S. S. Raman, N. H. Asvadi, S. Siripongsakun, R. M. Hicks, J. Chen, A. Worakitsitisatorn, J. McWilliams, M. J. Tong, R. S. Finn, V. G. Agopian, R. W. Busuttil, and D. S. K. Lu, "Radiofrequency ablation of hepatocellular carcinoma as bridge therapy to liver transplantation: A 10-year intention-to-treat analysis," *Hepatology*, vol. 65, no. 6, pp. 1979–1990, 2017.
4. M. Moche, H. Busse, J. J. Futterer, C. A. Hinestrosa, D. Seider, P. Brandmaier, M. Kolesnik, S. Jenniskens, R. Blanco Sequeiros, G. Komar, M. Pollari, M. Eibisberger, H. R. Portugaller, P. Voglreiter, R. Flanagan, P. Mariappan, and M. Reinhardt, "Clinical evaluation of in silico planning and real-time simulation of hepatic radiofrequency ablation (ClinicIMPPACT Trial)," *Eur Radiol*, pp. 1–9, 2019.
5. V. Lopresto, R. Pinto, L. Farina, and M. Cavagnaro, "Treatment planning in microwave thermal ablation: Clinical gaps and recent research advances," *Int J Hyperthermia*, vol. 33, no. 1, pp. 83–100, 2017.
6. E. Li, G. R. Liu, V. Tan, and Z. C. He, "Modeling and simulation of bioheat transfer in the human eye using the 3D alpha finite element method (αFEM)," *Int J Numer Method Biomed Eng*, vol. 26, no. 8, pp. 955–976, 2010.
7. E. Li, G. R. Liu, and V. Tan, "Simulation of hyperthermia treatment using the edge-based smoothed finite-element method," *Numer Heat Transfer A: Appl*, vol. 57, no. 11, pp. 822–847, 2010.
8. P. Rattanadecho, and P. Keangin, "Numerical study of heat transfer and blood flow in two-layered porous liver tissue during microwave ablation process using single and double slot antenna," *Int J Heat Mass Transfer*, vol. 58, no. 1–2, pp. 457–470, 2013.
9. C. Rieder, T. Kroger, C. Schumann, and H. K. Hahn, "GPU-based real-time approximation of the ablation zone for radiofrequency ablation," *IEEE Trans Vis Comput Graph*, vol. 17, no. 12, pp. 1812–1821, 2011.
10. P. C. Johnson, and G. M. Saidel, "Thermal model for fast simulation during magnetic resonance imaging guidance of radio frequency tumor ablation," *Ann Biomed Eng*, vol. 30, no. 9, pp. 1152–1161, 2002.
11. M. Schwenke, J. Georgii, and T. Preusser, "Fast numerical simulation of focused ultrasound treatments during respiratory motion with discontinuous motion boundaries," *IEEE Trans Biomed Eng*, vol. 64, no. 7, pp. 1455–1468, 2017.
12. G. Kalantzis, W. Miller, W. Tichy, and S. LeBlang, "A GPU accelerated finite differences method of the bioheat transfer equation for ultrasound thermal ablation," *Software Engineering, Artificial Intelligence, Networking and Parallel/Distributed Computing*, Roger Lee, Ed. pp. 45–55: Springer, Switzerland, 2016.
13. J. Zhang, J. Hills, Y. Zhong, B. Shirinzadeh, J. Smith, and C. Gu, "Gpu-accelerated finite element modeling of bio-heat conduction for simulation of thermal ablation," *Journal of Mechanics in Medicine and Biology*, vol. 18, no. 07, p. 1840012, 2018.
14. J. Zhang, J. Hills, Y. Zhong, B. Shirinzadeh, J. Smith, and C. Gu, "Modeling of soft tissue thermal damage based on GPU acceleration," *Comput Assist Surg (Abingdon)*, vol. 24, no. supl, pp. 5–12, 2019.

15. P. Mariappan, P. Weir, R. Flanagan, P. Voglreiter, T. Alhonnoro, M. Pollari, M. Moche, H. Busse, J. Futterer, H. R. Portugaller, R. B. Sequeiros, and M. Kolesnik, "GPU-based RFA simulation for minimally invasive cancer treatment of liver tumours," *Int J Comput Assist Radiol Surg*, vol. 12, no. 1, pp. 59–68, 2017.
16. Z.-Z. He, and J. Liu, "An efficient parallel numerical modeling of bio-heat transfer in realistic tissue structure," *Int J Heat Mass Trans*, vol. 95, pp. —843–852, 2016.
17. G. Carluccio, D. Erricolo, S. Oh, and C. M. Collins, "An approach to rapid calculation of temperature change in tissue using spatial filters to approximate effects of thermal conduction," *IEEE Trans Biomed Eng*, vol. 60, no. 6, pp. 1735–1741, 2013.
18. J. Zhang, and S. Chauhan, "Fast explicit dynamics finite element algorithm for transient heat transfer," *Int J Therm Sci*, vol. 139, pp. 160–175, 2019.
19. J. Zhang, and S. Chauhan, "Real-time computation of bio-heat transfer in the fast explicit dynamics finite element algorithm (FED-FEM) framework," *Numer Heat Transfer B: Fundament*, vol. 75, no. 4, pp. 217–238, 2019.
20. J. L. Dillenseger, and S. Esneault, "Fast FFT-based bioheat transfer equation computation," *Comput Biol Med*, vol. 40, no. 2, pp. 119–23, 2010.
21. M. E. Kowalski, and J. M. Jin, "Model-order reduction of nonlinear models of electromagnetic phased-array hyperthermia," *IEEE Trans Biomed Eng*, vol. 50, no. 11, pp. 1243–1254, 2003.
22. J. H. Indik, R. A. Indik, and T. C. Cetas, "Fast and efficient computer modeling of ferromagnetic seed arrays of arbitrary orientation for hyperthermia treatment planning," *Int J Radiat Oncol Biol Phys*, vol. 30, no. 3, pp. 653–662, 1994.
23. R. A. Indik, and J. H. Indik, "A new computer method to quickly and accurately compute steady-state temperatures from ferromagnetic seed heating," *Med Phys*, vol. 21, no. 7, pp. 1135–1144, 1994.
24. G. C. Bourantas, M. Ghommem, G. C. Kagadis, K. Katsanos, V. C. Loukopoulos, V. N. Burganos, and G. C. Nikiforidis, "Real-time tumor ablation simulation based on the dynamic mode decomposition method," *Med Phys*, vol. 41, no. 5, p. 053301, 2014.
25. J. Zhang, Y. Zhong, and C. Gu, "Neural network modelling of soft tissue deformation for surgical simulation," *Artif Intell Med*, vol. 97, pp. 61–70, 2019.
26. J. Zhang, Y. Zhong, and C. Gu, "Soft tissue deformation modelling through neural dynamics-based reaction-diffusion mechanics," *Med Biol Eng Comput*, vol. 56, no. 12, pp. 2163–2176, 2018.
27. J. Zhang, Y. Zhong, J. Smith, and C. Gu, "Cellular neural network modelling of soft tissue dynamics for surgical simulation," *Technol Health Care*, vol. 25, no. S1, pp. 337–344, 2017.
28. J. Zhang, Y. Zhong, J. Smith, and C. Gu, "ChainMail based neural dynamics modeling of soft tissue deformation for surgical simulation," *Technol Health Care*, vol. 25, no. S1, pp. 231–239, 2017.

29. J. C. Chedjou, and K. Kyamakya, "A universal concept based on cellular neural networks for ultrafast and flexible solving of differential equations," *IEEE Trans Neural Netw Learn Syst*, vol. 26, no. 4, pp. 749–762, 2015.
30. L. O. Chua, and L. Yang, "Cellular neural networks: Theory," *IEEE Trans Circuit Syst*, vol. 35, no. 10, pp. 1257–1272, 1988.
31. L. O. Chua, and L. Yang, "Cellular neural networks: Applications," *IEEE Trans Circuit Syst*, vol. 35, no. 10, pp. 1273–1290, 1988.
32. Á. Zarándy, C. Rekeczky, P. Szolgay, and L. O. Chua, "Overview of CNN research: 25 years history and the current trends," pp. 401–404.
33. A. Slavova, *Cellular Neural Networks: Dynamics and Modelling*: Springer Science & Business Media, Dordrecht, Netherlands, 2003.
34. T. Roska, L. O. Chua, D. Wolf, T. Kozek, R. Tetzlaff, and F. Puffer, "Simulating nonlinear waves and partial differential equations via CNN. I. Basic techniques," *IEEE Trans Circuit Syst I: Fundament Theory Appl*, vol. 42, no. 10, pp. 807–815, 1995.
35. T. Kozek, L. O. Chua, T. Roska, D. Wolf, R. Tetzlaff, F. Puffer, and K. Lotz, "Simulating nonlinear waves and partial differential equations via CNN. II. Typical examples," *IEEE Tran Circuit Syst I: Fundament Theory Appl*, vol. 42, no. 10, pp. 816–820, 1995.
36. P. Szolgay, G. Voros, and G. Eross, "On the applications of the cellular neural network paradigm in mechanical vibrating systems," *IEEE Trans Circuit Syst I: Fundament Theory Appl*, vol. 40, no. 3, pp. 222–227, 1993.
37. L. O. Chua, M. Hasler, G. S. Moschytz, and J. Neirynck, "Autonomous cellular neural networks: A unified paradigm for pattern formation and active wave propagation," *IEEE Trans Circuit Syst I: Fundament Theory Appl*, vol. 42, no. 10, pp. 559–577, 1995.
38. Y. Zhong, B. Shirinzadeh, G. Alici, and J. Smith, "A cellular neural network methodology for deformable object simulation," *IEEE Trans Inf Technol Biomed*, vol. 10, no. 4, pp. 749–762, 2006.
39. J. Zhang, Y. Zhong, J. Smith, and C. Gu, "Neural dynamics-based Poisson propagation for deformable modelling," *Neur Comput Appl*, vol. 31, no. S2, pp. 1091–1101, 2017.
40. J. H. Niu, H. Z. Wang, H. X. Zhang, J. Y. Yan, and Y. S. Zhu, "Cellular neural network analysis for two-dimensional bioheat transfer equation," *Med Biol Eng Comput*, vol. 39, no. 5, pp. 601–604, 2001.
41. J. Zhang, and S. Chauhan, "Neural network methodology for real-time modelling of bio-heat transfer during thermo-therapeutic applications," *Artif Intell Med*, vol. 101, p. 101728, 2019.
42. P. Liu, J. Qin, B. Duan, Q. Wang, X. Tan, B. Zhao, P. L. Jonnathan, C. K. Chui, and P. A. Heng, "Overlapping radiofrequency ablation planning and robot-assisted needle insertion for large liver tumors," *Int J Med Robot*, vol. 15, no. 1, p. e1952, 2019.
43. T. Williamson, S. Everitt, and S. Chauhan, "Automated geometric optimization for robotic HIFU treatment of liver tumors," *Comput Biol Med*, vol. 96, pp. 1–7, 2018.

44. C. W. Huang, M. K. Sun, B. T. Chen, J. Shieh, C. S. Chen, and W. S. Chen, "Simulation of thermal ablation by high-intensity focused ultrasound with temperature-dependent properties," *Ultrason Sonochem*, vol. 27, pp. 456–465, 2015.
45. S. Haddadi, and M. T. Ahmadian, "Numerical and experimental evaluation of high-intensity focused ultrasound-induced lesions in liver tissue ex vivo," *J Ultrasound Med*, vol. 37, no. 6, pp. 1481–1491, 2018.
46. H. H. Pennes, "Analysis of tissue and arterial blood temperatures in the resting human forearm," *J Appl Physiol*, vol. 1, no. 2, pp. 93–122, 1948.
47. M. C. Kolios, A. E. Worthington, M. D. Sherar, and J. W. Hunt, "Experimental evaluation of two simple thermal models using transient temperature analysis," *Phys Med Biol*, vol. 43, no. 11, p. 3325, 1998.
48. E. H. Wissler, "Pennes' 1948 paper revisited," *J Appl Physiol*, vol. 85, no. 1, pp. 35–41, 1998.
49. E. H. Ooi, K. W. Lee, S. Yap, M. A. Khattab, I. Y. Liao, E. T. Ooi, J. J. Foo, S. R. Nair, and A. F. Mohd Ali, "The effects of electrical and thermal boundary condition on the simulation of radiofrequency ablation of liver cancer for tumours located near to the liver boundary," *Comput Biol Med*, vol. 106, pp. 12–23, 2019.
50. W. Karaki, Rahul, C. A. Lopez, D. A. Borca-Tasciuc, and S. De, "A continuum thermomechanical model of in vivo electrosurgical heating of hydrated soft biological tissues," *Int J Heat Mass Transf*, vol. 127, no. Pt A, pp. 961–974, 2018.
51. P. Gupta, and A. Srivastava, "Numerical analysis of thermal response of tissues subjected to high intensity focused ultrasound," *Int J Hyperthermia*, vol. 35, no. 1, pp. 419–434, 2018.
52. B. Prasad, J. K. Kim, and S. Kim, "Role of simulations in the treatment planning of radiofrequency hyperthermia therapy in clinics," *J Oncol*, vol. 2019, p. 9685476, 2019.
53. P. Thiran, G. Setti, and M. Hasler, "An approach to information propagation in 1-D cellular neural networks-Part I: Local diffusion," *IEEE Trans Circuit Syst I: Fundament Theory Appl*, vol. 45, no. 8, pp. 777–789, 1998.
54. G. Setti, P. Thiran, and C. Serpico, "An approach to information propagation in 1-D cellular neural networks. II. Global propagation," *IEEE Trans Circuit Syst I: Fundament Theory Appl*, vol. 45, no. 8, pp. 790–811, 1998.
55. D. R. Croft, and D. G. Lilley, *Heat Transfer Calculations Using Finite Difference Equations*: Applied science publishers, London, 1977.
56. M. Ciesielski, and B. Mochnacki, "Hyperbolic model of thermal interactions in a system biological tissue—protective clothing subjected to an external heat source," *J Numer Heat Transfer A: Appl*, vol. 74, no. 11, pp. 1685–1700, 2018.
57. J. Zhang, Y. Zhong, J. Smith, and C. Gu, "Energy propagation modeling of nonlinear soft tissue deformation for surgical simulation," *Simulation*, vol. 94, no. 1, pp. 3–10, 2017.

58. J. Gu, and Y. Jing, "Modeling of wave propagation for medical ultrasound: A review," *IEEE Trans Ultrason Ferroelectr Freq Control*, vol. 62, no. 11, pp. 1979–1993, 2015.
59. B. E. Treeby, and B. T. Cox, "Modeling power law absorption and dispersion for acoustic propagation using the fractional Laplacian," *J Acoust Soc Am*, vol. 127, no. 5, pp. 2741–2748, 2010.
60. S. Chauhan, H. Amir, G. Chen, A. Hacker, M. S. Michel, and K. U. Koehrmann, "Intra-operative feedback and dynamic compensation for image-guided robotic focal ultrasound surgery," *Comput Aided Surg*, vol. 13, no. 6, pp. 353–368, 2008.
61. A. Häcker, S. Chauhan, K. Peters, R. Hildenbrand, E. Marlinghaus, P. Alken, and M. S. Michel, "Multiple high-intensity focused ultrasound probes for kidney-tissue ablation," *J Endourol*, vol. 19, no. 8, pp. 1036–1040, 2005.
62. J. Zhang, J. Hills, Y. Zhong, B. Shirinzadeh, J. Smith, and C. Gu, "Temperature-dependent thermomechanical modeling of soft tissue deformation," *Journal of Mechanics in Medicine and Biology*, vol. 18, no. 08, p. 1840021, 2019.
63. R. H. Abhilash, S. Chauhan, M. V. Che, C. C. Ooi, R. A. Bakar, and R. H. Lo, "Quantitative study on the effect of abnormalities on respiration-induced kidney movement," *Ultrasound Med Biol*, vol. 42, no. 7, pp. 1681–1688, 2016.
64. R. A. Lencioni, H. P. Allgaier, D. Cioni, M. Olschewski, P. Deibert, L. Crocetti, H. Frings, J. Laubenberger, I. Zuber, H. E. Blum, and C. Bartolozzi, "Small hepatocellular carcinoma in cirrhosis: Randomized comparison of radio-frequency thermal ablation versus percutaneous ethanol injection," *Radiology*, vol. 228, no. 1, pp. 235–240, 2003.
65. T. Livraghi, F. Meloni, M. Di Stasi, E. Rolle, L. Solbiati, C. Tinelli, and S. Rossi, "Sustained complete response and complications rates after radiofrequency ablation of very early hepatocellular carcinoma in cirrhosis: Is resection still the treatment of choice?," *Hepatology*, vol. 47, no. 1, pp. 82–89, 2008.
66. S. B. Solomon, T. L. Nicol, D. Y. Chan, T. Fjield, N. Fried, and L. R. Kavoussi, "Histologic evolution of high-intensity focused ultrasound in rabbit muscle," *Invest Radiol*, vol. 38, no. 5, pp. 293–301, 2003.
67. C. X. Zhang, S. Zhang, Z. Zhang and Y. Z. Chen, "Effects of Large Blood Vessel Locations during High Intensity Focused Ultrasound Therapy for Hepatic Tumors: a finite element study," *2005 IEEE Engineering in Medicine and Biology 27th Annual Conference*, Shanghai, China, 2005, pp. 209-212, doi: 10.1109/IEMBS.2005.1616380.
68. R. H. Abhilash, and S. Chauhan, "Empirical modeling of renal motion for improved targeting during focused ultrasound surgery," *Comput Biol Med*, vol. 43, no. 4, pp. 240–247, 2013.
69. R. H. Abhilash, and S. Chauhan, "Respiration-induced movement correlation for synchronous noninvasive renal cancer surgery," *IEEE Trans Ultrason Ferroelectr Freq Control*, vol. 59, no. 7, pp. 1478–1486, 2012.

70. M. Ries, B. D. de Senneville, S. Roujol, Y. Berber, B. Quesson, and C. Moonen, "Real-time 3D target tracking in MRI guided focused ultrasound ablations in moving tissues," *Magn Reson Med*, vol. 64, no. 6, pp. 1704–1712, 2010.
71. T. Williamson, W. Cheung, S. K. Roberts, and S. Chauhan, "Ultrasound-based liver tracking utilizing a hybrid template/optical flow approach," *Int J Comput Assist Radiol Surg*, vol. 13, no. 10, pp. 1605–1615, 2018.
72. J. Zhang, Y. Zhong, and C. Gu, "Energy balance method for modelling of soft tissue deformation," *Comp. Aid. Des.*, vol. 93, pp. 15–25, 2017.
73. J. Zhang, Y. Zhong, and C. Gu, "Deformable models for surgical simulation: A survey," *IEEE Rev Biomed Eng*, vol. 11, pp. 143–164, 2018.
74. J. Zhang, and S. Chauhan, "Fast computation of soft tissue thermal response under deformation based on fast explicit dynamics finite element algorithm for surgical simulation," *Comput Methods Programs Biomed*, vol. 187, p. 105244, 2019.

CHAPTER 5

Ensembles of Convolutional Neural Networks with Different Activation Functions for Small to Medium-Sized Biomedical Datasets

Filippo Berno, Loris Nanni, and Gianluca Maguolo
University of Padua
Padua, Italy

Sheryl Brahnam
Missouri State University
Springfield, Missouri

CONTENTS

5.1 INTRODUCTION

In artificial intelligence, neural networks have been in and out of popularity since the 1940s, but in the last decade, deep learning with artificial neural networks has been a game-changer in many engineering application areas [1,2] and in basic science [3–5]. Deep learners, such as Convolutional Neural Networks (CNNs), have consistently obtained state-of-the-art results in many computer vision tasks such as image classification [1,6], object detection [7], face recognition [8], and machine translation [9]. CNNs also have been proven to be more accurate than humans in many recognition tasks, including recognizing traffic signs [10], faces [11,12], handwritten digits [10,13], and the 1,000 classes of the ImageNet dataset [14,15].

Since activation functions play a critical role in the training dynamics and task performance of deep neural networks, the development of more efficient and better-performing activation functions has been the focus of a large number of researchers. Until recently, the sigmoid and hyperbolic tangent were among the most widely used activation functions in neural networks. Although the hyperbolic tangent has the advantage of having a derivative that is steeper than the sigmoid function, they both suffer from the vanishing gradient problem and do a poor job training at deep neural networks, in part because gradients rapidly decrease as the modulus of the input goes to infinity. There is increasing evidence, however, that other nonlinearities improve the performance of neural networks. Glorot et al. [16], for example, demonstrated the superiority of Rectified Linear Units (ReLU) to train deep networks. ReLU is an activation function that is equal to the identity function when the input is positive but zero when it is negative [17]. Even though this function is not differentiable, it nonetheless enabled AlexNet to win the ImageNet competition in 2012 [1].

Due to the success of ReLU and the fact that this activation is fast, effective, and simple to evaluate, many researchers in deep learning began to explore the properties of other rectifying nonlinearities. For example, Leaky ReLU, proposed by Mass [18], is an activation function that, like ReLU, is equivalent to the identity function for positive values but has a hyperparameter $\alpha > 0$ for negative inputs. This hyperparameter guarantees that the gradient of the activating function is never zero, thereby making it less likely that the optimization process will get stuck in local minima. Another advantage of Leaky ReLU is that it alleviates problems caused by hard zero activations of ReLU, which can produce cases where a unit never activates, significantly slowing training when networks have excessive constant zero gradients. Another rectifying nonlinearity is Exponential Linear Units (ELU), proposed by Clevert et al. [19], which is similar to Leaky ReLU but exponentially decreases to the limit point α as the input goes to minus infinity, thereby always producing a positive gradient. However, unlike Leaky ReLU, ELU saturates on its left side. The Scaled Exponential Linear Unit (SELU), proposed by Klambauer et al. [20], was also developed to mitigate the vanishing gradient problem. SELU is the same as ELU but multiplied by the constant $\lambda > 1$ to preserve the mean and the variance of the input features.

In the past, activation functions were handcrafted and only modified the weights and biases in neural networks, with no part of the function depending on learnable parameters. This situation changed in 2015 with the proposal of Parametric ReLU (PReLU) by He et al. [14]. PReLU is a modified Leaky ReLU where the slope of the negative part is a learnable parameter. PReLU works best with extremely large datasets since the additional learnable parameter increases the likelihood of overfitting. Many learnable activations have since been proposed [21,22]. Related to this work is the Adaptive Piecewise Linear Unit (APLU), proposed by Agostinelli et al. [21]. APLU is a piecewise linear function whose slopes and points of nondifferentiability are learned independently for each neuron using gradient descent during the training phase.

A simple way to define learnable activations is to start with multiple fixed activations, as in the work of Manessi and Rozza [23], who generated a learnable activation function that automatically learned different combinations of the base activation functions tanh, ReLU, and the identity function. Jin et al. used an S-shaped Rectified Linear Activation Unit (SReLU) to learn both convex and nonconvex functions, imitating, as a result, two fundamental laws: the Webner–Fechner law and the Stevens law. Ramachandran et al. [24] harnessed reinforcement learning to discover novel scalar activation functions. One of the best performing functions they discovered is Swish, defined as $f(x) = x\sigma(\beta x)$, where $\sigma(\cdot)$ is the sigmoid activation function and β is a trainable parameter. As β approaches infinity, the sigmoid activation approaches the ReLU function. When β is zero, the Swish becomes the scaled linear function $f(x) = x/2$ According to the authors, Swish can be viewed as a smooth function that nonlinearly interpolates between the linear function and the ReLU function. In experiments, Swish consistently outperformed ReLU and other nonlinearities.

Another learnable activation function is the Mexican ReLU (MeLU), proposed by Maguolo et al. [25], so named because its shape is similar to the famous Mexican hat wavelet. MeLU is a piecewise linear activation function that is the sum of PReLU and multiple Mexican hat functions. This piecewise function has many parameters (collectively considered a hyperparameter) that range from zero to infinity and possess many desirable properties: (1) its gradient is rarely flat, (2) saturation does not occur in any direction, (3) it can approximate every continuous function on a compact set as the number of parameters goes to infinity, and (4) modifying a single parameter changes the activation only on a small interval, thereby making the optimization process simpler.

In this chapter, we propose a new activation function based on MeLU, a Gaussian type learning unit that we call (GaLU) since it is a piecewise linear activation function that is the sum of PReLU and multiple Gaussian wavelets of the first order. We compare several state-of-the-art activation functions with GaLU, using three different CNN architectures (Vgg16 [26], ResNet50 [27], and DenseNet201 [28]) on 13 small to medium-sized biomedical datasets, showing that an ensemble of activation functions strongly outperforms each individual function.

The remainder of this chapter is organized as follows. In Section 5.2, we describe the eight state-of-the-art activation functions tested in this work as well as the novel method proposed here. In Section 5.3, we evaluate all nine activation functions on 13 different datasets. Finally, in Section 5.4, we conclude by offering some suggestions for future research.

5.2 ACTIVATION FUNCTIONS FOR THE THREE CNNs

To compare our method with some of the best performing activation functions proposed in the literature, we substitute them into three well-known CNNs: Vgg16 [26], ResNet50 [27], and DenseNet201 [28] pretrained on ImageNet. ResNet50 is a CNN with 50 layers and is known for its skip connections [6], which directly connect the given layer n to some $n+x$ layer. Unlike the standard CNN that has a convolution followed by an activation, in the skip connection, the input of a block is summed to its output, a procedure that promotes gradient propagation. DenseNet201 [28] is similar to ResNet, but each of the layers is interconnected, an architecture that also results in strong gradient flow. VGG16 [26] is a CNN where the input passes through blocks composed of stacked convolutional filters, which have the same effect as larger convolutional filters but are more efficient since fewer parameters are involved.

The nine activation functions compared in this study are the eight briefly mentioned in the Introduction (ReLU [16], Leaky ReLU [29], ELU [19], SELU [20], PReLU [14], APLU [21], SReLU [30], and MeLU [25]) and the method proposed here, GaLU. These activation functions are detailed in the remainder of this section.

5.2.1 ReLu

ReLU [16] (see Figure 5.1) is defined as

$$y_i = f(x_i) = \begin{cases} 0, & x_i < 0 \\ x_i, & x_i \geq 0. \end{cases}$$

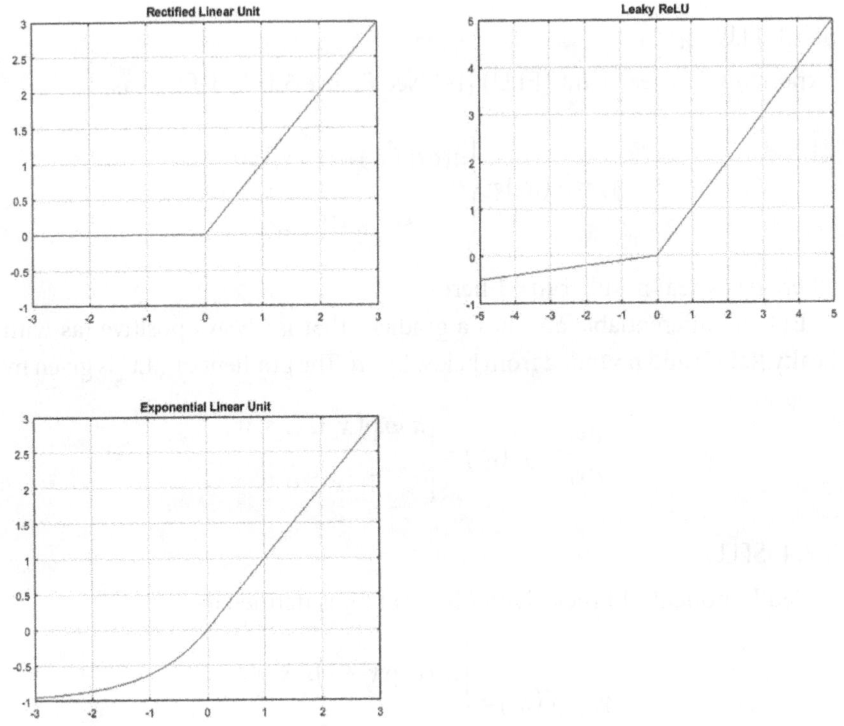

FIGURE 5.1 ReLu (a), Leaky ReLu (b), and ELU (c).

The gradient of ReLU is

$$\frac{dy_i}{dx_i} = f'(x_i) = \begin{cases} 0, & x_i < 0 \\ 1, & x_i \geq 0. \end{cases}$$

5.2.2 Leaky ReLU

Leaky ReLU [18] (see Figure 5.1) is defined as

$$y_i = f(x_i) = \begin{cases} ax_i, & x_i < 0 \\ x_i, & x_i \geq 0 \end{cases},$$

where a is a small real number ($a = 0.01$ here). As noted in the Introduction, this function, unlike ReLu, has no point with a null gradient:

$$\frac{dy_i}{dx_i} = f'(x_i) = \begin{cases} a, & x_i < 0 \\ 1, & x_i \geq 0 \end{cases}$$

5.2.3 ELU

Exponential Linear Unit (ELU) [19] (see Figure 5.1) is defined as

$$y_i = f(x_i) = \begin{cases} a(\exp(x_i) - 1), & x_i < 0 \\ x_i, & x_i \geq 0 \end{cases},$$

where a is a real number ($a = 1$ here).

ELU is differentiable and has a gradient that is always positive (as with Leaky ReLU) and bounded from below by $-a$. The gradient of ELU is given by

$$\frac{dy_i}{dx_i} = f'(x_i) = \begin{cases} a\exp(x_i), & x_i < 0 \\ 1, & x_i \geq 0 \end{cases}$$

5.2.4 SELU

Scaled Exponential Linear Unit (SELU) [20] is defined as

$$y_i = f(x_i) = \begin{cases} sa(\exp x_i - 1), & x_i < 0 \\ sx_i, & x_i \geq 0 \end{cases}$$

where both a and s are real numbers (a=1.6733 and s=1.0507 here; these are the same values used in Ref. [20] and were selected to map a random variable of null mean and unit variance in a random variable with null mean and unit variance).

Note that SELU is basically the same as ELU but is multiplied by the additional scaled parameter s to prevent the gradient from vanishing or exploding. The gradient of SELU is given by

$$\frac{dy_i}{dx_i} = f'(x_i) = \begin{cases} sa\exp(x_i), & x_i < 0 \\ s, & x_i \geq 0 \end{cases}$$

5.2.5 PReLU

Parametric ReLU (PreLU) [14] is defined as

$$y_i = f(x_i) = \begin{cases} a_c x_i, & x_i < 0 \\ x_i, & x_i \geq 0 \end{cases}$$

where a_c includes real numbers that are different for every channel of the input. PreLU is the same as Leaky ReLU except that the parameters a_c are learnable.

The gradients of PReLU are

$$\frac{dy_i}{dx_i} = f'(x_i) = \begin{cases} a_c, & x_i < 0 \\ 1, & x_i \geq 0 \end{cases} \quad \text{and} \quad \frac{dy_i}{da_c} = \begin{cases} x_i, & x_i < 0 \\ 0, & x_i \geq 0 \end{cases}$$

Note that the slopes of the left-hand sides are all initialized to 0.

5.2.6 SReLU

S-Shaped ReLU (SReLU) [30] is composed of three piecewise linear functions that are expressed by four learnable parameters, thus

$$y_i = f(x_i) = \begin{cases} t^l + a^l\left(x_i - t^l\right), & x_i < t^l \\ x_i, & t^l \leq x_i \leq t^r \\ t^r + a^r\left(x_i - t^r\right), & x_i > t^r \end{cases},$$

where t^l, t^r, a^l and a^r are the four learnable real number parameters (initialized as $a^l=0$, $t^l=0$, and $t^r=maxInput$, where $maxInput$ is a hyper-parameter). SReLU's rather large number of parameters results in high representation power.

The gradients of SReLU are given by

$$\frac{dy_i}{dx_i} = f'(x_i) = \begin{cases} a^l, & x_i < t^l \\ 1, & t^l \le x_i \le t^r \\ a^r, & x_i > t^r \end{cases},$$

$$\frac{dy_i}{da^l} = \begin{cases} x_i - t^l, & x_i < t^l \\ 0, & x_i \ge t^l \end{cases}, \text{ and}$$

$$\frac{dy_i}{dt^l} = \begin{cases} 1 - a^l, & x_i < t^l \\ 0, & x_i \ge t^l \end{cases}.$$

5.2.7 APLU

Adaptive Piecewise Linear Unit (APLU) [21] is defined as

$$y_i = \text{ReLU}(x_i) + \sum_{c=1}^{n} a_c \max(0, -x_i + b_c)$$

where a_c and b_c are real numbers, each different for each channel of the input. *APLU* is a linear piecewise function able to approximate, as noted in the Introduction, any continuous function on a compact set.

The gradient of APLU is given by the sum of the gradients of ReLU and of the functions contained in the sum. With respect to the parameters, a_c and b_c, the gradients are

$$\frac{df(x,a)}{da_c} = \begin{cases} -x + b_c, & x < b_c \\ 0, & x \ge b_c \end{cases} \quad \text{and} \quad \frac{df(x,a)}{db_c} = \begin{cases} -a_c, & x < b_c \\ 0, & x \ge b_c \end{cases}$$

In this study, the parameters a_c were initialized to 0, while the points were randomly initialized. Added was a 0.001 L^2 -penalty on the norm of the parameters a_c. Thus, another term was included in the loss function, which is defined as

$$L^{reg} = \sum_{c=1}^{n} |a_c|^2 \; L^{reg} = \sum_{c=1}^{n} |a_c|^2$$

A relative learning rate was also added to these parameters: *maxInput* times the smallest used for the rest of the network. Thus, if λ is the global learning rate, the learning rate λ^* of the parameters a_c would be

$$\lambda^* = \frac{\lambda}{maxInput} \; \lambda^* = \frac{\lambda}{maxInput}.$$

5.2.8 MeLU

To understand the Mexican ReLU (MeLU) [25], let $\phi^{a,\lambda}(x) = \max(\lambda - |x-a|, 0)$ be a "Mexican hat type" function, where a and λ are real numbers. When $|x-a| > \lambda$, the function $\phi^{a,\lambda}(x)$ is null but constantly increases with a derivative of 1 and between a and a–λ and decreases with a derivative of –1 between a and $a+\lambda$.

The aforementioned functions serve as the building blocks of MeLU, which is defined as

$$y_i = \text{MeLU}(x_i) = \text{PReLU}^{c_0}(x_i) + \sum_{j=1}^{k-1} c_j \; \phi^{a_j,\lambda_j}(x_i),$$

where k is the number of learnable parameters for each channel (one parameter for PReLU and k–1 parameters for the coefficients in the sum of the Mexican hat functions; k=4, 8 here), c_j are the learnable parameters, c_0 is the vector of parameters in PReLU, and a_j and λ_j are both fixed and chosen recursively.

Initially, the parameter *maxInput* is set. The first Mexican hat function has its maximum in $2 \cdot maxInput$ and is equal to zero in 0 and $4 \cdot maxInput$. The next two functions are chosen to be zero outside the interval [0, $2 \cdot maxInput$] and [$2 \cdot maxInput$, $4 \cdot maxInput$], with the requirement being that they have their maximum in *maxInput* and $3 \cdot maxInput$ (Table 5.1).

Since Mexican hat functions are continuous and piecewise differentiable, so is MeLU. If all the c_i learnable parameters are initialized to zero,

TABLE 5.1 Fixed Parameters of MeLU with *maxInput*=256

j	1	2	3	4	5	6	7
a_j	512	256	768	128	384	640	896
λ_j	512	256	256	128	128	128	128

MeLU coincides with ReLU, a property that is helpful in transfer learning when the network is pretrained with ReLU (in which case MeLU can simply be substituted; of course, MeLU can also be substituted for networks trained with Leaky ReLU and PReLU). Another important property derives from the fact that the Mexican hat functions are a Hilbert basis on a compact set with the L^2 norm; thus, they can approximate every function in $L^2([0, 1{,}024])$ as k goes to infinity.

MeLU is similar to SReLU and APLU in having multiple learnable parameters, but this number is larger in APLU. MeLU is also similar to APLU in that it can approximate the same set of piecewise linear functions equal to identity when x is large enough, but how this is done is different for each function. Given the right choice of the parameters, APLU can be equal to any piecewise linear function because the points of nondifferentiability are learnable, but MeLU is more efficient because it can represent every piecewise linear function by exploiting only the joint optimization of the weight matrix and the biases. Moreover, the gradients of the two activations with respect to the learnable parameters are different. The optimization of a neural network depends in large part on two factors: the output of every hidden layer and the gradient of that output with respect to the parameters.

Unlike APLU, MeLU changes the activation where it is needed, making optimization easier. The difference between the basis functions of MeLU and APLU is illustrated in Figure 5.2. Moreover, as noted in Section 5.2.7, the coefficients in APLU must be regularized with an L^2 penalty and benefits from a low learning rate; MeLU does not need any regularization.

In this study, the learnable parameters in MeLU are initialized to zero, so the activation starts off as ReLU, thereby exploiting all the nice properties of ReLU at the beginning.

5.2.9 GaLU

Gaussian ReLU (GaLU), proposed here, is based on MeLU and possesses the same desirable properties. To define GaLU, let $\phi_g^{a,\lambda}(x) = \max(\lambda - |x-a|, 0) + \min\left(|x-a-2\lambda| - \lambda, 0\right)$ be a Gaussian

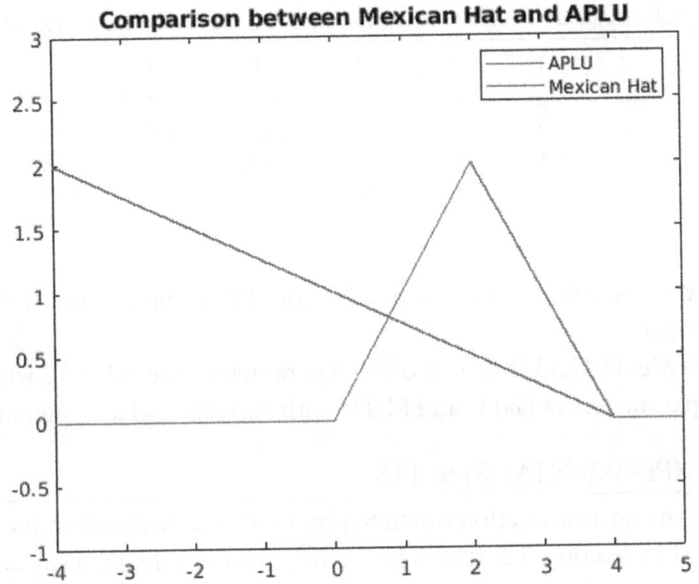

FIGURE 5.2 Partial derivatives of MeLU and APLU.

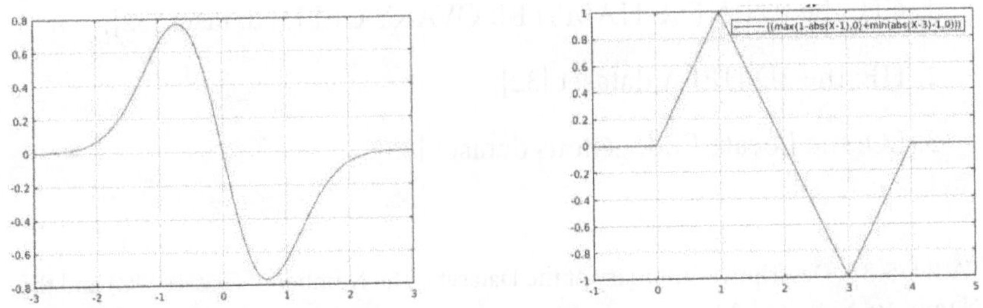

FIGURE 5.3 Gaussian wavelet (a) and our Gaussian type (b).

type function, where a and λ are real numbers. In Figure 5.3, a standard Gaussian wavelet function is compared with a Gaussian type with $a=1, \lambda=1$.

GaLU is defined, similarly to MeLU, as

$$y_i = \text{GaLU}(x_i) = \text{PReLU}^{c_0}(x_i) + \sum_{j=1}^{k-1} c_j \ \phi_g^{a_j, \lambda_j}(x_i).$$

As shown in Ref. [31], piecewise linear odd functions constructed of many linear pieces approximate nonlinear functions better than ReLU does.

TABLE 5.2 Comparison of the Fixed parameters of GaLU and MeLU with $maxInput=1$

	j	1	2	3	4	5	6	7
MeLU	a_j	2	1	3	0.5	1.5	2.5	3.5
	λ_j	2	1	1	0.5	0.5	0.5	0.5
GaLU	a_j	1	0.5	2.5	0.25	1.25	2.25	3.25
	λ_j	1	0.5	0.5	0.25	0.25	0.25	0.25

The rationale behind GaLU is to add more linear pieces than is the case with MeLU.

Like MeLU, GaLU has a set of fixed parameters (see Table 5.2 where the fixed parameters of GaLU and MeLU with $maxInput=1$ are compared).

5.3 EXPERIMENTAL RESULTS

GaLU, the novel activation function proposed here, is tested on the CNNs detailed in Section 5.2 across 13 publicly available biomedical datasets. Details of the datasets are summarized in Table 5.3. The 13 datasets are the following:

1. CH: the CHINESE HAMSTER OVARY CELLS dataset [32];
2. HE: the 2D HELA dataset [32];
3. LO: the Locate Endogenous dataset [33];

TABLE 5.3 Descriptive Summary of the Datasets: The Number of Classes (#C) and the Number of Samples (#S)

Dataset	#C	#S	URL for Download
CH	5	327	http://ome.grc.nia.nih.gov/iicbu2008/hela/index.html#cho
HE	10	862	http://ome.grc.nia.nih.gov/iicbu2008/hela/index.html
LO	10	502	http://locate.imb.uq.edu.au/downloads.shtml
TR	11	553	http://locate.imb.uq.edu.au/downloads.shtml
RN	10	200	http://ome.grc.nia.nih.gov/iicbu2008/rnai/index.html
TB	7	970	https://ome.grc.nia.nih.gov/iicbu2008
LY	3	375	https://ome.grc.nia.nih.gov/iicbu2008
MA	4	237	https://ome.grc.nia.nih.gov/iicbu2008
LG	2	265	https://ome.grc.nia.nih.gov/iicbu2008
LA	4	529	https://ome.grc.nia.nih.gov/iicbu2008
CO	8	5,000	https://zenodo.org/record/53169#.WaXjW8hJaUm
BGR	3	300	https://zenodo.org/record/834910#.Wp1bQ-jOWUl
LAR	3	1,320	https://zenodo.org/record/1003200#.WdeQcnBx0nQ

4. TR: the LOCATE TRANSFECTED dataset [33];
5. RN: the FLY CELL dataset [34];
6. MA: Muscle aging [34], a dataset that includes images of *C. elegans* muscles at four ages;
7. TB: Terminal bulb aging [34] dataset of images of *C. elegans* terminal bulb at seven ages;
8. LY: Lymphoma dataset [34];
9. LG: Liver gender [34], a dataset of liver tissue sections from 6-month male and female mice on a caloric restriction diet, the two classes representing the gender of the mice;
10. LA: Liver aging [34], a dataset of liver tissue sections from female mice on an ad libitum diet;
11. CO: histological images of human colorectal cancer [35];
12. BGR: breast grading carcinoma [36];
13. LAR: Laryngeal dataset [37].

Unless specified, the protocol used on the above datasets is five-fold cross-validation, and the Wilcoxon signed rank test [38] was used to validate the experiments.

In Tables 5.4–5.6, the performances of the different activation functions considering Vgg16, ResNet50, and DenseNet201 are respectively reported. Bold text means that the classifier is the best among the ones we tested. All the networks are trained with a batch size (BS) of 30 and a learning rate (LR) of 0.0001 for 30 epochs. These settings were selected to reduce the computation time. Random reflection on both axes and two independent random rescales of both axes by two factors uniformly sampled in Refs. [1,2] were applied for data augmentation (the vertical and horizontal proportions of the new image were thus rescaled).

Several ensembles are reported in Tables 5.4 and 5.5:

1. ENS, sum rule of all methods, except smallGaLU and GaLU, with a given *MaxInput* of a given CNN;
2. eENS, sum rule of all methods, except smallGaLU and GaLU, of a given CNN.

TABLE 5.4 Performance Obtained Using ResNet

	Activation	CH	HE	LO	TR	RN	TB	LY	MA	LG	LA	CO	BG	LAR	Avg
Resnet50	MeLU (k=8)	92.92	86.40	91.80	82.91	25.50	56.29	67.47	76.25	91.00	82.48	94.82	89.67	88.79	78.94
MaxInput=1	Leaky ReLu	89.23	87.09	92.80	84.18	34.00	57.11	70.93	79.17	93.67	82.48	95.66	90.33	87.27	80.30
	ELU	90.15	86.74	94.00	85.82	48.00	60.82	65.33	85.00	96.00	90.10	95.14	89.33	89.92	82.79
	MeLU (k=4)	91.08	85.35	92.80	84.91	27.50	55.36	68.53	77.08	90.00	79.43	95.34	89.33	87.20	78.76
	PReLU	92.00	85.35	91.40	81.64	33.50	57.11	68.80	76.25	88.33	82.10	95.68	88.67	89.55	79.26
	SReLU	91.38	85.58	92.60	83.27	30.00	55.88	69.33	75.00	88.00	82.10	95.66	89.00	89.47	79.02
	APLU	92.31	87.09	93.20	80.91	25.00	54.12	67.20	76.67	93.00	82.67	95.46	90.33	88.86	78.98
	ReLu	93.54	89.88	95.60	90.00	55.00	58.45	**77.87**	90.00	93.00	85.14	94.92	88.67	87.05	84.54
	SmallGaLU	92.31	87.91	93.20	91.09	52.00	60.00	72.53	90.00	95.33	87.43	95.38	87.67	88.79	84.12
	GaLU	92.92	88.37	92.20	90.36	41.50	57.84	73.60	89.17	92.67	88.76	94.90	90.33	90.00	83.27
	ENS	**95.38**	89.53	97.00	89.82	**59.00**	62.78	76.53	86.67	96.00	**91.43**	**96.60**	**91.00**	89.92	86.28
	ENS_G	93.54	**90.70**	**97.20**	**92.73**	56.00	**63.92**	77.60	**90.83**	**96.33**	**91.43**	96.42	90.00	**90.00**	**86.67**
Resnet50	MeLU (k=8)	94.46	89.30	94.20	92.18	54.00	61.86	75.73	89.17	97.00	88.57	95.60	87.67	88.71	85.26
MaxInput=255	MeLU (k=4)	92.92	90.23	95.00	91.82	57.00	59.79	78.40	87.50	97.33	85.14	95.72	89.33	88.26	85.26
	SReLU	92.31	89.42	93.00	90.73	56.50	59.69	73.33	91.67	**98.33**	**88.95**	95.52	**89.67**	87.88	85.15
	APLU	**95.08**	89.19	93.60	90.73	47.50	56.91	75.20	89.17	97.33	87.05	95.68	**89.67**	89.47	84.35
	ReLu	93.54	89.88	95.60	90.00	55.00	58.45	77.87	90.00	93.00	85.14	94.92	88.67	87.05	84.54
	SmallGaLU	93.54	87.79	95.60	89.82	55.00	63.09	76.00	90.42	95.00	85.33	95.08	**89.67**	**89.77**	85.08
	GaLU	92.92	87.21	92.00	91.27	47.50	60.10	74.13	87.92	96.00	86.86	95.56	89.33	87.73	83.73
	ENS	93.85	**91.28**	**96.20**	93.27	59.00	63.30	77.60	91.67	98.00	87.43	96.30	89.00	89.17	86.62
	ENS_G	**95.08**	**91.28**	**96.20**	**94.18**	**63.00**	**64.85**	**78.67**	**92.50**	97.67	87.62	**96.54**	**89.67**	**89.77**	**87.46**
eENS		94.77	**91.40**	**97.00**	92.91	60.00	64.74	77.87	88.75	**98.00**	90.10	96.50	**90.00**	89.77	87.06
eENS_G		**95.08**	91.28	96.80	**93.45**	**62.50**	**65.26**	**78.93**	**91.67**	96.67	**90.48**	**96.60**	89.33	**89.85**	**87.53**
ENS_MeLU		**94.46**	**90.93**	**97.00**	93.45	57.50	63.92	78.40	90.00	**97.67**	87.62	96.18	**90.00**	89.32	86.65
ENS_MG		**94.46**	**90.93**	96.60	**94.55**	**58.50**	**64.23**	**79.47**	**92.92**	96.33	**88.38**	**96.44**	89.33	**90.30**	**87.11**

TABLE 5.5 Performance Obtained Using Vgg16

	Activation	CH	HE	LO	TR	RN	TB	LY	MA	LG	LA	CO	BG	LAR	Avg
Vgg16 *MaxInput*=1	MeLU (*k*=8)	**99.69**	92.09	98.00	92.91	59.00	60.93	78.67	87.92	**86.67**	93.14	95.20	89.67	90.53	86.49
	Leaky ReLu	99.08	91.98	98.00	93.45	66.50	61.13	80.00	92.08	**86.67**	91.81	95.62	91.33	88.94	87.43
	ELU	98.77	93.95	97.00	92.36	56.00	59.69	81.60	90.83	78.33	85.90	95.78	93.00	90.45	85.66
	MeLU (*k*=4)	99.38	91.16	97.60	92.73	64.50	62.37	81.07	89.58	86.00	89.71	95.82	89.67	93.18	87.13
	PReLU	99.08	90.47	97.80	94.55	64.00	60.00	81.33	**92.92**	78.33	91.05	95.80	92.67	90.38	86.79
	SReLU	99.08	91.16	97.00	93.64	65.50	60.62	82.67	90.00	79.33	93.33	96.10	94.00	92.58	87.30
	APLU	99.08	92.33	97.60	91.82	63.50	62.27	77.33	90.00	82.00	92.38	96.00	91.33	90.98	86.66
	ReLu	**99.69**	93.60	98.20	93.27	69.50	61.44	80.80	85.00	85.33	88.57	95.50	93.00	91.44	87.33
	SmallGaLU	98.46	91.63	97.80	91.35	64.50	59.79	80.53	89.58	77.33	92.76	95.70	91.67	91.97	86.39
	GaLU	98.46	94.07	97.40	92.36	65.00	59.07	81.07	92.08	75.67	93.71	95.68	88.67	91.74	86.53
	ENS	99.38	93.84	98.40	**95.64**	68.00	**65.67**	85.07	92.08	85.00	96.38	**96.74**	94.33	**92.65**	89.47
	ENS_G	**99.69**	**94.65**	**99.00**	95.45	**72.00**	64.95	**86.93**	92.50	83.33	**97.14**	96.72	**94.67**	**92.65**	**89.97**
Vgg16 *MaxInput*=255	MeLU (*k*=8)	**99.69**	92.09	97.40	93.09	59.50	60.82	80.53	88.75	80.33	88.57	95.94	90.33	88.33	85.79
	MeLU (*k*=4)	99.38	91.98	98.60	92.55	66.50	59.59	84.53	91.67	**88.00**	94.86	95.46	93.00	**93.03**	88.39
	SReLU	98.77	93.14	97.00	92.18	65.00	62.47	77.60	89.58	76.00	96.00	95.84	94.33	89.85	86.75
	APLU	98.77	92.91	97.40	93.09	63.00	57.32	82.67	90.42	77.00	90.67	94.90	93.00	91.21	86.33
	ReLu	**99.69**	93.60	98.20	93.27	69.50	61.44	80.80	85.00	85.33	88.57	95.50	93.00	91.44	87.33
	SmallGaLU	99.38	92.91	97.00	92.73	50.50	62.16	78.40	90.42	73.00	94.48	95.32	92.00	90.98	85.32
	GaLU	98.77	92.91	97.60	93.09	66.50	59.48	83.47	90.83	95.00	85.52	95.96	91.67	93.41	88.01
	ENS	99.38	93.84	98.80	95.27	68.50	64.23	84.53	92.50	81.33	**96.57**	96.66	95.00	92.20	89.13
	ENS_G	99.38	**94.88**	98.80	95.64	70.50	**65.88**	85.87	93.75	81.67	96.38	**96.70**	**95.67**	92.80	**89.84**
eENS		99.38	94.07	98.80	**95.64**	69.00	**65.88**	85.87	**93.33**	82.67	96.57	**96.88**	**95.33**	**92.50**	89.68
eENS_G		**99.69**	94.65	**99.00**	95.27	**71.00**	65.57	**86.93**	92.92	**83.33**	**97.71**	96.82	95.00	92.42	**90.02**
ENS_MeLU		**99.69**	93.72	98.80	**95.09**	71.00	63.61	**86.93**	91.25	**85.33**	95.24	96.48	93.00	92.95	89.46
ENS_MG		**99.69**	**94.88**	**99.00**	**95.09**	**72.50**	**64.12**	86.40	**92.92**	84.67	**96.57**	**96.68**	**95.00**	**93.48**	**90.07**

TABLE 5.6 Performance Obtained Using DenseNet

	Activation	CH	HE	LO	TR	RN	TB	LY	MA	LG	LA	CO	BG	LAR	Avg
DenseNet *MaxInput*=1	MeLU (*k*=8)	93.23	93.02	96.60	95.27	55.00	60.82	80.53	90.00	85.67	84.38	95.60	88.67	90.00	85.29
	Leaky ReLu	92.92	92.44	95.80	93.45	50.50	62.58	75.47	89.17	81.33	76.38	95.48	91.33	90.98	83.67
	ELU	78.77	79.07	91.80	91.64	34.00	39.07	63.73	72.50	**97.00**	84.95	89.34	81.67	82.27	75.83
	MeLU (*k*=4)	89.85	91.05	96.00	94.18	52.50	62.99	79.73	89.58	81.00	77.52	95.52	89.33	90.98	83.86
	PReLU	93.85	92.44	96.40	92.18	58.00	61.03	80.27	89.58	77.00	81.90	95.80	87.67	90.15	84.32
	SReLU	93.85	89.88	97.00	94.91	63.50	65.15	79.47	92.08	78.67	87.24	95.95	90.00	90.68	86.02
	APLU	93.54	92.44	97.00	92.73	54.50	60.82	78.13	90.83	79.33	85.14	95.00	88.67	92.12	84.63
	ReLu	96.92	91.63	95.80	93.82	59.00	59.18	82.93	87.92	87.33	73.71	94.90	86.00	91.21	84.64
	SmallGaLU	90.77	92.21	96.20	92.91	51.00	61.03	75.47	86.67	81.00	81.71	95.00	87.33	90.83	83.24
	GaLU	88.00	92.44	96.40	92.18	49.50	60.00	75.73	91.25	80.33	84.38	96.00	89.33	90.98	83.57
	ENS	**96.62**	94.65	**98.20**	96.18	**71.00**	67.01	87.73	93.33	86.33	91.81	96.52	92.33	92.27	89.53
	ENS_G	**96.92**	**95.12**	98.00	**96.55**	69.50	**67.73**	**88.53**	93.33	86.33	**91.81**	**96.56**	**92.33**	**92.58**	**89.63**
DenseNet *MaxInput*=255	MeLU (*k*=8)	93.85	90.23	96.60	93.45	41.50	62.16	80.53	87.08	81.67	78.67	95.72	89.00	91.59	83.23
	MeLU (*k*=4)	91.08	90.47	96.00	94.73	55.00	61.03	75.73	89.17	81.33	80.95	95.40	90.67	88.79	83.87
	SReLU	92.31	89.88	96.40	93.45	54.00	65.36	77.33	89.17	**85.00**	75.81	90.20	88.67	92.05	83.81
	APLU	95.69	93.26	97.20	95.09	48.00	60.93	77.60	91.25	70.33	87.62	95.20	89.67	91.74	84.12
	ReLu	96.92	91.63	95.80	93.82	59.00	59.18	82.93	87.92	87.33	73.71	94.90	86.00	91.21	84.64
	SmallGaLU	92.92	91.51	97.20	94.18	54.00	61.44	77.07	89.58	84.33	85.14	95.40	89.33	91.44	84.88
	GaLU	94.66	90.93	96.40	94.91	52.00	62.27	73.87	90.00	77.33	78.10	95.40	88.00	90.83	83.43
	ENS	**97.85**	94.53	98.20	96.73	**67.50**	66.08	**84.80**	90.83	82.33	87.62	**96.06**	92.00	92.80	88.25
	ENS_G	**97.85**	**95.12**	**98.60**	**96.91**	**67.50**	**66.49**	84.53	90.83	82.67	**88.57**	**96.06**	91.67	**92.95**	**88.44**
eENS		**97.23**	**95.12**	**98.40**	**96.91**	**72.50**	**68.45**	**88.80**	**92.08**	**85.33**	**91.24**	96.60	**92.00**	92.35	**89.77**
eENS_G		**97.23**	**95.12**	**98.40**	**96.91**	70.50	67.53	86.93	**92.08**	85.00	90.86	**96.62**	91.33	**92.65**	89.32
ENS_MeLU		**97.54**	94.53	98.00	96.36	**66.50**	**66.08**	85.07	90.42	**85.67**	86.67	96.54	91.00	91.97	88.18

3. ENS_G, sum rule of all methods with a given MaxInput of a given CNN;
4. eENS_G, sum rule of all methods of a given CNN.
5. ENS_MeLU, sum rule of all methods based on MeLU with ReLu.
6. ENS_MG, sum rule of all methods based on MeLU, smallGaLU, and GaLU with ReLu.

In Table 5.7, the performance on some datasets obtained by choosing optimal values for BS and LR are reported for ReLU. It will be noted that with BS and LR optimized for ReLU, the performance of ENS is higher than that obtained of ReLU. Results in Table 5.7 are similar to those in Tables 5.4–5.6.

Examining the results reported in Tables 5.4–5.7, the following conclusions can be drawn:

- ENS/ENS_G and eENS/eENS_G outperform (*P*-value of 0.05) all the stand-alone activation functions, including ReLu. The most important finding of this work is the performance of eENS/eENS_G, which outperforms ReLu (*P*-value of 0.05) on all three CNN topologies;
- eENS and eENS_G obtain similar performance, but ENS_G many times outperforms ENS;
- MeLU obtains the best average performance considering all the CNNs;

TABLE 5.7 Performance with Optimized BS and LR

	Activation	CH	LA		MA
Resnet50	MeLU (k=8)	98.15	98.48	Vgg16	90.42
MaxInput=255	MeLU (k=4)	98.15	98.67	*MaxInput*=255	87.08
BS=10	SReLU	99.08	96.00	BS=50	88.33
LR=0.001	APLU	98.46	98.48	LR=0.0001	**93.75**
	ReLu	97.23	96.57		92.08
	SmallGaLU	97.54	93.90		90.00
	GaLU	**99.38**	96.38		88.75
	ENS	**99.38**	**99.05**		**93.75**
	ENS_G	**99.38**	98.67		93.33
	ENS_MeLU	**99.38**	**99.05**		91.67
	ENS_MG	99.08	98.86		93.33

- ENS_MeLU outperforms ReLu on all three CNN topologies, but ENS_MG outperforms ENS_MeLU on all three CNN topologies;
- Different behavior occurs in the different topologies; in ResNet50 and DenseNet201, there is a clear performance difference between *MaxInput* = 1, 255, while in Vgg16, similar performance is obtained with *MaxInput* = 1, 255.
- Also, by optimizing BS and LR for ReLU, similar conclusions are obtained: ENS and ENS_G outperform other activation functions, including ReLU.

5.4 CONCLUSION

In this chapter, an evaluation of the performance of an ensemble of CNNs generated by changing the activation functions in three famous pretrained networks: Vgg16, ResNet50, and DenseNet201 is presented. The performance of eight activation functions, including a novel activation function, GaLU, on 13 challenging datasets is reported. The most interesting result is that in all the three CNN topologies, the proposed ensembles strongly outperform each single CNN, as well as those based on the standard ReLu.

Experiments show that an ensemble of multiple CNNs that differ only in their activation functions outperforms the results of the single CNNs with the nine different activation functions. Experiments also demonstrate that no single activation performs consistently better than any other across the 13 datasets. In particular, we see that MeLU is competitive with the other activation functions in the literature. MeLU also seems to be the best performing activation when k=4, in particular on VGG16. Notice that we only tested MeLU with k=4, 8; in other words, we did not cherry-pick the best performing parameters of k on the testing set.

In future work, we plan on generating larger ensembles of CNNs to ascertain the degree to which the performances of a single CNN can be boosted by different activation functions. The difficulty of studies involving ensembles of CNNs lies in the enormous speed and memory resources required to conduct such experiments.

ACKNOWLEDGMENT

We gratefully acknowledge the support from the NVIDIA Corporation for the "NVIDIA Hardware Donation Grant" of a Titan X used in this research.

BIBLIOGRAPHY

[1] A. Krizhevsky, I. Sutskever, and G. E. Hinton, ImageNet classification with deep convolutional neural networks, in *Advances in Neural Information Processing Systems*, F. Pereira, C. J. C. Burges, L. Bottou, and K. Q. Weinberger, Eds. Red Hook, NY: Curran Associates, Inc., 2012, pp. 1097–1105.

[2] A. Y. Hannun et al., Deep speech: scaling up end-to-end speech recognition, *ArXiv*, vol. abs/1412.5567, 2014.

[3] P. Di Lena, K. Nagata, and P. Baldi, Deep architectures for protein contact map prediction, *Bioinformatics*, vol. 28, no. 19, pp. 2449–2457, 2012.

[4] A. Lusci, G. Pollastri, and P. Baldi, Deep architectures and deep learning in chemoinformatics: the prediction of aqueous solubility for drug-like molecules, *Journal of Chemical Information and Modeling*, vol. 53, no. 7, pp. 1563–1575, 2013.

[5] P. Baldi, P. Sadowski, and D. Whiteson, Searching for exotic particles in high-energy physics with deep learning, *Nature Communications*, vol. 5, no. 1, p. 4308, 2014.

[6] K. He, X. Zhang, S. Ren, and J. Sun, Deep residual learning for image recognition, *2016 IEEE Conference on Computer Vision and Pattern Recognition (CVPR)*, pp. 770–778, 2015.

[7] S. Ren, K. He, R. B. Girshick, and J. Sun, Faster R-CNN: towards real-time object detection with region proposal networks, *IEEE Transactions on Pattern Analysis and Machine Intelligence*, vol. 39, pp. 1137–1149, 2015.

[8] F. Schroff, D. Kalenichenko, and J. Philbin, FaceNet: a unified embedding for face recognition and clustering, *2015 IEEE Conference on Computer Vision and Pattern Recognition (CVPR)*, pp. 815–823, 2015.

[9] D. Bahdanau, K. Cho, and Y. Bengio, Neural machine translation by jointly learning to align and translate, *CoRR*, vol. abs/1409.0473, 2014.

[10] D. C. Ciresan, U. Meier, and J. Schmidhuber, Multi-column deep neural networks for image classification, *2012 IEEE Conference on Computer Vision and Pattern Recognition*, pp. 3642–3649, 2012.

[11] Y. Sun, X. Wang, and X. Tang, Deep learning face representation by joint identification-verification, presented at the NIPS, Montreal, 2014.

[12] Y. Taigman, M. Yang, M. A. Ranzato, M. Yang, and L. Wolf, DeepFace: closing the gap to human-level performance in face verification, *2014 IEEE Conference on Computer Vision and Pattern Recognition*, pp. 1701–1708, 2014.

[13] L. Wan, M. D. Zeiler, S. Zhang, Y. LeCun, and R. Fergus, Regularization of neural networks using dropconnect, in *ICML*, 2013.

[14] K. He, X. Zhang, S. Ren, and J. Sun, Delving deep into rectifiers: surpassing human-level performance on imagenet classification, *2015 IEEE International Conference on Computer Vision (ICCV)*, pp. 1026–1034, 2015.

[15] O. Russakovsky et al., ImageNet large scale visual recognition challenge, ARXIV:1409.0575, 2014.

[16] X. Glorot, A. Bordes, and Y. Bengio, Deep sparse rectifier neural networks, in *AISTATS*, 2011.

[17] V. Nair and G. E. Hinton, Rectified Linear Units Improve Restricted Boltzmann Machines, *Presented at the 27 th International Conference on Machine Learning*, Haifa, Israel, 2010.

[18] A. L. Maas, Rectifier nonlinearities improve neural network acoustic models, 2013.

[19] D.-A. Clevert, T. Unterthiner, and S. Hochreiter, Fast and accurate deep network learning by exponential linear units (ELUs), *CoRR*, vol. abs/1511.07289, 2015.

[20] G. Klambauer, T. Unterthiner, A. Mayr, and S. Hochreiter, Self-normalizing neural networks, *Presented at the 31st Conference on Neural Information Processing Systems (NIPS 2017)*, Long Beach, CA, 2017.

[21] F. Agostinelli, M. D. Hoffman, P. J. Sadowski, and P. Baldi, Learning Activation Functions to Improve Deep Neural Networks, *CoRR*, vol. abs/1412.6830, 2014.

[22] S. Scardapane, S. V. Vaerenbergh, and A. Uncini, Kafnets: kernel-based non-parametric activation functions for neural networks, *Neural Networks: The Official Journal of the International Neural Network Society*, vol. 110, pp. 19–32, 2017.

[23] F. Manessi and A. Rozza, Learning Combinations of Activation Functions, *2018 24th International Conference on Pattern Recognition (ICPR)*, pp. 61–66, 2018.

[24] P. Ramachandran, B. Zoph, and Q. V. Le, Searching for Activation Functions, *ArXiv*, vol. abs/1710.05941, 2017.

[25] G. Maguolo, L. Nanni, and S. Ghidoni, Ensemble of convolutional neural networks trained with different activation functions, Cornell University, *arXiv.org*, 2019.

[26] K. Simonyan and A. Zisserman, Very deep convolutional networks for large-scale image recognition, Cornell University, *arXiv:1409.1556v6*, 2014.

[27] K. He, X. Zhang, S. Ren, and J. Sun, Deep residual learning for image recognition, *Presented at the 2016 IEEE Conference on Computer Vision and Pattern Recognition (CVPR)*, Las Vegas, NV, 2016.

[28] G. Huang, Z. Liu, L. Van Der Maaten, and K. Q. Weinberger, Densely connected convolutional networks, *CVPR*, vol. 1, no. 2, p. 3, 2017.

[29] B. Geraldo Junior, S. V. da Rocha, M. Gattass, A. C. Silva, and A. C. de Paiva, A mass classification using spatial diversity approaches in mammography images for false positive reduction, *Expert System with Applications*, vol. 40, no. 18, pp. 7534–7543, 2013.

[30] X. Jin, C. Xu, J. Feng, Y. Wei, J. Xiong, and S. Yan, Deep learning with S-shaped rectified linear activation units, *Presented at the Proceedings of the Thirtieth AAAI Conference on Artificial Intelligence*, Phoenix, AZ, 2016.

[31] A. Nicolae, PLU: the piecewise linear unit activation function, *ArXiv*, vol. abs/1809.09534, 2018.

[32] M. V. Boland and R. F. Murphy, A neural network classifier capable of recognizing the patterns of all major subcellular structures in fluorescence microscope images of HeLa cells, *BioInformatics*, vol. 17, no. 12, pp. 1213–223, 2001.

[33] N. Hamilton, R. Pantelic, K. Hanson, and R. D. Teasdale, Fast automated cell phenotype classification, *BMC Bioinformatics*, pp. 8–110, 2007.

[34] L. Shamir, N. V. Orlov, D. M. Eckley, and I. Goldberg, IICBU 2008: a proposed benchmark suite for biological image analysis, *Medical & Biological Engineering & Computing*, vol. 46, no. 9, pp. 943–947, 2008.

[35] J. N. Kather et al., Multi-class texture analysis in colorectal cancer histology, *Scientific Reports*, vol. 6, p. 27988, 2016.

[36] K. Dimitropoulos, P. Barmpoutis, C. Zioga, A. Kamas, K. Patsiaoura, and N. Grammalidis, Grading of invasive breast carcinoma through Grassmannian VLAD encoding, *PLoS One*, vol. 12, pp. 1–18, 2017.

[37] S. Moccia et al., Confident texture-based laryngeal tissue classification for early stage diagnosis support, *Journal of Medical Imaging (Bellingham)*, vol. 4, no. 3, p. 34502, 2017.

[38] J. Demšar, Statistical comparisons of classifiers over multiple data sets, *Journal of Machine Learning Research*, vol. 7, pp. 1–30, 2006.

CHAPTER 6

Analysis of Structural MRI Data for Epilepsy Diagnosis Using Machine Learning Techniques

Seyedmohammad Shams
and Esmaeil Davoodi-Bojd
Henry Ford Health System
Detroit, Michigan

Hamid Soltanian-Zadeh
Henry Ford Health System
Detroit, Michigan
University of Tehran
Tehran, Iran

CONTENTS

6.1 INTRODUCTION

Epilepsy, characterized by spontaneous and recurrent seizures, is one of the major neurological disorders affecting 0.5%–2% of the population, and based on the World Health organization's report, more than three million Americans suffer from it [1,2]. According to the new classification identified by the International League Against Epilepsy (ILAE), seizures can be categorized into generalized and focal epileptic seizures [3]. Of those, focal epilepsy is more common than generalized [4]. It has been shown that epilepsy with focal seizures in the temporal lobe, which is termed temporal lobe epilepsy (TLE), is the most probable one with local seizures, and about 60% of all adult and adolescent epileptic patients suffer from this type of focal epilepsy. The mesial temporal lobe epilepsy (mTLE) with hippocampal sclerosis, identified by ILAE due to its prevalence, is the most common and intractable TLE [5,6] and more often refractory to medical treatment in adults.

A drug-resistant patient who fails more than two optimal trials of antiepileptics and has at least one seizure per month is considered a candidate for epilepsy surgery. In this case, a resection surgery can be an efficacious option and will be performed if an epileptic focus is localized with confidence [7,8]. Obviously, the success of surgical treatment in these cases is thoroughly dependent on the localization/lateralization accuracy provided by imaging, electrocortical, and neuropsychological testing. Congruent EEG, seizure semiology, and imaging studies in determining epileptogenic mesial temporal lobe can sufficiently satisfy the requirement of a successful epilepsy resective surgery, while in the presence of incongruent lateralization, patients may undergo intracranial electrode implantation, which has a major medical risk and financial cost [9].

Hence, the determination of the primary origin of a patient's seizure by advanced structural imaging techniques is one of the active areas in epilepsy research, due to its noninvasive nature. Among abnormality syndromes, mesial temporal sclerosis (MTS) is the best predictor of mTLE [10–12]. Several structural imaging modalities have been utilized to diagnose MTS and reduce the error and uncertainty in the lateralization of mTLE, as the most operated form of epilepsy. In this direction, the following neuroimaging modalities have been widely used for determining structural features that are well-suited to distinguish patients with right and left mTLE as well as patients with unilateral and bilateral abnormality: anatomical magnetic resonance imaging (T1-weighted MRI), fluid-attenuated inversion recovery (FLAIR), and diffusion tensor imaging (DTI) [13].

Hippocampal sclerosis (HS) is the most frequent pathology encountered in patients with intractable TLE and has been recognized for at least 190 years [14,15]. Hardening or sclerosis of the hippocampus refers to severe neuronal cell loss and gliosis in the different hippocampal subfields, e.g., CA1 and CA4 [16]. The incidence rate of HR in mTLE has been reported to be 56% and has been widely used as the first feature in determining the most affected side, i.e., lateralization [17–19]. Hippocampal sclerosis has been characterized on MRI by the use of volume loss on T1-weighted imaging, hyperintensity on T2-weighted imaging, and signal intensity change on FLAIR.

Although the aforementioned structural changes in the hippocampus have been reported in up to 70% of cases, in several cases, these changes are undetectable, or the laterality of the epileptic focus merely based on them does not provide sufficient certainty for a successful surgery [20,21]. Hence, alterations in some adjacent structures, e.g., amygdala, have been added to these quantitative analyses to strengthen the classification. To document structural changes attributed to mTLE beyond alterations in the hippocampus and amygdala, several studies have been conducted and a variety of abnormalities associated with mTLE in gray matter and white matter were reported [20]. Among them, abnormalities in the entorhinal cortex, piriform cortex, thalamus, cingulum, fornix, and corpus callosum are well-known.

It is widely assumed that neuronal cell loss and gliosis are associated with an increase in the free water in the tissue. Therefore, FLAIR, which provides a measure of free water in the tissue, has been considered as a standard technique for the investigation of neuronal cell gliosis and localization of focal epilepsy, especially in mTLS patients. However, many studies have shown that FLAIR lacks sufficient sensitivity in the lateralization of mTLE patients and should be accompanied by other imaging features to achieve satisfactory results.

Since some studies have reported that a recognizable portion of mTLE patients with pathologically confirmed hippocampal sclerosis did not show clear abnormality symptoms on T1-weighted and FLAIR MRI [21], there has been a compelling need to employ other imaging techniques. To this end, it has been shown that DTI-based tractography can detect microstructural alterations in brain tissues before any abnormalities can be seen on anatomical MRI. DTI can play a specific role in investigating alterations in the white matter tracts due to neuronal loss in the epileptic focus and in the extralimbic structures due to widespread neural firing.

In the following sections, we describe five recent studies, which have used the above MRI modalities to provide a set of effective features that can be used in a machine learning approach to diagnose epilepsy.

6.2 LATERALIZATION INDICES/FEATURES EXTRACTED FROM STRUCTURAL MRI

The hypothesis behind the studies that focus on lateralization using structural MRI is that the need for intracranial electroencephalography (iEEG), i.e., phase II, can be minimized by optimizing the lateralization of mTLE using a set of optimal imaging features and a model for laterality classification. To lateralize mTLE, MRI has been widely used to extract several effective features to detect MTS *in vivo* [22]. MTS is characterized by neuronal loss, gliosis/sclerosis, granule cell dispersion, and mossy fiber sprouting in hippocampal specimens [23]. Hippocampal volume reduction based on T1-weighted images and increase in signal intensity in T2-weighted and FLAIR MRI have been the dominant features used for the quantification of MTS [17,24–29]. It has been shown that these features successfully lateralize the origin of epilepsy in up to 70% of the cases, although in 15%–30% of the confirmed unilateral mTLE patients, a significant hippocampal asymmetry has not been reported, i.e., subtle or even no evidence of asymmetry is reported [8,17,30]. In such cases, additional structural features may be needed to provide sufficient certainty in laterality declaration.

The second category of MRI features has been assessed by texture analysis. Texture features provide information about signal intensity patterns in tissues and have also been used in psychological disorders, like Alzheimer's, multiple sclerosis, and schizophrenia [31]. These signal patterns and their alterations relative to histological changes in the hippocampus and other regions of interest have been used as a complementary set of features for detecting hippocampal sclerosis as well as focal cortical dysplasia [32–34]. In Ref. [31], several image intensity features of the hippocampal body—mean, standard deviation, and wavelet-based texture features—extracted from the FLAIR images were used to lateralize the site of epileptogenicity. The authors trained a linear classifier based on the right to left ratios of the aforementioned features to establish laterality. They showed that, in 75% of the cases, the mean and standard deviation of FLAIR intensities successfully lateralized the site of epileptogenicity. They also reported 64% and 75% success rates in lateralization based on the wavelet texture features and the hippocampal volumetric features, respectively.

Although hippocampal texture analysis is an image analysis tool for MTS diagnosis, variance of the features extracted from the hippocampus has yielded an uncertainty in epilepsy lateralization, especially in the condition of incompatible electroencephalographic (EEG) lateralization. In cases with a lack of hippocampal imaging asymmetry, features extracted from neighboring structures, such as the amygdala, have been suggested and investigated as alternatives in many studies. These suggestions were based on the studies that showed, in the presence of an intact hippocampus, amygdala sclerosis (AS) in a subgroup of patients with mTLE [35]. Determination of amygdala atrophy as an indicator of neuronal loss and gliosis of the amygdala (AS) based on MRI is a challenging task, due to the small size and lack of structural distinction [35,36]. In Ref. [37], the mean signal and standard deviation of the FLAIR signal intensity in the amygdala have been proposed as complementary features that improved the accuracy of lateralization in mTLE patients.

Some studies have indicated that the mentioned structural measures—T1-weighted, FLAIR—did not determine the side of epileptogenicity in several mTLE patients or misclassified them in bilateral epilepsy while the intracranial EEG (icEEG) clearly showed unilateral epileptogenicity in these patients. For example, Aghakhani et al. [38] reported that icEEG investigations found unilateral epileptogenicity in 73% of patients (1,026 out of 1,403) who had been categorized under bilateral mTLE. These pieces of evidence have encouraged many research groups to examine alternative noninvasive neuroimaging modalities, e.g., DTI, to detect and quantify the epilepsy-related alterations in neuronal microstructures to consequently improve lateralization of epilepsy patients [20,39].

It has been hypothesized that hardening or sclerosis at the seizure focus in mTLE causes alterations in white matter tracts of the focus, which may be detected through white matter tractography [40]. For example, some studies have shown that connectivity of the default mode network (DMN) regions diminishes in mTLE patients [41–43]. DTI techniques, which measure molecular diffusion—diffusivity and directionality—in the brain, can detect epilepsy-associated microstructural alterations in epileptogenic areas earlier than they can be detected on structural MRI modalities [44–47].

6.2.1 Study Population

The following research studies were conducted at Henry Ford Health System (HFHS) and approved by the Institutional Review Board (IRB). All imaging data were de-identified before processing according to a protocol approved by the IRB. Patients whose data were analyzed in these studies had been diagnosed with mTLE including bilateral and unilateral cases. To establish the conditions, the patients underwent a standard investigation protocol including inpatient scalp video-EEG, MRI, neurophysiological testing, and intracarotid amobarbital study.

Bilateral cases were selected among the patients who entered the phase II study and had bilaterality confirmation by icEEG. The unilateral cases were selected among the patients who underwent the resection of mesial temporal structure and achieved an Engle class I outcome, as defined by the Engel classification [10].

Patients without all three imaging modalities—T1-weighted and FLAIR, and DTI—were excluded from the following comparison studies. Some other patients were also excluded due to a high level of artifact contamination or insufficient resolution. For instance, an acceptable MRI segmentation result from FreeSurfer [48] was an inclusion criterion for the studies reviewed in this chapter.

The majority of the cases used in the following studies achieved an Engel class Ia outcome (more than 92%) following surgical resection at the Henry Ford Hospital between 1996 and 2014 [10]. For all cases analyzed in these studies, amygdalohippocampectomy and inferior temporopolar topectomy formed the resection surgery. Also, about 49% of the unilateral cases underwent extraoperative electrocorticography (eECoG), due to uncertainty in the non-invasive determination of the side of epileptogenicity.

It should be noted that the excised tissues, especially the hippocampus, were studied to qualitatively examine hippocampal sclerosis and to investigate the correlation between MRI characteristics, i.e., hippocampal volume loss on T1-weighted images and signal hyperintensity on FLAIR images, and HS identified by neuroradiologists. According to many reports regarding pathologically confirmed HS in the absence of any abnormalities on T1-weighted and FLAIR imaging (about 30%), both hippocampal sclerosis positive (HS-P) and hippocampal sclerosis negative (HS-N) were included in the studies.

Some alterations in the imaging features (e.g., FLAIR intensity, diffusion anisotropy, and volumetric features) may be due to natural physiological variations. Therefore, imaging features of a reliable control group, i.e., nonepileptic subjects, may be investigated to take into account the natural variability in imaging features among healthy individuals. In this direction, in the selected studies, nonepileptic subjects were used to form a control group.

6.2.2 MRI Acquisition

For every patient, MRI scans—coronal T1-weighted using the IRSPGR protocol and coronal T2-weighted using the FLAIR protocol—were acquired on a 1.5T or a 3.0T MRI system (Signa, GE, Milwaukee, USA) preoperatively. T1-weighted imaging parameters for the 1.5 T scanner were TR/TI/TE=7.6/1.7/500 ms, flip angle=20°, voxel size=$0.781\times0.781\times2.0\,mm^3$, and FLAIR imaging parameters were TR/TI/TE=10,002/2,200/119 ms, flip angle=90°, and voxel size=$0.781\times0.781\times3.0\,mm^3$. For the 3.0 T MRI, T1-weighted imaging parameters were TR/TI/TE=10.4/4.5/ 300 ms, flip angle=15°, and voxel size=$0.39\times0.39\times2.00\,mm^3$ and FLAIR imaging parameters were TR/TI/TE=9,002/2,250/124 ms, flip angle=90°, and voxel size=$0.39\times0.39\times3.00\,mm^3$. DTI images (b-value of 1,000 s/mm^2) in 25 diffusion gradient directions along with a set of null images (b-value of 0 s/mm^2) were acquired using echo planar imaging (EPI) with TR/TI/TE=10,000/0/76 ms, flip angle=90°, and voxel size=$1.96\times1.96\times2.6\,mm^3$.

6.2.3 Image Processing

The first processing step for the studies in the field of structural MRI analysis is to segment a region of interest (ROI), e.g., the hippocampus, using T1-weighted MRI (Figure 6.1). This step is a key step since all features are extracted based on the results of this step, especially when T1-weighted and FLAIR image sets are coregistered subsequently (studies I, II, and III). In *study I*, the segmentation was performed manually by the experts, and multiple verifications were performed. To avoid human error, automated segmentation tools, such as FreeSurfer [48], were used in other studies. The second step is the coregistration of the imaging modalities in the feature extraction phase, e.g., coregistration of T1-weighted and FLAIR images.

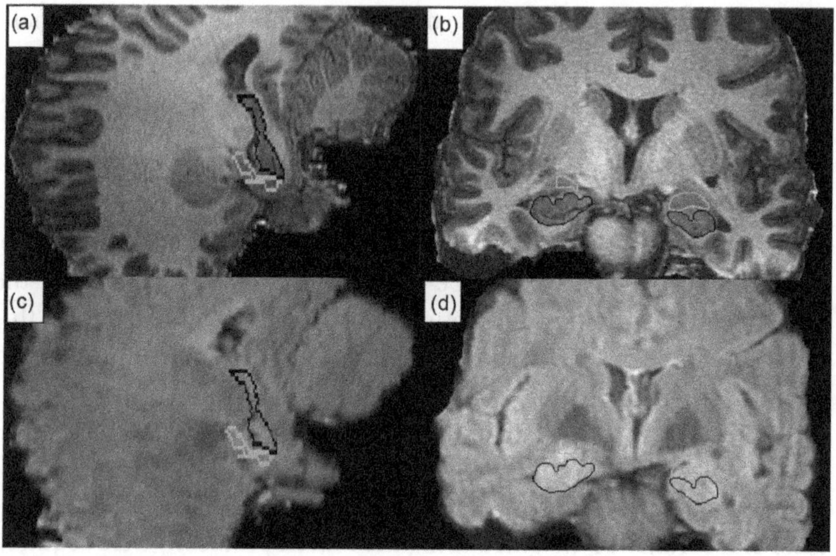

FIGURE 6.1 (a and b): Sample sagittal and coronal T1-weighted images with segmented amygdala and segmented hippocampus shown. (c and d): Sample coronal and sagittal FLAIR images with segmented amygdala and segmented hippocampus shown.

6.2.4 Feature Analysis and Classification

In the following, we focus on the methods used for feature analysis—feature extraction, selection, and reduction—as well as the methods used for classification in the five selected studies.

Study I: T1-Weighted and FLAIR Features: A Hippocampus Study

It has been shown in several studies that hippocampal volume reduction correlates with the side of mTLE in a significant portion of the patients. Thus, this volume reduction has been widely used for mTLE lateralization. In addition to the hippocampal volume reduction, the presence of an increased FLAIR signal has been used as a feature for lateralization. An increase in hippocampal FLAIR signal intensity has been assumed to represent hippocampal gliosis and consequently probable focal epileptogenicity. The third set of image features were extracted using wavelet transform. Wavelet transform is a well-known tool for revealing the local frequency contents of an image and expressing the texture properties of an image. In Ref. [31], volumetric feature, mean and standard deviation of the

FLAIR images, and wavelet-based features were extracted from the two MRI modalities, as described below.

1. For the volumetric feature, the whole hippocampus volume in each hemisphere was examined. The volume of an ROI, e.g., hippocampus, was calculated by the summation of all voxels' volumes in the ROI, i.e., pixel size×slice thickness. The volumetric feature was calculated by the ratio of the volume of the right hippocampus to the left hippocampus. This was a normalized feature and well-suited for the classification of unilateral epilepsy.
2. Two features were extracted from the FLAIR images—mean ratio and standard deviation ratio. Each feature was expressed as a ratio of the two values obtained from the two hippocampi, i.e., right and left hippocampi. Using these ratios instead of the original values facilitates the lateralization by feature reduction and normalization.
3. For each hippocampus, two levels of wavelet transform were calculated, and so seven subband images were produced for each hippocampus. Daubechies' wavelet bases were used for extracting the subband images. Each subband image characterized the frequency content (i.e., texture properties) at a predefined scale. Thus, the energy feature (i.e., the sum of the square intensities) for each subband was used as a texture feature:

$$E_K = \frac{1}{MN} \tag{6.1}$$

where $I_k^2(i,j)$ is an $M \times N$ image in the k-th subband. The choice of an equivalent rectangular image is indeed an important issue that may impact the results of the wavelet analysis since a segmented hippocampus is not rectangular. In Ref. [31], this problem was overcome by filling the background areas in the segmented image using an inpainting technique, i.e., repetitive dilations [49]. Through this method, each slice of the hippocampus was assigned seven energy features and an average over all hippocampus slices produced seven energy features for the whole hippocampus.

The above features were then represented in a feature vector and used to develop a *linear classification* algorithm for categorizing the epilepsy patients into the right-sided and left-sided groups. In this study, a boundary domain was introduced using two lines parallel to the discriminator line, which provided a variation of 0.25 standard deviation (SD) from the discriminator line. Through these boundary lines, the classifier had an uncertainty group, and the accuracy was provided with and without considering the uncertainty group (see Table 6.1). Due to the limited number of patients, all feature vectors were used for developing a linear discriminator function. The ideal approach to avoid any bias in the estimated accuracy would be to divide the data into the training and testing sets, construct the linear classifier by using the training set only, and then test the trained classifier using the testing set. The results of using these hippocampus features are presented in the Results section.

Study II: Hippocampal and Amygdalar Study: FLAIR and Volumetric Features

It has been shown that in about 10% of the mTLE patients, alterations in amygdalar volume and T2 relaxometry do not accompany changes in the hippocampus, cerebral cortex, cerebellum, and thalamus [35,36,50,51]. This restricted histopathological distribution led the researchers to use changes in amygdalar volume and FLAIR intensity as the supplementary features in mTLE lateralization. In Ref. [37], the mean and the standard deviation of the FLAIR signal in the amygdala were added to the features investigated in Study I to improve the results of classification. Accordingly, four features related to the FLAIR images—mean and standard deviation ratios for amygdala and hippocampus and two features related to the hippocampal volumetry—were used for mTLE lateralization.

Segmentation of the amygdala and hippocampus, which are used in the downstream analysis, was performed manually on the T1-weighted images (Figure 6.1). The hippocampus and amygdala segmentations were then mapped to the FLAIR images, after rigidly registering the T1-weighted image to the FLAIR image for each subject separately. The FLAIR mean and standard deviation were then calculated for each structure, i.e., hippocampus and amygdala, in each hemisphere, and then the right to left ratios of the mean and the standard deviation for each structure were used as features for the lateralization of mTLE.

Similar to Study I, the means and standard deviations of the FLAIR signal intensity in the hippocampus and amygdala were calculated. To reduce the bias imposed by the use of a different scanner, an intensity inhomogeneity correction was applied and then the right/left ratios were used as features.

In Ref. [37], three linear classifiers distinguishing laterality were trained separately using hippocampal volumetry and amygdalar and hippocampal FLAIR features. Also, a boundary/uncertainty region was established for each linear classifier using two parallel lines between which 95% of the control subjects laid. To examine whether adding the amygdalar FLAIR features improved the lateralization process, the McNemar's test was applied.

Study III: DTI-Based Response-Driven Modeling

DTI can detect microstructural alterations induced by epilepsy through segmentation and fiber tracking. In Ref. [20], microstructural changes in the cingulum, fornix, and corpus callosum were exploited using DTI analysis to lateralize mTLE and distinguish unilateral and bilateral cases. The preprocessing algorithm included: (1) establishment of white matter structures—cingulum, corpus callosum, fornix, and their subregions—using DTI and (2) segmentation of the hippocampus and co-registering T1-weighted image to FLAIR to calculate the mean and standard deviation of the FLAIR intensity within the hippocampus.

Before the establishment of the white matter structures, the DTI images were interpolated to provide a homogenous voxel size. For segmentation, in addition to fractional anisotropy (FA) and mean diffusivity (MD), the eigenvector associated with the largest eigenvalue of the diffusion tensor was calculated as the principal diffusion direction. Next, cingulum, corpus callosum, fornix, and their subregions were defined using seed-based segmentation and fiber tracking [52,53]. A typical segmentation result for these fibers is shown in Figure 6.2. For all the cohorts (i.e., right and left unilateral mTLE, bilateral mTLE, and control groups), FA and MD of 15 subregions (including left and right of anteroinferior, superior, and posteroinferior of the cingulum; the genu, rostral body, anterior midbody, posterior midbody, isthmus, and splenium of the corpus callosum; and the anterior body, and left and right crus of the fornix) were estimated. The set of features used to lateralize mTLE and detect unilaterality were:

1. hippocampal volumetry,
2. hippocampal mean and standard deviation of FLAIR intensity, and
3. FA in corpus callosum, cingulum, and fornix regions.

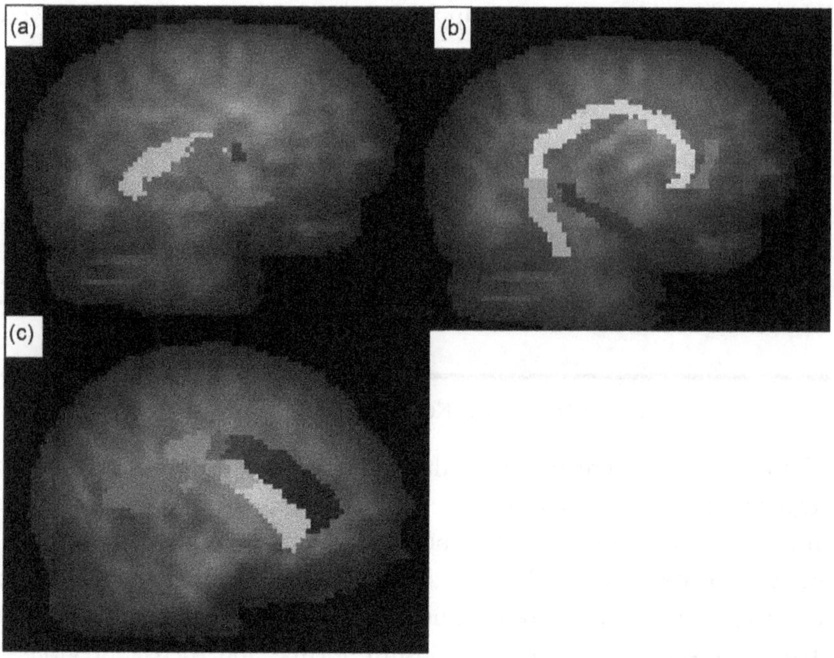

FIGURE 6.2 Typical segmentation of fornix, cingulum, and corpus callosum overlaid on 3D rendered FA maps. (a): Fornix segmented into the anterior body and left and right crus. (b): Cingulum segmented into the left and right antero-inferior, superior, and posteroinferior. (c): Corpus callosum segmented into the left and right genu, rostral body, anterior midbody, posterior midbody, isthmus, and splenium.

Using the *t*-test and two-way repeated measures analysis of variance, the relationships between the above features—15 features for FA of the above subregions and 6 features for hippocampal volumetry and FLAIR mean and SD of intensity—and mTLE laterality were examined. This can be considered as the *feature selection* step in machine learning terminology.

Next, multinomial logistic regression [54] was used to develop three different models based on the above features as the independent variables and the laterality labels—right mTLE, left mTLE, bilateral mTLE, and control—as the dependent variables. These models include:

1. Right vs. left mTLE,
2. Unilateral vs. bilateral mTLE, and
3. Right mTLE vs. Left mTLE vs. Bilateral mTLE vs. Control.

Due to the small sample size of the data set (54 cases), the authors used the leave-one-out procedure to perform a cross-validation accuracy estimation. To this end, 54 training-testing trials were performed. Each training was assessed by multinomial logistic function regression through the following formula:

$$\ln\left(\frac{Pr(Y_i = T \mid M_k)}{Pr(Y_i = N \mid M_k)}\right) = \beta_T^K \tag{6.2}$$

where X_i and β_i are the observation feature vector and the vector of regression coefficients, respectively, and $\Pr(Y_i = T \mid M_k)$ is the posterior probability of the label Y_i, which was set to 0 or 1 depending on the decision made by the model. Through multinomial logistic regression, the regression coefficients were estimated for each of the three regression models. Subsequently, the accuracy of the estimated models was assessed by using β_i for the testing data.

Study IV: Texture Features of the Whole Brain

Since epilepsy may affect the structural features of the entire brain, this study hypothesized that the textural features—first and second-order statistical features—might be used to identify epileptic patients. To this end, the second-order statistical features were obtained based on a volumetric gray-level occurrence matrix (GLCM). These features were extracted from the brain tissue segmentation results. Here, two tissue segmentation methods were exploited: Gram–Schmidt orthogonalization [55] and unified segmentation method [56]. The results of the two methods were compared quantitatively. The features were calculated for the brain tissues—CSF, gray matter, and white matter—defined by the above segmentation methods. In addition, the hippocampi were segmented in all subjects using the FSL-FIRST software [57], and their texture features were calculated.

The first-order features including mean, variance, skewness, and kurtosis were derived using voxel-based MRI analysis based on the intensity of each voxel and the probability of occurrence of that intensity in the brain, e.g., skewness is defined as $\sum_{i=0}^{G-1} (i-\mu)^3 P(i)$. For a complete set of definitions, see [58].

For extracting the second-order features, i.e., structural features and three-dimensional extensions of the features [59], (1) energy, (2) entropy, (3) correlation, (4) contrast, (5) sum average, (6) dissimilarity, (7) texture variance, (8) cluster shade, (9) cluster tendency, (10) homogeneity, (11) maximum probability, and (12) inverse texture variance were used. To extract features from 3D images, three different displacement vectors were exploited—d1 = (0,1,0), d2 = (1,1,0), and d3 = (0,1,–1)—each of which captures one direction across the three principal axes. For each region/tissue, 4 first-order features and 36 (3×12) second-order features were extracted from each modality. Thus, 120 features were extracted for the three main brain tissues. Therefore, there was a clear need for a comprehensive feature reduction.

To reduce the dimensionality of the feature vectors, three main steps were applied. The first step (feature selection) discarded the irrelevant features based on a Relief algorithm [60]. The second step reduced the number of features in two steps: (1) clustering the features according to their similarity in the voxel space using *k*-means clustering and (2) selecting the highest Relief score in each cluster and discarding the remaining features in the cluster. In the final step, sequential floating forward selection was used to combinatorically select the prominent features according to the least classification error. In each condition, the authors extracted the features, selected the best features based on the above explanations, and then trained and tested an SVM classifier, using the leave-one-out procedure. The results of feature selection and classifier training are presented in the Results section (Section 3.4).

Study V: Multi-Structural Volume Features

In the above studies, as well as most of the studies conducted in this field, several structural features have been proposed to quantitatively provide evidence for lateralization. However, it is still a matter of debate whether such incorporation is associated with improvement of the lateralization and indeed beneficial. The aim of the study presented in Ref. [61] was to identify the contribution of the neuroanatomical sites/regions in lateralization and establish a robust classifier with the optimal number of features. The feature space included 53 volumetric features extracted from 53 hemispherically paired neuroanatomical regions using Eq. (6.3). A list of these regions segmented by FreeSurfer is available in Ref. [61]. The volume differences of paired structures were normalized to the total volume of the paired structures:

$$f_i = \frac{v_{Li} - v_{Ri}}{v_{Li} + v_{Ri}} \tag{6.3}$$

where v_{Li} and v_{Ri} denote the segmented volumes of the i-th region in the left and right hemispheres, respectively. To avoid human variability, the structures were segmented automatically using FreeSurfer [48]. The premise behind the use of the volume-based features is that the recurrent excitations can result in cell death and consequently atrophy in the hippocampus and other related sites in the brain. Thus, the side-related volume changes may correlate with the side of the epileptogenicity and their use may improve the lateralization accuracy.

In Ref. [61], the feature selection step, which provides an optimal subset of the features, was performed by the wrapper subset evaluation proposed by Kohavi and John in 1997 [62]. This approach found the most distinctive subset of features with the highest mTLE lateralization accuracy. The wrapper subset evaluation method used a supervised learning algorithm to find the optimal subset among the possible feature subsets. Next, logistic regression (LR) and support vector machine (SVM), as two robust and widely used supervised classifiers, were employed and compared in terms of accuracy in the identification of the side of epileptogenicity of mTLE patients. The ridge estimator was used in the multinomial logistic regression implementation to prevent any overfitting. The following multinomial logistic regression kernel model computed the *a posteriori* probability of class j given feature vectors, i.e., $\left[f_1, f_2, \ldots, f_m\right]$.

$$Pr\left[j \mid \left[f_1, f_2, \ldots, f_m\right]\right] = \frac{e^{\beta_0^j + \beta_1^j f_1 + \beta_2^j f_2 + \cdots + \beta_m^j f_m}}{1 + \sum_{j=1}^{k-1} e^{\beta_0^j + \beta_1^j f_1 + \beta_2^j f_2 + \cdots + \beta_m^j f_m}} \tag{6.4}$$

where k was the number of classes and $\beta_0^j, \beta_1^j, \beta_2^j, \ldots, \beta_m^j$ denote the coefficients that were obtained through the training process. Besides, the SVM was used to learn a hyperplane, i.e., an m-dimensional hyperplane model, with the maximum margins as a linear function of feature vectors. To implement the SVM classifier, Pegasos was used as a simple and effective stochastic sub-gradient descent algorithm [63].

6.2.5 Summary of Machine Learning for mTLE Lateralization

To establish a machine learning algorithm for mTLE lateralization, a retrospective comparative assessment was undertaken. In this manner, the patients who underwent resective surgery and without seizures postoperatively were chosen for these types of studies to establish and test a single feature or multiple features for laterality determination. While various machine learning algorithms were used for automated identification of the side of epileptogenicity, those used in the studies presented in this chapter are summarized in Table 6.1. For illustration, the methods used for feature analysis are summarized along with the methods used for classification. We also briefly described the patients' categories, population types, and imaging modalities in Table 6.1.

6.3 RESULTS

6.3.1 Study I: Hippocampal Study – FLAIR Intensity Texture Analysis, and Volumetry

In study I, three sets of features were extracted from the segmented hippocampus in the two hemispheres: mean and standard deviation of FLAIR intensity, wavelet energy features, and hippocampal volumetric features. In this study, linear discriminator line/plane as a classifier was trained for each set of features and the ratio of the number of the correctly classified to the whole number of the subjects was considered as the *classification accuracy*. Considering the uncertain boundaries on each side of the discriminator line, two different accuracies were calculated for each set of features. Uncertain boundaries were placed on the 0.25 standard deviation (SD) separation from and in parallel with the discriminator line.

The accuracy of using seven different combinations of the features was examined and reported separately in this study: (1) mean of the hippocampal FLAIR intensity, (2) standard deviation of the hippocampal FLAIR intensity, (3) mean and standard deviation of the hippocampal FLAIR intensity, (4) two wavelet signatures using db4 (*E1*, *E2*), (5) two wavelet signatures using db6 (*E1*, *E2*), (6) two wavelet signatures using db8 (*E1*, *E2*), and (7) hippocampal volume (right/left). The combination of the mean and the standard deviation (SD) of the hippocampal FLAIR signal intensity provided the most accurate classifiers, which yielded 75% accuracy when correctly classified subjects placed within the uncertain boundaries are considered misclassified and 98% accuracy when considering them as correctly classified. Taking into account the uncertain boundaries, the accuracies were 72% (58%) if the SD (mean) of the hippocampal FLAIR

TABLE 6.1 A Summary of the Studies Reviewed in This Chapter

Study	Imaging Sets	Population of the Study	Feature Sets	Machine Learning Algorithm	Results
Jafari et al. [31]	1. T1-weighted MRI 2. FLAIR (1.5T scanner)	1. Right-sided epilepsy: 16 subjects 2. Left-sided epilepsy: 20 subjects 3. Control group: 25 subjects	1. Mean and SD of hippocampal FLAIR intensity 2. Wavelet energy ratio 3. Hippocampal volume	Linear Discriminant Analysis (LDA)	Accuracy with an uncertain region → accuracy without an uncertain region 1. 75% → 98% 2. 64% → 94% 3. 75% → 83%
Jafari et al. [37]	1. T1-weighted MRI 2. FLAIR 1.5T & 3T scanner	1. Right-sided epilepsy: 26 subjects 2. Left-sided epilepsy: 43 subjects 3. Control group: 46 subjects	1. Mean and SD of hippocampal FLAIR intensity 2. Mean and SD of amygdalar FLAIR intensity 3. Hippocampal volume 4. Amygdalar volume	Linear Discriminant Analysis (LDA)	Accuracy with an uncertain region → accuracy without an uncertain region 1. 70% → 87% 2. 29% → 78% 3. 67% → 75%
Nazem-Zadeh et al. [20]	1. T1-weighted MRI 2. FLAIR 1.5T & 3T scanner 3. DTI	1. Right-sided epilepsy: 11 subjects 2. Left-sided epilepsy: 13 subjects 3. Bilateral: 7 subjects 4. Control group: 23 subjects	FA in: 1. Cingulate subregions 2. Callosal subregions 3. Forniceal subregions	Multinomial logistic model in a leave-one-out manner	Model 1: R vs. L a. 100% accuracy: FA in cingulum b. 100% accuracy: FA in cingulum and corpus callosum Model 2: U vs. B 100% accuracy: FA in corpus callosum and cingulum Model 2: R vs. L vs. B vs. C 100% accuracy: FA in corpus callosum and cingulum

(*Continued*)

TABLE 6.1 (*Continued*) A Summary of the Studies Reviewed in This Chapter

Study	Imaging Sets	Population of the Study	Feature Sets	Machine Learning Algorithm	Results
Sahebzamani et al. [58]	1. T1-weighted MRI 2. FLAIR (3T scanner) 3. T2-weighted image 4. Proton density	1. Unilateral sided epilepsy: 5 subjects 2. Left-sided epilepsy: 5 subjects 3. Control group: 7 subjects	A complete set of first and second-order texture features extracted from FLAIR and T1-weighted images: whole brain and hippocampus	Support vector machine (SVM) in a leave one out manner: epileptic vs. nonepileptic	94% accuracy using FLAIR textural features of white matter 82.3% accuracy using T2 textural features of the hippocampus
Mahmoudi et al. [61]		1. 68 unilateral epileptic patients 2. 2–46 control patients	53 volumetric features extracted for 53 regions segmented using T1 images	**Feature selection**: wrapper algorithm and hill-climbing strategy **Classification**: logistic regression (LR) and support vector machine (SVM)	Selected features: normalized volumetric features of hippocampus, amygdala, and thalamus LR & L-1-O: 98.5% in all patients LR & five-fold CV: 92.6% in all patients

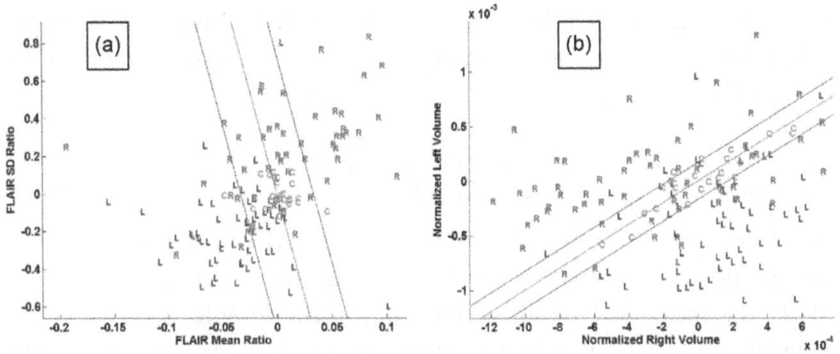

FIGURE 6.3 (a): Scatter plot of the mean and standard deviation (SD) ratios of hippocampal FLAIR intensities using data of nonepileptic subjects (shown by C), right mTLE patients (shown by R), and left mTLE patients (shown by L). (b): Scatter plot of the normalized right and left hippocampal volumes using data of nonepileptic subjects (shown by C), right mTLE patients (shown by R), and left mTLE patients (shown by L).

signal intensity was solely used for classification (Figure 5 in Ref. [31] shows the corresponding scatter plots). We produced a scatter plot for the combination of mean and SD ratios of the hippocampal FLAIR intensities in Figure 6.3a. This scatter plot was generated using a more complete dataset than that reported in Ref. [31]. Further examination revealed that the mean ratio and standard deviation ratio of the hippocampal FLAIR intensity were different among the right-sided, left-sided, and control groups with P-values less than 4.0×10^{-6} and 10^{-12}, respectively.

The above study reported that the classification based on the texture features extracted using Daubechies' wavelet bases with 2, 4, and 6 lengths resulted in 64% accuracy. This was achieved by using energy features of subbands 1 and 2 (right/left ratios) and a linear classifier. In addition, when considering the correctly classified subjects within the uncertain boundaries as misclassified subjects, the maximum accuracy was 64%, which was obtained by using the db8 wavelet.

Classification based on the hippocampal volumetric analysis resulted in 75% accuracy, which was similar to the accuracy of using SD and mean ratio. When considering the correctly classified subjects within the uncertain boundaries as correctly classified, the accuracy of using volumetric features rises to 83% while the accuracy of using SD and mean ratio rises to 98%. The linear scatter plots corresponding to the use of the normalized right and left hippocampal volumes (RHV and LHV) are presented in Figure 6.3b. The discriminator line in this figure is specified by RHV = LHV.

6.3.2 Study II: Hippocampal and Amygdalar Study – FLAIR Intensity and Volumetry

Since alterations in amygdalar volume and FLAIR intensity have often been found to accompany alterations in the hippocampus in cases of mTLE, the mean and standard deviation of the FLAIR intensity in the amygdala were examined for lateralization of epileptogenicity along with the ones from the hippocampus. For lateralization based on FLAIR, two linear classifiers were derived by linear discriminant analysis using the amygdalar and hippocampal FLAIR features for the right and left mTLE.

In the first step, the use of two different scanners, i.e., 3 T and 1.5 T, was found to make no significant difference between amygdalar FLAIR features in control subjects. The results also showed that the linear classifier based on the amygdalar FLAIR intensity-ratio features, i.e., mean and SD ratios, correctly lateralized 78% of the cases while only 29% of these cases were outside the uncertain region. The linear classifier based on the hippocampal FLAIR intensity features was successful to lateralize the epileptogenicity at the rate of 87% while a 70% accuracy was obtained when considering the correctly classified subjects placed within the uncertain region as misclassified subjects (uncertain group). As expected, a significant correlation between hippocampal and amygdalar FLAIR mean intensity ratios was detected ($P < 10^{-18}$). In addition, classification using hippocampal and amygdalar FLAIR mean intensity ratios resulted in similar laterality for 74% of the patients. Interestingly, four patients (6%) who are placed within the uncertain region based on the hippocampal mean intensity ratio were correctly lateralized using the amygdalar mean intensity ratio. This showed that amygdalar and hippocampal FLAIR intensity provided complementary information.

The lateralization based on the hippocampal volumetric feature resulted in 75% accuracy, which decreased to 67% when considering the uncertain region. The lateralization based on the amygdalar volumetric feature alone was about 29% accurate.

6.3.3 Study III: DTI-Based Response-Driven Modeling

In Ref. [20], the significance of differences between all pairs of the mTLE laterality—right, left, and bilateral—was tested using the FA extracted from 15 subregions: left and right of anteroinferior, superior, and posteroinferior of cingulum; genu, rostral body, anterior midbody, posterior midbody, isthmus, and splenium of the corpus callosum; and anterior body, and left and right crus of the fornix. The results showed significant differences between:

1. Control subjects and right mTLE cases for FA in all callosal subregions, in both left and right superior cingulate subregions, and in forniceal crura
2. Right and left mTLE cases for FA in callosal genu, rostral body, and splenium and the right posteroinferior and superior cingulate subregions
3. Control subjects and left mTLE cases in FA of the callosal isthmus
4. Right and bilateral mTLE cases in FA of the rostral and midbody callosal subregions and isthmus

Using FA in cingulate, callosal, and forniceal subregions, three models were constructed to distinguish between unilateral and bilateral cases and also to determine the side of epileptogenicity in the unilateral mTLE. For model 1, i.e., detecting the side of the epileptogenicity in unilateral mTLE cases, the multinomial logistic classifier using FA in the cingulum subregions reached an accuracy of 100% with 7.3 deviance. By incorporating FA in the corpus callosum, the deviance of the fit dropped to 0.7. To distinguish between unilateral and bilateral cases, i.e., model 2, an integration of FA in the corpus callosum and cingulum provided 100% accuracy. This integration also achieved an accuracy of 100% in model 3 (right mTLE vs. left mTLE vs. bilateral mTLE vs. control). This accuracy (100%) was also achieved when the cingulate features were reduced to two features, i.e., those of the left and right posteroinferior cingulum.

6.3.4 Study IV: Texture Features Extracted from Whole Brain MRI

First-order and second-order texture features were extracted from T1-weighted, FLAIR, T2-weighted, and proton-density-weighted images of the hippocampus, white matter, and gray matter. The segmentations were performed using two methods: Gram–Schmidt and unified. Applying the three-step feature selection procedure on the whole-brain segmented by unified segmentation resulted in four features: contrasts of white matter for FLAIR images in three different directions (d1, d2, and d3) and sum average of white matter in the FLAIR images in the d2 direction. Using these four features, a trained SVM classifier achieved 94% accuracy in distinguishing mTLE patients from control subjects. The same feature selection procedure on the whole-brain segmented by Gram–Schmidt segmentation resulted in three dissimilarity features for gray matter in three different directions (d1, d2, and d3) and an SVM classifier achieved 82.3% accuracy.

For unified segmentation, extracting the first and second-order texture features from the segmented hippocampi and applying a feature selection procedure provided two features: cluster tendency of gray matter on the T2-weighted images in two directions (d1 and d2). These features achieved 82.3% accuracy in classifying mTLE patients and control subjects while the hippocampus segmentation provided by Gram–Schmidt achieved 76.4% accuracy.

6.3.5 Study V: Multi-Structural Vomuletric Features

Here, 53 normalized volumetric features were extracted from the brain MRI segmented using FreeSurfer [48]. The normalized features were used as an input set to a wrapper algorithm with logistic regression. The best feature subset resulted from the wrapper algorithm included ten brain structures: hippocampus, amygdala, thalamus, putamen, cerebral white matter, entorhinal cortex, inferior temporal gyrus, paracentral lobule, postcentral gyrus, and parahippocampal gyrus. However, a feature vector with a dimension of 10 was not suitable for classifying 68 subjects. Therefore, the hill-climbing strategy was exploited to find the most promising features among these ten features. The results presented in Ref. [61] demonstrated that the volumetric features extracted from the hippocampus, amygdala, and thalamus provided the highest level of accuracy in lateralization using logistic regression and SVM. The results also demonstrated that adding putamen as the fourth volumetric feature did not increase the accuracy of the LR method while decreasing that of SVM.

Investigating the absolute volumetric features—the mean and standard deviation—of the structures revealed that these features were not distinctive enough for lateralization neither in patients with hippocampus sclerosis (HS-P) nor in patients without it (HS-N). Conversely, normalized volumetric feature, obtained by Eq. (6.3), for the hippocampus showed no overlap between the right- and left-sided patients within the HS-P group. Thus, the normalized volumetric feature of the hippocampus, i.e., hippocampus atrophy, could successfully lateralize the mTLE in the HS-P patients with an accuracy of 100%. However, the normalized volumetric feature did not fully distinguish between the right- and left-sided patients within the HS-N group.

In general, the results of investigating the relationships between each structure's atrophy and the side of epileptogenicity indicated that normalized volumetric feature of each of the structures—hippocampus, amygdala, and thalamus—could not solely identify the side of epileptogenicity.

In Ref. [61], mTLE lateralization based on multi-structural volumetric features was performed using a simplified version of the logistic probability function shown in Eq. (6.4). The results of estimating the parameters and the location of 68 patients are illustrated in Figure 6.4a.

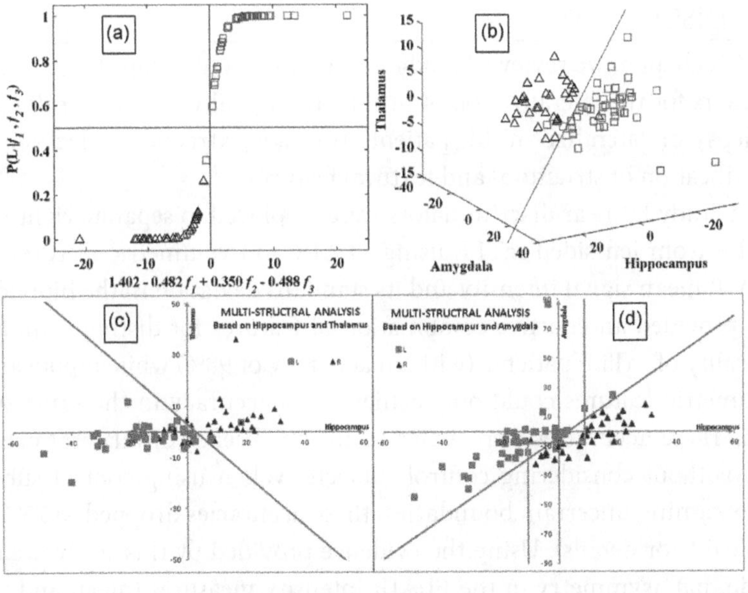

FIGURE 6.4 Illustration of logistic regression of multi-structural volumetric features for mTLE lateralization. (a): Left lateralization probability based on Eq. (6.4) for all mTLE cases (left mTLE cases shown by blue rectangles and right mTLE by red triangles). (b): Scatter plot of the mTLE patients in the three-dimensional feature space defined by the volumetric features of hippocampus, amygdala, and thalamus. Since the decision plane is parallel to the view angle, it is seen as a line. (c and d): Decision plane projected onto the two-dimensional feature spaces defined by the volumetric features of the hippocampus and amygdala, and hippocampus and thalamus, respectively.

The discriminator threshold was set such that the logistic probability function was equal to 0.5:

$$Pr\left[L\middle|\left[f_1, f_2, f_3\right]\right] = \frac{e^{\beta_0^L+\beta_1^L f_1+\beta_2^L f_2+\beta_3^L f_3}}{1+e^{\beta_0^L+\beta_1^L f_1+\beta_2^L f_2+\beta_3^L f_3}} = 0.5 \tag{6.5}$$

which resulted in a plane in the three-dimensional feature space, i.e., $\beta_0^L+\beta_1^L f_1+\beta_2^L f_2+\beta_3^L f_3=0$. This plane can be projected in two-dimensional feature spaces, e.g., the hippocampus–amygdala and hippocampus–thalamus spaces. Figure 6.4b shows the scatter plot of the left and right TLE patients on the three-dimensional feature space along with the decision plane. For further illustration, the decision planes projected into the corresponding two-dimensional feature spaces are shown in Figure 6.4c and d.

6.4 DISCUSSION

In this chapter, we reviewed studies that aimed to develop structural biomarkers for the lateralization of mTLE. Their goal was to either diagnose epilepsy or lateralize mTLE patients through extraction, selection, and modification of structural and textural features.

In Study I, linear discriminators were employed to separate right-sided mTLE from left-sided mTLE using FLAIR and volumetric features. The FLAIR mean signal intensity and its standard deviation in the hippocampus provided an effective combination of features for distinguishing the laterality of mTLE patients (with an accuracy of 98%) while hippocampal volumetric features could only achieve 83% accuracy in the same situation. These accuracies were achieved in the absence of bilateral patients and without considering control subjects. When using control subjects for obtaining uncertain boundaries, these accuracies dropped to 75% (see Table 6.1 for details). Using the evidence provided by this study, we conclude that asymmetry in the FLAIR intensity measures (mean and standard deviation) of the hippocampus may provide additional biomarkers, besides hippocampal volume asymmetry, for hippocampal sclerosis (HS) and side of epileptogenicity.

In addition to the mean and standard deviation of the hippocampus, four conventional texture features—co-occurrence matrix, run-length matrix, absolute gradient, and histogram—of the FLAIR intensity were extracted to be investigated in this study. The wavelet transform energy features defined by Eq. (6.1) correctly classified unilateral hippocampal sclerosis into right- and left-sided mTLE with an accuracy of 94%. This indicates that wavelet-based feature extraction has the capability to be used for mTLE lateralization. Three issues may be raised about this study: (1) the small sample size of 36 patients (20 left-sided and 16 right-sided), (2) not using bilateral cases as an additional category, and (3) dependency on the segmentation accuracy.

In Study II [37], amygdalar FLAIR intensity features were used for epileptic lateralization in the absence of hippocampal atrophy through volumetric and FLAIR features. By using solely the amygdalar features, the side of epileptogenicity could achieve only 29% accuracy while 70% accuracy was achieved by similar features from the hippocampus, but it would be of interest to know that 22% of the cases that could not be lateralized with confidence using hippocampal FLAIR features were classified with confidence using amygdalar FLAIR features. This could be good evidence for a previous report [64]. Moreover, the results indicated that the automated segmentation of the amygdala was sufficient for this study and all wrongly lateralized patients fell within the uncertain boundaries. Since the data used in this study were acquired by different scanners (1.5T and 3T), the scanner variability could have affected the results if the intensity inhomogeneity of the FLAIR images had not been corrected.

Similar to Study I, the bilateral cases were not investigated in this study, since the study focused on the patients with the Engel Ia outcomes. This means that one of the limitations of the previous study (lack of bilateral category) remained unaddressed while the other two were addressed adequately. Another limitation of this study was that it did not investigate the amygdalar volumetric changes associated with mTLE.

The comprehensive study reported in Ref. [20] showed that the FA in the white matter structures affected by mTLE (cingulum, fornix, and corpus callosum) expressed distinctive patterns in unilateral and bilateral mTL relative to nonepileptic subjects. The results showed that FA in the subregions of the fornix, cingulum, and corpus callosum could determine the side of the epileptogenicity in all unilateral mTLE cases. In addition, the volumetric and FLAIR intensity changes in the hippocampus indicated that although these features were useful for lateralization, they did not distinguish unilateral from bilateral mTLE cases.

The data used in this study were collected using a single scanner. This clearly reduced the undesirable variability and provided stable classification results. However, the capability of the proposed model in the case of multi-scanner/multi-center studies should be verified. In addition, the small sample size of the subjects, especially for the bilateral cohort, can be considered as a limitation for this study.

Study IV compared the accuracy of differentiating mTLE subjects from the control subjects based on the segmentations obtained by the unified segmentation and the Gram–Schmidt method. The results showed that the texture features of the regions segmented by the unified method were more discriminative than those of the Gram–Schmidt method. They found the three-dimensional texture features successfully in detecting mTLE cases. Moreover, whole-brain texture features outperformed those of the hippocampus.

In the last study discussed in this chapter [61], normalized volumes of three neuroanatomical regions were found to be optimal for mTLE lateralization. The study showed that a combination of the normalized volumetric features of the hippocampus and amygdala resulted in 94.1% accuracy in mTLE lateralization. Without integrating amygdalar volumetric features, hippocampal volumetric features generated 82.4% accuracy. Moreover, integrating thalamic volumetric features increased the accuracy of the mTLE lateralization to 98.5%.

In all of the above studies, the patients used in the training phase were diagnosed to have mTLE. Thus, the proposed machine learning models are applicable to the mTLE patients. They may not be applicable to patients with other types of epilepsy, e.g., extra-temporal epilepsy. Also, the performance of the proposed features and classification models should be studied for patients with lateral, neocortical TLE.

6.5 CONCLUSION

The features used in the presented studies can be clustered in four groups: (1) volumetric features including single and multi-structural volumes used in Studies I–V; (2) first- and second-order texture features used in Study IV; (3) DTI features used in Study III; and (4) FLAIR intensity features including single and multi-structural features used in Studies I–III. We described the roles of these features in the lateralization of drug-resistant mTLE patients.

The multi-structural approaches proposed in Ref. [37,61] offered high reliability in the prediction of the side of the epilepsy at a reduced cost and risk to the patients. Based on these results, it can be concluded that an integration of the FLAIR intensity features, like those presented in Ref. [37] and the tri-structural imaging biomarker proposed in Ref. [61], may further improve the lateralization accuracy. However, these methods have not been validated in the case of bilateral epilepsy. To include bilateral cases, future work may extend the methods in an approach similar to that of Ref. [20].

REFERENCES

1. D. Hirtz, D. J. Thurman, K. Gwinn-Hardy, M. Mohamed, A. R. Chaudhuri, and R. Zalutsky, "How common are the 'common' neurologic disorders?," *Neurology*, vol. 68, no. 5, pp. 326–337, Jan. 2007.
2. G. S. Bell, A. Neligan, and J. W. Sander, "An unknown quantity – The worldwide prevalence of epilepsy," *Epilepsia*, vol. 55, no. 7, pp. 958–962, 2014.
3. A. T. Berg, et al., "Revised terminology and concepts for organization of seizures and epilepsies: Report of the ILAE Commission on Classification and Terminology, 2005–2009," *Epilepsia*, vol. 51, no. 4, pp. 676–685, 2010.
4. A. M. Harriott and W. O. Tatum, *Electroclinical Syndromes: Adolescent Onset*, Swaiman's Pediatric Neurology, 6th ed.: Elsevier Inc., 2017.
5. R. D. G. Blair, "Temporal lobe epilepsy semiology," *Epilepsy Res. Treat.*, vol. 2012, pp. 1–10, 2012.
6. J. A. Hill and N. Venna, *Human Herpesvirus 6 and the Nervous System*, 1st ed., vol. 123: Elsevier B.V., 2014.
7. F. J. Rugg-Gunn, et al., "Diffusion tensor imaging in refractory epilepsy," *Lancet*, vol. 359, no. 9319, pp. 1748–1751, 2002.
8. R. P. Carne, et al., "MRI-negative PET-positive temporal lobe epilepsy: A distinct surgically remediable syndrome," *Brain*, vol. 127, no. 10, pp. 2276–2285, 2004.
9. J. C. Bulacio, et al., "Long-term seizure outcome after resective surgery in patients evaluated with intracranial electrodes," *Epilepsia*, vol. 53, no. 10, pp. 1722–1730, 2012.
10. Engel J Jr, Van Ness PC, Rasmussen T, et al. Outcome with respect to epileptic seizures. In: Engel J Jr, editor. *Surgical Treatment of the Epilepsies.* 2nd ed. New York: Raven Press; 1993:609–622..
11. E. Achten, P. Boon, T. Van De Kerckhove, J. Caemaert, J. De Reuck, and M. Kunnen, "Value of single-voxel proton MR spectroscopy in temporal lobe epilepsy," *Am. J. Neuroradiol.*, vol. 18, no. 6, pp. 1131–1139, 1997.
12. J. De Tisi, et al., "The long-term outcome of adult epilepsy surgery, patterns of seizure remission, and relapse: A cohort study," *Lancet*, vol. 378, no. 9800, pp. 1388–1395, 2011.
13. G. D. Cascino, "Neuroimaging in partial epilepsy: Structural magnetic resonance imaging," *J. Epilepsy*, vol. 11, no. 3, pp. 121–129, 1998.
14. M. Thom, "Review: Hippocampal sclerosis in epilepsy: A neuropathology review," *Neuropathol. Appl. Neurobiol.*, vol. 40, no. 5, pp. 520–543, 2014.
15. M. Thom, "Hippocampal sclerosis: Progress since sommer," *Brain Pathol.*, vol. 19, no. 4, pp. 565–572, 2009.
16. I. Blümcke, et al., "International consensus classification of hippocampal sclerosis in temporal lobe epilepsy: A Task Force report from the ILAE Commission on Diagnostic Methods," *Epilepsia*, vol. 54, no. 7, pp. 1315–1329, 2013.

17. G. D. Jackson, R. I. Kuzniecky, and G. D. Cascino, "Hippocampal sclerosis without detectable hippocampal atrophy," *Neurology*, vol. 44, no. 1, pp. 42–42, Jan. 1994.
18. I. Blümcke, M. T. Mrcpath, and D. Wiestler, "Blümcke, Mrcpath, Wiestler_ Ammon's Horn Sclerosis A Maldevelopmental Disorder Associated with Temporal Lobe Epilepsy.pdf," vol. 1, 2002.
19. I. Blümcke, R. Coras, H. Miyata, and C. Özkara, "Defining clinico-neuropathological subtypes of mesial temporal lobe epilepsy with hippocampal sclerosis," *Brain Pathol.*, vol. 22, no. 3, pp. 402–411, 2012.
20. M. R. Nazem-Zadeh, et al., "DTI-based response-driven modeling of mTLE laterality," *NeuroImage Clin.*, vol. 11, pp. 694–706, 2016.
21. P. F. Yang, et al., "Long-term epilepsy surgery outcomes in patients with PET-positive, MRI-negative temporal lobe epilepsy," *Epilepsy Behav.*, vol. 41, no. 2014, pp. 91–97, 2014.
22. S. Treit, et al., "Regional hippocampal diffusion abnormalities associated with subfield-specific pathology in temporal lobe epilepsy," *Epilepsia Open*, no. August, pp. 544–554, 2019.
23. M. Mishto, et al., "Immunoproteasome expression is induced in mesial temporal lobe epilepsy," *Biochem. Biophys. Res. Commun.*, vol. 408, no. 1, pp. 65–70, 2011.
24. R. S. Briellmann, R. M. Kalnins, S. F. Berkovic, and G. D. Jackson, "Hippocampal pathology in refractory temporal lobe epilepsy," *Neurology*, vol. 58, no. 2, pp. 265–271, Jan. 2002.
25. F. Cendes, et al., "MRI of amygdala and hippocampus in temporal lobe epilepsy," *J. Comput. Assist. Tomogr.*, vol. 17, no. 2, pp. 206–210, 1993.
26. C. R. Jack, et al., "Temporal lobe seizures: Lateralization with MR volume measurements of the hippocampal formation," *Radiology*, vol. 175, no. 2, pp. 423–429, May 1990.
27. C. R. Jack, "Hippocampal T2 relaxometry in epilepsy: Past, present, and future," *AJNR. Am. J. Neuroradiol.*, vol. 17, no. 10, pp. 1811–1814, 1996.
28. C. R. Jack, et al., "Mesial temporal sclerosis: Diagnosis with fluid-attenuated inversion-recovery versus spin-echo MR imaging," *Radiology*, vol. 199, no. 2, pp. 367–373, May 1996.
29. J. H. Kim, R. D. Tien, G. J. Felsberg, A. K. Osumi, and N. Lee, "MR measurements of the hippocampus for lateralization of temporal lobe epilepsy: Value of measurements of the body vs the whole structure," *Am. J. Roentgenol.*, vol. 163, no. 6, pp. 1453–1457, 1994.
30. W. Van Paesschen, "Quantitative MRI of mesial temporal structures in temporal lobe epilepsy," *Epilepsia*, vol. 38, no. SUPPL. 10, pp. 3–12, 1997.
31. K. Jafari-Khouzani, K. Elisevich, S. Patel, B. Smith, and H. Soltanian-Zadeh, "FLAIR signal and texture analysis for lateralizing mesial temporal lobe epilepsy," *Neuroimage*, vol. 49, no. 2, pp. 1559–1571, 2010.
32. L. Bonilha, et al., "Texture analysis of hippocampal sclerosis," *Epilepsia*, vol. 44, no. 12, pp. 1546–1550, Dec. 2003.
33. S. B. Antel, et al., "Automated detection of focal cortical dysplasia lesions using computational models of their MRI characteristics and texture analysis," *Neuroimage*, vol. 19, no. 4, pp. 1748–1759, Aug. 2003.

34. A. Bernasconi, et al., "Texture analysis and morphological processing of magnetic resonance imaging assist detection of focal cortical dysplasia in extra-temporal partial epilepsy," *Ann. Neurol.*, vol. 49, no. 6, pp. 770–775, Jun. 2001.
35. L. A. Miller, R. S. McLachlan, M. S. Bouwer, L. P. Hudson, and D. G. Munoz, "Amygdalar sclerosis: Preoperative indicators and outcome after temporal lobectomy," *J. Neurol. Neurosurg. Psychiatry*, vol. 57, no. 9, pp. 1099–1105, 1994.
36. L. P. Hudson, D. G. Munoz, L. Miller, R. S. McLachlan, J. P. Girvin, and W. T. Blume, "Amygdaloid sclerosis in temporal lobe epilepsy," *Ann. Neurol.*, vol. 33, no. 6, pp. 622–631, Jun. 1993.
37. K. Jafari-Khouzani, K. Elisevich, V. S. Wasade, and H. Soltanian-Zadeh, "Contribution of quantitative amygdalar MR FLAIR signal analysis for lateralization of mesial temporal lobe epilepsy," *J. Neuroimag.*, vol. 28, no. 6, pp. 666–675, 2018.
38. Y. Aghakhani, X. Liu, N. Jette, and S. Wiebe, "Epilepsy surgery in patients with bilateral temporal lobe seizures: A systematic review," *Epilepsia*, vol. 55, no. 12, pp. 1892–1901, Dec. 2014.
39. J. Zhang, et al., "Identifying the affected hemisphere with a multimodal approach in MRI-positive or negative, unilateral or bilateral temporal lobe epilepsy," *Neuropsychiatr. Dis. Treat.*, vol. 10, pp. 71–80, 2014.
40. C. Scanlon, S. G. Mueller, I. Cheong, M. Hartig, M. W. Weiner, and K. D. Laxer, "Grey and white matter abnormalities in temporal lobe epilepsy with and without mesial temporal sclerosis," *J. Neurol.*, vol. 260, no. 9, pp. 2320–2329, 2013.
41. S. Chiang and Z. Haneef, "Graph theory findings in the pathophysiology of temporal lobe epilepsy," *Clin. Neurophysiol.*, vol. 125, no. 7, pp. 1295–1305, Jul. 2014.
42. M. N. DeSalvo, L. Douw, N. Tanaka, C. Reinsberger, and S. M. Stufflebeam, "Altered structural connectome in temporal lobe epilepsy," *Radiology*, vol. 270, no. 3, pp. 842–848, Nov. 2013.
43. M. J. Vaessen, et al., "White matter network abnormalities are associated with cognitive decline in chronic epilepsy," *Cereb. Cortex*, vol. 22, no. 9, pp. 2139–2147, Oct. 2011.
44. M. Liu, Z. Chen, C. Beaulieu, and D. W. Gross, "Disrupted anatomic white matter network in left mesial temporal lobe epilepsy," *Epilepsia*, vol. 55, no. 5, pp. 674–682, May 2014.
45. A. Hufnagel, et al., "Brain diffusion after single seizures," *Epilepsia*, vol. 44, no. 1, pp. 54–63, Jan. 2003.
46. Y. Nakasu, S. Nakasu, S. Morikawa, S. Uemura, T. Inubushi, and J. Handa, "Diffusion-weighted MR in experimental sustained seizures elicited with kainic acid," *Am. J. Neuroradiol.*, vol. 16, no. 6, pp. 1185–1192, 1995.
47. M. B. Parekh, P. R. Carney, H. Sepulveda, W. Norman, M. King, and T. H. Mareci, "Early MR diffusion and relaxation changes in the parahippocampal gyrus precede the onset of spontaneous seizures in an animal model of chronic limbic epilepsy," *Exp. Neurol.*, vol. 224, no. 1, pp. 258–270, Jul. 2010.

48. B. Fischl, et al., "Whole brain segmentation: Automated labeling of neuroanatomical structures in the human brain," *Neuron*, vol. 33, no. 3, pp. 341–355, 2002.
49. A. Criminisi, P. Perez, and K. Toyama, "Region filling and object removal by exemplar-based image inpainting," *IEEE Trans. Image Process.*, vol. 13, no. 9, pp. 1200–1212, 2004.
50. B. E. Swartz, U. Tomiyasu, A. V Delgado-Escueta, M. Mandelkern, and A. Khonsari, "Neuroimaging in temporal lobe epilepsy: Test sensitivity and relationships to pathology and postoperative outcome," *Epilepsia*, vol. 33, no. 4, pp. 624–634, Jul. 1992.
51. C. Guerreiro, et al., "Clinical patterns of patients with temporal lobe epilepsy and pure amygdalar atrophy," *Epilepsia*, vol. 40, no. 4, pp. 453–461, Apr. 1999.
52. M.-R. Nazem-Zadeh, C. H. Chapman, T. L. Lawrence, C. I. Tsien, and Y. Cao, "Radiation therapy effects on white matter fiber tracts of the limbic circuit," *Med. Phys.*, vol. 39, no. 9, pp. 5603–5613, Sep. 2012.
53. M.-R. Nazem-Zadeh, et al., "Segmentation of corpus callosum using diffusion tensor imaging: Validation in patients with glioblastoma," *BMC Med. Imaging*, vol. 12, no. 1, p. 10, 2012.
54. D. Böhning, "Multinomial logistic regression algorithm," *Ann. Inst. Stat. Math.*, vol. 44, no. 1, pp. 197–200, 1992.
55. H. Soltanian-Zadeh, D. J. Peck, J. P. Windham, and T. Mikkelsen, "Brain tumor segmentation and characterization by pattern analysis of multispectral NMR images," *NMR Biomed.*, vol. 11, no. 4–5, pp. 201–208, 1998.
56. J. Ashburner and K. J. Friston, "Unified segmentation," *Neuroimage*, vol. 26, no. 3, pp. 839–851, 2005.
57. B. Patenaude, S. M. Smith, D. N. Kennedy, and M. Jenkinson, "A Bayesian model of shape and appearance for subcortical brain segmentation," *Neuroimage*, vol. 56, no. 3, pp. 907–922, Jun. 2011.
58. G. Sahebzamani, M. Saffar, and H. Soltanian-Zadeh, "Machine learning based analysis of structural MRI for epilepsy diagnosis," in *2019 4th International Conference on Pattern Recognition and Image Analysis (IPRIA)*, 2019, pp. 58–63.
59. E. Ben Othmen, M. Sayadi, and F. Fniaech, "3D gray level co-occurrence matrices for volumetric texture classification," in *3rd International Conference on Systems and Control*, 2013, pp. 833–837.
60. I. Kononenko, "Estimating attributes: Analysis and extensions of RELIEF," *Lect. Notes Comput. Sci. (including Subser. Lect. Notes Artif. Intell. Lect. Notes Bioinformatics)*, vol. 784 LNCS, pp. 171–182, 1994.
61. F. Mahmoudi, et al., "Data mining MR image features of select structures for lateralization of mesial temporal lobe epilepsy," *PLoS One*, vol. 13, no. 8, pp. 1–19, 2018.
62. R. Kohavi and G. H. John, "Wrappers for feature subset selection," *Artif. Intell.*, vol. 97, no. 1–2, pp. 273–324, Dec. 1997.

63. S. Shalev-Shwartz, Y. Singer, N. Srebro, and A. Cotter, "Pegasos: Primal estimated sub-gradient solver for SVM," *Math. Program.*, vol. 127, no. 1, pp. 3–30, 2011.
64. H. G. Wieser, "Mesial temporal lobe epilepsy versus amygdalar epilepsy: Late seizure recurrence after initially amygdalotomy and regained seizure control following hippocampectomy," *Epileptic Disord.*, vol. 2, no. 3, pp. 141–152, Oct. 2000.

CHAPTER 7

Artificial Intelligence-Powered Ultrasound for Diagnosis and Improving Clinical Workflow

Zeynettin Akkus

Mayo Clinic

Rochester, Minnesota

CONTENTS

7.1 INTRODUCTION

Artificial intelligence (AI) could be considered as a system that has the ability to observe its environment and takes actions to maximize the success of achieving its goals. Some examples of such a system that has the ability of sensing, reasoning, engaging, and learning are computer vision for understanding digital images, natural language processing for interaction between human and computer languages, voice recognition for recognition and translation of spoken languages, robotics and motion,

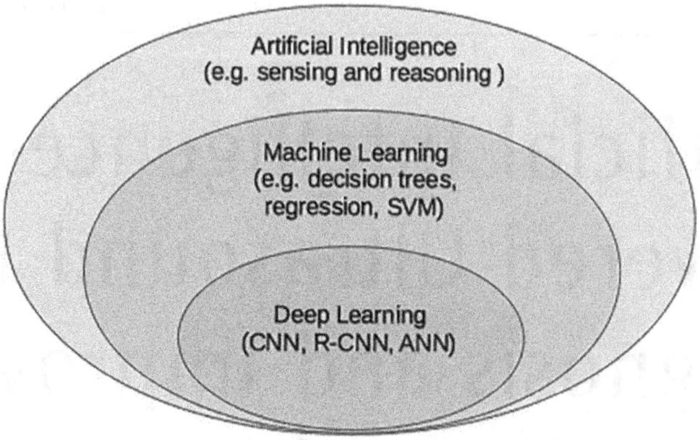

FIGURE 7.1 The context of artificial intelligence, machine learning, and deep learning.

planning and organization, and knowledge capture. Machine learning (ML) is a subsection of AI that covers the ability of a system to learn about data using supervised or unsupervised statistical and ML methods such as regression, support vector machines, decision trees, and neural networks. Deep learning (DL), which is a subclass of ML, learns a sequential chain of pivotal features from images that maximizes the success of learning process with its self-learning ability. This is different from statistical ML algorithms that require handcrafted feature selection [1] (Figure 7.1). In this chapter, we will start with a brief background on ultrasound imaging and DL and will continue with a summary of the advances in ultrasound (US) powered with AI. These advances could potentially allow evaluating US data objectively, improving clinical workflow, and cutting healthcare costs. Subsequently, we present currently available AI-powered US applications in radiology and cardiology, go into challenges of current AI applications, and present our view on future trends in US powered with AI.

7.1.1 Ultrasound Imaging

US imaging has been commonly used in routine clinical practice for diagnosis and visualization of internal organs (e.g. liver, kidney, and heart) and superficial structures (e.g. thyroid, breast, carotid artery, and muscles). An US transducer uses a piezoelectric material that converts electrical energy to mechanical movement, which transmits and receives sound waves with frequencies higher than human hearing. It generates US waves and transmits into the tissue and listens to receive the reflected sound wave (echo). The reflected echo signal is recorded in order to construct an image of the interrogated region. The sound waves travel through a soft tissue medium with approximately 1,540 m/s. The time of flight between the transmitted and received sound waves is used to locate objects and construct an image of the probed area. US has several advantages compared to magnetic resonance (MR), computed tomography (CT), and positron emission tomography (PET) imaging modalities. US is unharmful as it does not use destructive ionizing radiations like X-ray, CT, and PET. It is considerably lower in cost, handy for point-of-care (POCUS) applications, and provides actual real-time imaging. Since it is handy, it can be carried to a patient's bedside for examining patients and monitoring changes over time. The disadvantages of US include operator dependability and being incapable of examining body areas that contain gas and bones.

Diverse image types are formed by using US (Figure 7.2). The most common types used in clinics are:

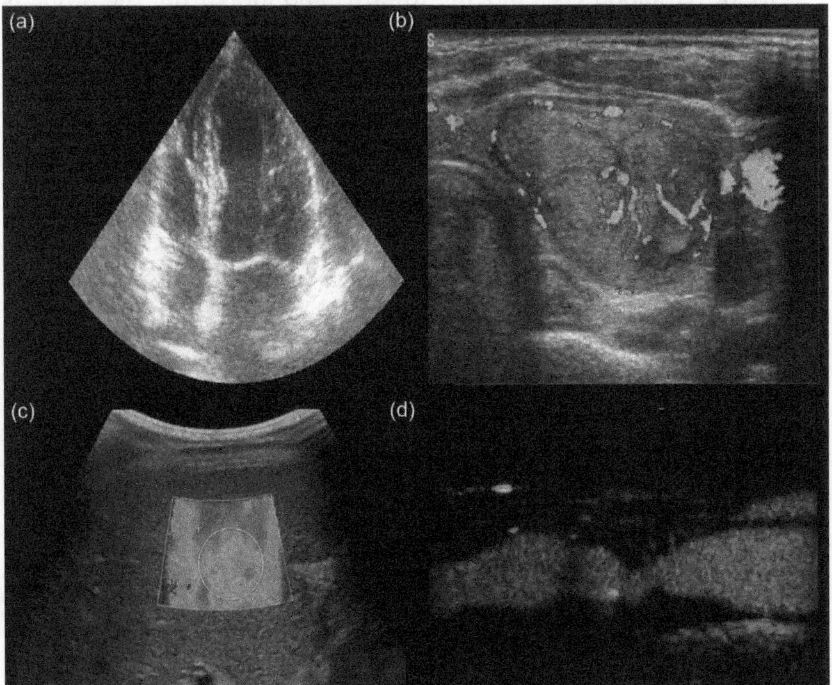

FIGURE 7.2 Sample US images showing different US modes. (a) A B-mode image of a heart: An apical four chamber view. (b) A color Doppler image of a thyroid nodule. (c) A Shear Wave Elastography map of a liver. (d) A CEUS image of a carotid artery.

B-mode ultrasound: It is also called as brightness mode (B-mode) and is the most well-known US image. An US beam is scanned across a tissue to construct a 2D cross-section image of the tissue.

M-mode ultrasound: Motion mode (M-mode) is used to examine motion over time. For example, it provides a single scan line of the heart and all of the reflectors along this line are shown along the time axis to measure the temporal resolution of the cardiac structures.

Doppler ultrasound: A change in the frequency of a wave occurs when the source and observer are moving relative to each other, and this is called the Doppler effect. An US wave is transmitted with a specific frequency through an US probe (the observer). The US waves that are reflected from moving objects (e.g. red blood cells in vessels) return to the probe with a frequency shift. This frequency shift is used to estimate the velocity of the moving object. In blood flow, the velocity of red blood cells moving towards and away from the probe is recorded to construct Doppler images. The velocity of information overlaid on top of B-mode anatomical images to show color Doppler images of blood flow.

Ultrasound Shear Wave Elastography (SWE): This technique provides a 2D stiffness map of tissue cross-sections. An acoustic radiation force generated with an US probe is used to induce a push force inside the tissue of interest and generates shear waves. The stiffness of a tissue can be measured from the speed of the resulting shear wave that travels through the medium. Therefore, SWE is able to characterize the mechanical and elastic properties of various body parts, and it can potentially be used in liver, musculoskeletal, thyroid, and breast imaging.

Contrast Enhanced Ultrasound (CEUS): CEUS is a functional imaging that suppresses anatomical details but visualizes blood flow information. It exploits the nonlinear response of US contrast agents (lipid-coated gas bubbles). Generally, two consecutive US signals are propagated through the same medium and their echo response is subtracted to obtain a contrast signal. Since the tissue generates linear echo response, the subtraction cancels out the tissue signal and only the difference signal from nonlinear responses of bubbles remains. This imaging technique is used to examine cardiac chamber cavities, assess carotid artery stenosis, and evaluate prostate and liver perfusion. It is useful to detect perfusion abnormalities in tissues and enhance the visibility of tissue boundaries.

7.1.2 Deep Learning

Artificial neural networks (ANN) that mimic biological neurons for creating representation for an input signal include many consecutive layers that learn a hierarchy of features from an input signal. ANN and the advance in graphics processing units (GPU) processing power have enabled the development of deep and complex DL models with multitasking at the same time. DL models can be trained with thousands or millions of samples to gain robustness to variations in data. The representation power of DL models is massive that can create representation for any given variation of a signal. Recent accomplishments of DL especially in image classification and segmentation applications made it very popular in data science community. Traditional ML methods use hand-crafted features extracted from data and process them in decomposable pipelines. This makes them more comprehensible as each component is explainable. On the other hand, they tend to be less generalizable and robust to variations in data. With DL models, we give up understandability in exchange for obtaining robustness and greater generalization ability, but generate complex and abstract features.

State-of-art DL models have been developed for a variety of tasks such as object detection and segmentation in computer vision, voice recognition, and genotype/phenotype prediction. There are different types of models that include convolutional neural networks (CNNs) [2], deep Boltzmann machines, stacked auto-encoders [3], and deep belief neural networks [4]. The most commonly used DL method for processing images is CNNs as fully connected ANN would be quite computationally heavy for 2D/3D images and require extensive GPU memory. CNNs share weights across each feature map or convolutional layers to alleviate this. Since their first introduction in 1989 [5], CNNs have been widely utilized for image classification and segmentation tasks with great success [2]. CNN approaches have gained enormous awareness when CNNs achieved impressive results in the ImageNet [6,7] competition in 2012 [2], which includes natural photographic images. They were utilized to classify a dataset of around a million images that comprise 1,000 diverse classes, achieving half the error rates of the most popular traditional ML approaches [2].

Training DL methods on a large amount of data resulted in remarkable results and robustness in ImageNet competition. DL methods are also gaining recognition in the field of medical image analysis [8] (e.g. lesion diagnosis [1,9–13], tissue and lesion segmentation [1,14–18], and histopathological analysis [19,20]). The architectures of state-of-art CNN models are increasingly dense, with some models having more than 100 layers. This means millions of weights and billions of connections between nodes. Typically, a CNN architecture comprises consecutive layers of convolution, max-pooling, and activation. Feature maps are generated by convolving a convolutional kernel across the output of the previous layer. Max-pooling is employed to down-sample feature maps by computing the maximum value of a predefined neighborhood. Alternatively, convolutions with stride larger steps could be used for down-sampling. In addition, activation functions are applied to layers to produce nonlinear output and suppress redundancy. The most widely employed activation function is rectified linear unit (ReLU) that nonlinearly transforms input signal by clipping any negative input values to zero and passes only positive input values to the output [21]. A number of other activation functions (e.g. leaky RELU, ELU, sigmoid, maxout, and hyperbolic tangent) have also been used in the literature. As the final layer, a softmax nonlinearity function, which normalizes output scores into a multinomial distribution over labels, is employed. The output scores of the final CNN layer are connected to the softmax layer to obtain a prediction probability for each class. Furthermore, an optimizer such as stochastic gradient descent (SGD) minimizes the error between prediction and ground truth labels through an error or loss function. Later, gradients of the loss function with respect to weights with backpropagation using chain rule are estimated. Gradients and learning rate are used to update weights in each iteration and this continues to train CNN architectures until it converges to a steady state (Figure 7.3). Since DL algorithms do better than ML algorithms in general and exploit the GPU processing power, it allows real-time processing of US images. We will only focus on DL applications of AI-powered US in radiology and cardiology in the rest of this chapter.

To assess the performance of ML models, data are generally split into training, validation, and test sets. The training set is used for learning about the data. The validation set is employed to establish the reliability of learning results and the test set is used to assess the generalizability of a trained model on unobserved data. When training samples are limited, k-fold cross-validation approaches (e.g. leave-one-out, five-fold, or ten-fold cross-validation) are utilized. In cross-validation, the data are divided randomly into k equal sized pieces. One piece is reserved for assessing the

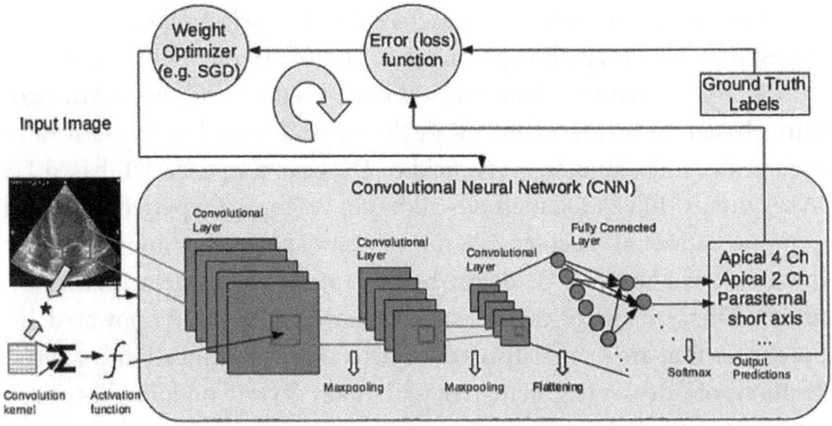

FIGURE 7.3 A framework of training a deep learning model for classification of echo views. Operations in between layers are shown with arrows.

performance of a model, and the remaining pieces (k–1) are utilized for training models. The training process is typically performed in a supervised way that involves ground truth labels for each input data and minimizes a loss function over training samples iteratively. Supervised learning is the most common training approach for a ML method but it requires a laborious ground truth label generation. In medical imaging, ground truth labels are generally obtained from clinical notes for a diagnosis or quantification. Furthermore, manual outlining of lesions or structures by experts is used to train ML models for segmentation tasks.

7.1.3 AI-Powered US in Radiology

As medical imaging data increase immensely with the advancing multimodality imaging technology (e.g. 2D/3D/4D anatomical and functional imaging US/CT/MR/PET/SPECT), there is a need for processing imaging data in an organized fashion to assist radiologists. Computer-aided detection and quantification (CAD) is an ongoing research subject in diagnostic radiology. CAD systems provide a second opinion to assist radiologists for image interpretation, which furthers the precision and consistency of diagnosis and decreases the image reading time. The greater part of CAD systems is based on traditional ML methods that employ texture features and involve several steps: image preprocessing, handcrafted feature extraction, selection of major features, and classification. Although CAD systems have shown great promise in assisting radiologists, they have several limitations (e.g. using limited datasets, subjective selection of a region of interest that includes pathology, and data obtained from a single vendor at a single medical center). Therefore, it is hard to adapt traditional ML algorithms based on textures difficult in the clinical workflow to assist radiologists. Recently, studies in the field of DL have proposed DL-based US CAD systems [10,22]. DL methods allow conveying an experience learned from one dataset at a center to a new dataset acquired at another center with a different brand of US device by fine-tuning the model with the new dataset. This process is called transfer learning. Many AI-powered US approaches that are primarily used for detection, quantification, and classifications of diseases (e.g. benign or malignant thyroid nodules) have been developed in the last 5 years.

Thyroid nodules, which are solid or fluid-filled lumps, are particularly frequent lesions that are found in 40%–50% of the adult population as shown in autopsy studies [23–26]. Fine needle aspiration (FNA) biopsy is the current and only nonsurgical test that differentiates a benign nodule from a malignant one in clinical practice. The overall frequency of cancer in patients with thyroid nodules selected for FNA is just about 10% as revealed in several studies [27,28]. Therefore, it is important to identify nodules that do not have a need of biopsy or surgery as the greater part of thyroid nodules are benign. A noninvasive and reliable diagnostic method will significantly cut healthcare costs and patient concerns about biopsy. To establish such a CAD system, sensitivity at or near 100% is desired to ensure that cancers are not missed with a reasonable specificity so that a good portion of benign lesions are not biopsied. Several studies have proposed DL approaches to classify and segment thyroid nodules from 2D US images. Assessing 2D cross-section images of thyroid nodules only is a limitation of current studies as cancer develops heterogeneously and 2D cross-sections might not be cutting through cancer developed within nodules. Therefore, 3D volume-based approaches would provide more accurate and reliable results than 2D imaging-based approaches. Recently, Ma et al. [29] proposed a DL method that employs the fusion of two customized CNN models for differentiating benign nodules from malignant nodules. The proposed model was trained on a large dataset of multi-US vendors collected from two hospitals (8,148 patients from hospital 1 + 4,782 patients from hospital 2 and in a total of 15,000 images) and accomplished an average accuracy of 83.02% $\mp$ 0.72% based on ten-fold cross-validation. Nevertheless, the receiver operating characteristic (ROC) curve shown in this study indicates that the proposed model generally misses some malignant patients and does not hit 100% sensitivity, which makes this model unreliable to use as a diagnostic tool. In another study, Ma et al. and his colleagues [30] developed two CNN models that are stacked to each other for the detection of nodules from B-mode US images. The model was evaluated using *k*-fold cross-validation and an average area under curve (AUC) of 98.51% was reported. Segmentation of nodules from B-mode US images is a challenging task due to fuzzy and missed nodule boundaries, which makes the precise automatic segmentation of nodules very difficult and unreliable. Li et al. [31] utilized a Faster R-CNN model for detection of benign and malignant regions of nodules in B-mode US images. A sensitivity of 93.5% and a specificity of 81.5% were achieved for the detection of papillary thyroid cancer. Another multi-cohort thyroid study with a large patient population that was collected from three hospitals was presented by Li et al. [32]. The study included in a total of 332,180 images of 45,644 patients. They assessed the sensitivity of their CNN model for cancer detection and compared the performance of the CNN model to a team of experienced radiologists. They concluded that their model's sensitivity in the detection of malignant nodules is as good as an experienced radiologist with a better specificity. In another study, Akkus et al. [11] trained inception and ResNet CNN models with an attention map, which enhances the nodule region, to identify malignant nodules B-mode US images. The model was trained on both transverse and longitudinal cross-section images of thyroid nodules. The model achieved 86% (sensitivity) and 90% (specificity) for detecting malignancy on a test set of 100 nodule images. Their ROC curve suggests that biopsies could be reduced by 52% without missing patients with malignant thyroid nodules when the threshold is set to 100% sensitivity. Choi et al. [22] utilized a commercial CAD system to classify 102 nodules obtained from 89 patients into benign or malignant (S-Detect for Thyroid from Samsung Medison Co.). The sensitivity of Samsung S-Detect CAD system was shown to be similar to the performance of an experienced radiologist. Differently from other studies, Pereira et al. [33] utilized DL approaches that process SWE images for thyroid nodule characterization. An accuracy of 83% was obtained on a test dataset by using their proposed method. Lastly, Chi et al. [12] presented a GoogleNet CNN model with a transfer learning approach that accomplished an accuracy of 98.29% on a test dataset of 61 patients for differentiating a benign nodule from a malignant one.

Breast cancer is one of the most common cancer types among women. It is also the leading cause of cancer-related deaths in females [34].

The breast imaging reporting and data system (BI-RADS) scoring system has been widely used to make consistent reporting and decrease confusion in the interpretation of breast B-mode US images. Yet, substantial intra- and inter-observer variability based on BI-RADS have been shown in a handful of studies [35,36]. Therefore, a CAD system that has high sensitivity and negative predictive value would not only reduce intra- and inter-variability but will also reduce the reading time and provide radiologists a second opinion. Most importantly, this will potentially help to cut unnecessary biopsies. Several studies have attempted to classify benign and malignant breast lesions from B-mode US images in an objective and reproducible manner. One of the first studies presented by Byra et al. [37] utilized transfer learning to differentiate breast lesions from benign and malignant lesions. They utilized the VGG19 [38] CNN model that is previously trained on publicly available ImageNet dataset and fine-tuned it on B-mode US images of breast masses. An AUC of 93.6% was achieved as the performance of their model on a test dataset of 150 cases. They inferred that the proposed model could potentially be used to aid radiologists in decision-making for classification of breast masses. In another study, a GoogleNet [39] model was trained on 7,408 breast US images by Han et al. [40]. The model was tested on a dataset of 829 images and 90% accuracy, 86% sensitivity, and 96% specificity were obtained. The proposed model is implemented as a part of the commercial S-Detect technology of Samsung Ultrasound System RS80A. A stacked denoising autoencoder model was utilized by Cheng et al. [10] to classify breast lesions. The average performance of the proposed model is an AUC of 89.6%, which overtakes traditional ML-based methods. The study presented by Zhang et al. [41] showed that a better performance can be obtained in classifying breast masses using SWE images and DL methods. DL has been also used to detect/segment breast lesions from US images [42,43]. Yet, segmentation of breast lesions is challenging due to low contrast and unclear boundaries of breast lesions.

Various liver diseases (e.g. chronic viral hepatitis and alcoholism, hemochromatosis, and fatty liver disease) are the end-stage manifestation of Cirrhosis. US is the widely used imaging modality to diagnose liver diseases as it supplies information about the structural changes of the liver and blood flow of portal venous, whereas liver biopsy is the gold standard in assessing cirrhosis, it is invasive and involves several limitations (e.g. imprecise localizations that result in sampling errors, bleeding, and infection). A number of studies used DL approaches to differentiate liver diseases using B-mode and SWE US images. Recently, a multicenter study was presented by Wang et al. [44] to stage the liver fibrosis with a DL method using US SWE images. In this study, it was found that staging fibrosis with DL using SWE images is more accurate than SWE measurements only in three liver fibrosis stages (AUC of 97% for cirrhosis, 98% for advanced fibrosis, and 85% for significant fibrosis) in patients with chronic hepatitis B. Early diagnosis is very important to prevent a disease. An AI model that detects early changes of liver parenchyma would be very useful in the treatment planning of patients. In another study, a fine-tuned VGGNet using transfer learning was introduced by Meng et al. [45] to detect the fibrosis stage of a liver. An accuracy of 93.90% was obtained with their proposed method. In another study, Liu et al. [46] used transfer learning, a CNN model that is pre-trained on an ImageNet dataset, to obtain features of liver capsule from B-mode US images and feed them into a support vector machine to distinguish an abnormal liver from a normal one. The model achieved an AUC of 96.8%, which is greater than the accuracy of the SVM model using hand-crafted texture features. Wu et al. [47] utilized a deep belief network model to classify focal liver lesions from CEUS images. They compared their method to traditional ML methods and achieved outperforming performance (accuracy: 86.36% vs. 66.67%–81.86%). Another study assessed fatty liver disease from B-mode US images using DL and achieved a performance greater than traditional ML methods (100% vs. 82%–92%) [48]. As shown above, DL methods could be utilized for the diagnosis of liver diseases from B-mode and SWE images and could hypothetically cut down unneeded liver biopsies and related healthcare costs.

Besides the applications of DL in the US mentioned above, many other AI-powered US applications have been investigated. Wu et al. [49] assessed the image quality of fetal US images using DL for accurate measurements. Chen et al. [50] and Yu et al. [52] utilized a DL model to detect standard imaging planes of a fetus. DL approaches were also used by Menchon-Lara et al. [51] to segment intima-media thickness (IMT), which provided results superior to traditional methods. In another study, a DL approach was introduced by Hetherington et al. [53] to identify a spine vertebra level from B-mode US images, which could help an anesthesiologist find the right site for the injection. Lekadir et al. [54] employed a CNN model to classify tissue components of a carotid plaque (e.g. lipid, fibrosis, and calcification), which outperformed an SVM model. Cheng and Malhi [55] used CNN to detect the anatomical location and abdominal imaging planes in US. Furthermore, DL approaches have also been used to improve image construction of portable US systems as they use a small number of transmit and receive elements to reduce the power consumption. There is an increasing demand for reconstructing good quality US images with fewer transmit/receive radio-frequency (RF) channels. Yoon et al. [56] used a DL-based approach for the reconstruction of US images with the same quality from sub-sampled RF data. This could also help improve the temporal resolution of 3D US volume acquisitions. DL-based approaches were also used for elastography image reconstruction [57], US beamforming [58,59], and image recovery [60].

7.1.4 AI-Powered US in Cardiology

Cardiac US, also known as echocardiography (echo), is currently the most widely used noninvasive imaging modality for the assessment of structures and functions of the heart (e.g. left ventricular ejection fraction, cardiac output, diastolic function, and valvular diseases). AI-powered echocardiography could be used for low-cost, serial, and automated evaluation of cardiac structures and function by experts and nonexperts in cardiology, primary, and emergency clinics. This would also allow triaging incoming patients with chest pain in an emergency department and longitudinal monitoring of patients with cardiovascular risk factors in a personalized manner. With the advancing US technology, the current clinical cart-based US systems could be replaced with portable point-of-care ultrasound (POCUS) systems. GE Vscan, Butterfly IQ, and Philips Lumify are popular POCUS devices. A single Butterfly IQ probe contains 9,000 micro-machined semiconductor sensors and emulates linear, phased, and curved array probes. While Butterfly IQ probe using US-on-chip technology could be used for imaging the whole body, Philips Lumify provides different probes for each organ (e.g. s4-1 phased array probe for cardiac applications). GE Vscan comes with two transducers placed in one probe and can be used for scanning deep and superficial structures. Using POCUS devices powered with cloud-based AI echo interpretation at point of care locations could significantly reduce the US cost and increase the utility of AI-powered echocardiography by nonexperts in primary and emergency departments (Figure 7.4). A number of promising studies using DL approaches have been published for the classification of standard echo views (e.g. apical and parasternal views), segmentation of heart structures (e.g. ventricle, atrium, septum, myocardium, and pericardium), and prediction of cardiac diseases (e.g. heart

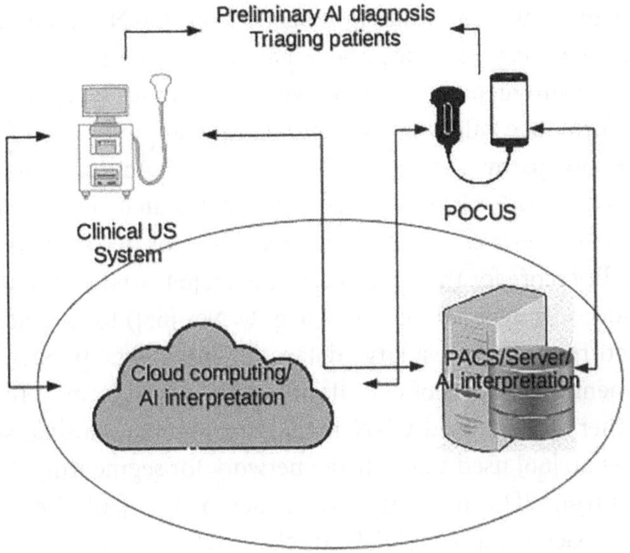

FIGURE 7.4 A schematic diagram of AI interpretation of echocardiography images for preliminary diagnosis and triaging patients in emergency and primary care clinics.

failure, hypertrophic cardiomyopathy, cardiac amyloidosis, and pulmonary hypertension) in recent years.

Echocardiography is an operator-dependent imaging modality that includes variability in data acquisition and evaluation. In addition to operator variability, it includes patient-specific variability (e.g. signal-to-noise ratio and limited acoustic window due to anatomical or body mass differences), and machine-specific variability (e.g. electronic noise and post-processing filters applied to acquired images. Image quality plays an important role in automated processing pipelines for accurate measurements. Suboptimal image quality could affect all measurements and results in misdiagnosis of patients.

Abdi et al. [61] trained a fully connected CNN with 6,916 end-diastolic echo images that were scored between 0 and 5 to assess the quality of apical four chamber (A4C) echo images. They reported an error comparable to intra-rater reliability (mean absolute error: 0.71 ∓ 0.58). Zhang et al. [62,63] presented a fully automated echo interpretation pipeline that includes 23 view classifications, segmentation of cardiac chambers in five common views, quantification of structure and function, and disease detection. Their results were evaluated on 8,666 echo images that have manual segmentation and measurements. Their CNN method accurately identified views (e.g. 96% for parasternal long axis) and obtained cardiac structure measurements comparable with values in study reports. The ROC curve performance values of their model for the prediction of hypertrophic cardiomyopathy, cardiac amyloidosis, and pulmonary hypertension are 0.93, 0.87, and 0.85, respectively. They calculated the averaged probability score of views classification across all videos in a study to define an image quality score for the study. Leclerc et al. [64] studied the state-of-art encoder–decoder type DL methods (e.g. U-Net [65]) for segmenting cardiac structures and made a large dataset (500 patients) publicly available with segmentation labels of end diastole and systole frames. In addition, several other studies used CNN models to segment cardiac structures. Carneiro et al. [66] used a deep belief network for segmenting the left ventricle (LV) from 2D echo images. Nascimento et al. [70] also employed a similar approach to segment LV. Jafari et al. [67] presented a recurrent fully CNN and optical flow for segmentation of the LV in echo images. Jafari et al. [68] also presented biplane ejection fraction estimation with POCUS using multi-task and learning and adversarial training. The performance of the proposed model for the segmentation of LV was an average Dice of 0.92 and for the automated ejection fraction was shown to be around an absolute error of 6.2%. Chen et al. [69] proposed an encoder–decoder type CNN with multi-view regularization to improve LV segmentation. The method was evaluated on 566 patients and achieved a Dice score of 92.7%. Oktay et al. [71] incorporated anatomical prior knowledge in their CNN model that allows following the global anatomical properties of the underlying anatomy. Mandani et al. [72] presented view classification of echo images using DL with 97.8% overall test accuracy.

7.2 DISCUSSION AND OUTLOOK

Automated image interpretation that mimics human vision with traditional machine learning has been existing for a long time. Recent advances in parallel processing with GPUs and DL algorithms, which extract patterns in images with their self-learning ability, changed the whole automated image interpretation practice with respect to computation speed, generalizability, and transferability of these algorithms. US powered with AI has been advancing and moving closer to be used in the routine clinical workflow in radiology and cardiology since there is an increased demand for standardizing acquisition and interpretation of US images. Even though DL-based methods for US provide promising results in diagnosis and quantification of diseases, US powered with AI is still far behind the advances in applications of AI in CT and MR imaging. High intra-/inter-variability in US make standardization of US image acquisition and interpretation challenging. AI could provide solutions to alleviate operator-dependent variability and interpretability but patient-dependent factors (e.g. obesity, limited acoustic window, artifacts, and signal drops) that affect image quality would still remain unsolved with US. Based on the outcome of DL applications presented above, the generalization ability of DL methods has been proven to be greater than conventional ML approaches. Therefore, DL methods are becoming more popular and replacing traditional ML methods.

Applications of DL in US are rapidly advancing as evidenced by the growing number of studies recently. DL models have enormous representation power and are hungry for a large amount of data in order to obtain generalization ability and stability. Creating databases with large datasets that are curated and have good quality data and labels is the most challenging and time-consuming part of the whole AI model development process. Although it has been shown that AI-powered US applications have superb performance compared to classical ML methods, small datasets were generally used for training and validation of AI models. It is important to train AI models on large multi-vendor and multi-center datasets to obtain generalization and validate on large multi-vendor datasets to increase the reliability of a proposed model. To overcome this limitation, several studies employed transfer learning and fine-tuning in their AI models but the knowledge obtained from optical images of ImageNet was generally used to initialize the AI models, as proposed in Ref. [37,45,55]. This might not be an appropriate way of using transfer learning and fine-tuning as US images are significantly different from natural optical images. An applicable way could be initializing AI models with the knowledge previously obtained from an US dataset and fine-tuning them on a new dataset obtained at a different center from multi-vendors. Another alternative way to overcome the limitation of having limited dataset would be augmenting the dataset with realistic transformations (e.g. scaling, horizontal flipping, translations, adding noise, tissue deformation, and enhancing image contrast) that could help improve the generalizability of AI models. On the other hand, realistic transformations need to be used to genuinely simulate variations in US images and transformations in applied images should not create artifacts. For example, flipping US images vertically will not be a convincing transformation as shadowing never shows up in the adverse course of the US beam travel through a medium. Alternatively, generative adversarial networks, which include a generator and a discriminator model, are trained until the model generates images that are not separable by the discriminator. This could be used to generate realistic US B-mode images of organs of interest. Introducing such transformations during the training process will make AI models more robust to small perturbations in input data space.

Making predictions based on only 2D cross-section images could be considered as a limitation of AI-powered US system. Two-dimensional cross-section images include limited information and do not constitute lesions entirely. Training AI models on 3D US data that include entire lesions or the structure of interest, multiple US views, or spatiotemporal data would potentially improve the diagnostic accuracy of an AI model. In addition, AI models that are trained on combined multi-mode US images (e.g. B-mode, Doppler, CEUS, and SWE), which complement each other, could also improve the diagnostic performance of AI models.

It is important to design AI models that are transparent for the prediction of any disease from medical images. The AI models developed for the diagnosis of a disease must elucidate the reasons and motivations behind their predictions in order to build trust in them. Comprehension of the inner mechanism of an AI model necessitates interpreting the activity of feature maps in each layer [73–75]. However, the extracted features are a combination of sequential layers and become complicated and conceptual in those layers. Therefore, the interpretation of these features becomes difficult compared to handcrafted imaging features in traditional ML methods. Traditional ML methods are designed with separable components that are more understandable. Each component of ML methods has an explanation but usually is not very accurate or robust. With DL-based AI models, the interpretability is given up for the robustness and complex imaging features with greater generalizability. Recently, a number of methods have been introduced about what DL models see and how to make their predictions. Several CNN architectures [38,65,76–78] employed techniques such as deconvolutional networks [79], gradient back-propagation [80], class activation maps (CAM) [81], gradient-weighted CAM [82], and saliency maps [83,84] to make CNN understandable. With these techniques, gradients of a model have been projected back to the input image space, which shows what parts in the input image contribute the most to the prediction outcome that maximizes the classification accuracy. Although making AI models understandable has been an active research topic in DL community, there are still a lot that needs to be done for that.

Developing AI models that standardize image acquisition and interpretation with less variability is essential considering that US is an operator and interpreter-dependent imaging modality. The AI guidance during data acquisition for the optimal angle, view, and measurements would make US less operator dependent and smarter and standardize data acquisition. Cost-effective and easy access to POCUS systems with AI capability would help clinicians and nonexperts perform swift initial examinations on patients and progress with vital and urgent decisions in emergency and primary care clinics. In the near future, POCUS systems with AI capability could replace the stethoscopes that doctors use in their daily practice to listen to patients' hearts. Clinical US or POCUS systems powered with AI, which can assess multi-mode data, steer sonographers during acquisition, and deliver objective qualifications, measurements, and diagnosis, will assist with decision making for diagnosis and treatments, improve US workflow in clinics, and cut healthcare cost.

REFERENCES

1. Z. Akkus, A. Galimzianova, A. Hoogi, D. L. Rubin, and B. J. Erickson, "Deep Learning for Brain MRI Segmentation: State of the Art and Future Directions," *J. Digit. Imaging*, vol. 30, pp. 449–459, 2017.
2. A. Krizhevsky, I. Sutskever, and G. E. Hinton, "ImageNet Classification with Deep Convolutional Neural Networks," in *Advances in Neural Information Processing Systems 25*, F. Pereira, C. J. C. Burges, L. Bottou, and K. Q. Weinberger, Eds. Curran Associates, Inc., Harrah's Lake Tahoe, Stateline, NV, 2012, pp. 1097–1105.
3. P. Vincent, H. Larochelle, I. Lajoie, Y. Bengio, and P.-A. Manzagol, "Stacked Denoising Autoencoders: Learning Useful Representations in a Deep Network with a Local Denoising Criterion," *J. Mach. Learn. Res.*, vol. 11, no. Dec, pp. 3371–3408, 2010.
4. G. E. Hinton, S. Osindero, and Y.-W. Teh, "A Fast Learning Algorithm for Deep Belief Nets," *Neural Comput.*, vol. 18, no. 7, pp. 1527–1554, Jul. 2006.
5. Y. LeCun et al., "Backpropagation Applied to Handwritten Zip Code Recognition," *Neural Comput.*, vol. 1, no. 4, pp. 541–551, 1989.
6. J. Deng et al., "ImageNet: A large-scale hierarchical image database," in *2009 IEEE Conference on Computer Vision and Pattern Recognition*, 2009, doi: 10.1109/cvprw.2009.5206848.
7. O. Russakovsky et al., "ImageNet Large Scale Visual Recognition Challenge," *Int. J. Comput. Vis.*, vol. 115, no. 3, pp. 211–252, 2015.
8. D. Lin, A. V. Vasilakos, Y. Tang, and Y. Yao, "Neural Networks for Computer-Aided Diagnosis in Medicine: A Review," *Neurocomputing*, vol. 216, pp. 700–708, Dec. 2016.
9. T. Kooi et al., "Large Scale Deep Learning for Computer Aided Detection of Mammographic Lesions," *Med. Image Anal.*, vol. 35, pp. 303–312, Jan. 2017.

10. J.-Z. Cheng et al., "Computer-Aided Diagnosis with Deep Learning Architecture: Applications to Breast Lesions in US Images and Pulmonary Nodules in CT Scans," *Sci. Rep.*, vol. 6, p. 24454, Apr. 2016.
11. Z. Akkus, A. Boonrod, M. Stan, R. Castro, and B. J. Erickson, "Reduction of thyroid nodule biopsies using deep learning," *Proc. SPIE Medical Imaging*, 2019, Image Processing, vol. 10949-31, in press.
12. J. Chi, E. Walia, P. Babyn, J. Wang, G. Groot, and M. Eramian, "Thyroid Nodule Classification in Ultrasound Images by Fine-Tuning Deep Convolutional Neural Network," *J. Digit. Imaging*, vol. 30, no. 4, pp. 477–486, Aug. 2017.
13. L. J. Brattain, B. A. Telfer, M. Dhyani, J. R. Grajo, and A. E. Samir, "Machine Learning for Medical Ultrasound: Status, Methods, and Future Opportunities," *Abdom Radiol (NY)*, vol. 43, no. 4, pp. 786–799, Apr. 2018.
14. Z. Akkus, P. Kostandy, A. K. Philbrick, and B. J. Erickson, "Robust Brain Extraction Tool for CT Images," *Neurocomputing*, in press.
15. Z. Akkus, P. Kostandy, K. Phillbrick, and B. J. Erickson, "Extraction of brain tissue from CT head images using fully convolutional neural networks," *in SPIE Medical Imaging*, Houston, TX, 2018.
16. G. Litjens et al., "A Survey on Deep Learning in Medical Image Analysis," *Med. Image Anal.*, vol. 42, pp. 60–88, Dec. 2017.
17. F. Milletari, N. Navab, and S. Ahmadi, "V-net: Fully convolutional neural networks for volumetric medical image segmentation," in *2016 Fourth International Conference on 3D Vision (3DV)*, 2016, pp. 565–571.
18. A. D. Weston et al., "Automated Abdominal Segmentation of CT Scans for Body Composition Analysis Using Deep Learning," *Radiology*, p. 181432, Dec. 2018.
19. G. Litjens et al., "Deep Learning as a Tool for Increased Accuracy and Efficiency of Histopathological Diagnosis," *Sci. Rep.*, vol. 6, p. 26286, May 2016.
20. A. Janowczyk and A. Madabhushi, "Deep Learning for Digital Pathology Image Analysis: A Comprehensive Tutorial with Selected Use Cases," *J. Pathol. Inform.*, vol. 7, p. 29, Jul. 2016.
21. K. He, X. Zhang, S. Ren, and J. Sun, "Delving deep into rectifiers: Surpassing human-level performance on ImageNet classification," in *2015 IEEE International Conference on Computer Vision (ICCV)*, 2015, doi: 10.1109/iccv.2015.123.
22. Y. J. Choi et al., "A Computer-Aided Diagnosis System Using Artificial Intelligence for the Diagnosis and Characterization of Thyroid Nodules on Ultrasound: Initial Clinical Assessment," *Thyroid*, vol. 27, no. 4, pp. 546–552, Apr. 2017.
23. K. D. Burman and L. Wartofsky, "CLINICAL PRACTICE. Thyroid Nodules," *N. Engl. J. Med.*, vol. 373, no. 24, pp. 2347–2356, Dec. 2015.
24. A. Jemal et al., "Cancer Statistics, 2005," *CA Cancer J. Clin.*, vol. 55, no. 1, pp. 10–30, Jan. 2005.
25. L. Hegedüs, "The Thyroid Nodule," *N. Engl. J. Med.*, vol. 351, no. 17, pp. 1764–1771, Oct. 2004.

26. American Thyroid Association (ATA) Guidelines Taskforce on Thyroid Nodules and Differentiated Thyroid Cancer et al., "Revised American Thyroid Association Management Guidelines for Patients with Thyroid Nodules and Differentiated Thyroid Cancer," *Thyroid*, vol. 19, no. 11, pp. 1167–1214, Nov. 2009.
27. M. C. Frates et al., "Management of Thyroid Nodules Detected at US: Society of Radiologists in Ultrasound Consensus Conference Statement," *Ultrasound Q.*, vol. 22, no. 4, pp. 231–238; discussion 239–240, Dec. 2006.
28. J. T. Guille, A. Opoku-Boateng, S. L. Thibeault, and H. Chen, "Evaluation and Management of the Pediatric Thyroid Nodule," *Oncologist*, vol. 20, no. 1, pp. 19–27, Jan. 2015.
29. J. Ma, F. Wu, J. Zhu, D. Xu, and D. Kong, "A Pre-Trained Convolutional Neural Network Based Method for Thyroid Nodule Diagnosis," *Ultrasonics*, vol. 73, pp. 221–230, Jan. 2017.
30. J. Ma, F. Wu, T. Jiang, J. Zhu, and D. Kong, "Cascade Convolutional Neural Networks for Automatic Detection of Thyroid Nodules in Ultrasound Images," *Med. Phys.*, vol. 44, no. 5, pp. 1678–1691, May 2017.
31. H. Li et al., "An Improved Deep Learning Approach for Detection of Thyroid Papillary Cancer in Ultrasound Images," *Sci. Rep.*, vol. 8, no. 1, p. 6600, Apr. 2018.
32. X. Li et al., "Diagnosis of Thyroid Cancer Using Deep Convolutional Neural Network Models Applied to Sonographic Images: A Retrospective, Multicohort, Diagnostic Study," *Lancet Oncol.*, Dec. 2018, doi: 10.1016/S1470-2045(18)30762-9.
33. C. Pereira, M. Dighe, and A. M. Alessio, "Comparison of machine learned approaches for thyroid nodule characterization from shear wave elastography images," in *Medical Imaging 2018: Computer-Aided Diagnosis*, 2018, vol. 10575, p. 105751X.
34. "WHO | Breast cancer," Sep. 2018.
35. F. Schwab, K. Redling, M. Siebert, A. Schötzau, C.-A. Schoenenberger, and R. Zanetti-Dällenbach, "Inter- and Intra-Observer Agreement in Ultrasound BI-RADS Classification and Real-Time Elastography Tsukuba Score Assessment of Breast Lesions," *Ultrasound Med. Biol.*, vol. 42, no. 11, pp. 2622–2629, Nov. 2016.
36. L. J. Grimm et al., "Interobserver Variability Between Breast Imagers Using the Fifth Edition of the BI-RADS MRI Lexicon," *AJR Am. J. Roentgenol.*, vol. 204, no. 5, pp. 1120–1124, May 2015.
37. M. Byra et al., "Breast Mass Classification in Sonography with Transfer Learning Using a Deep Convolutional Neural Network and Color Conversion," *Med. Phys.*, Dec. 2018, doi: 10.1002/mp.13361.
38. K. Simonyan and A. Zisserman, "Very deep convolutional networks for large-scale image recognition," *arXiv [cs.CV]*, 04-Sep-2014.
39. C. Szegedy et al., "Going deeper with convolutions," in *2015 IEEE Conference on Computer Vision and Pattern Recognition (CVPR)*, 2015, pp. 1–9.

40. S. Han et al., "A Deep Learning Framework for Supporting the Classification of Breast Lesions in Ultrasound Images," *Phys. Med. Biol.*, vol. 62, no. 19, pp. 7714–7728, Sep. 2017.
41. Q. Zhang et al., "Deep Learning Based Classification of Breast Tumors with Shear-Wave Elastography," *Ultrasonics*, vol. 72, pp. 150–157, Dec. 2016.
42. M. H. Yap et al., "Automated Breast Ultrasound Lesions Detection Using Convolutional Neural Networks," *IEEE J. Biomed. Health Inform.*, vol. 22, no. 4, pp. 1218–1226, Jul. 2018.
43. V. Kumar et al., "Automated and Real-Time Segmentation of Suspicious Breast Masses Using Convolutional Neural Network," *PLoS One*, vol. 13, no. 5, p. e0195816, May 2018.
44. K. Wang et al., "Deep Learning Radiomics of Shear Wave Elastography Significantly Improved Diagnostic Performance for Assessing Liver Fibrosis in Chronic Hepatitis B: A Prospective Multicentre Study," *Gut*, May 2018, doi: 10.1136/gutjnl-2018-316204.
45. D. Meng, L. Zhang, G. Cao, W. Cao, G. Zhang, and B. Hu, "Liver Fibrosis Classification Based on Transfer Learning and FCNet for Ultrasound Images," *IEEE Access*, vol. 5, pp. 5804–5810, 2017.
46. X. Liu, J. L. Song, S. H. Wang, J. W. Zhao, and Y. Q. Chen, "Learning to Diagnose Cirrhosis with Liver Capsule Guided Ultrasound Image Classification," *Sensors*, vol. 17, no. 1, Jan. 2017, doi: 10.3390/s17010149.
47. K. Wu, X. Chen, and M. Ding, "Deep Learning Based Classification of Focal Liver Lesions with Contrast-Enhanced Ultrasound," *Optik*, vol. 125, no. 15, pp. 4057–4063, Aug. 2014.
48. M. Biswas et al., "Symtosis: A Liver Ultrasound Tissue Characterization and Risk Stratification in Optimized Deep Learning Paradigm," *Comput. Methods Programs Biomed.*, vol. 155, pp. 165–177, Mar. 2018.
49. L. Wu, J.-Z. Cheng, S. Li, B. Lei, T. Wang, and D. Ni, "FUIQA: Fetal Ultrasound Image Quality Assessment with Deep Convolutional Networks," *IEEE Trans. Cybern.*, vol. 47, no. 5, pp. 1336–1349, May 2017.
50. H. Chen et al., "Ultrasound Standard Plane Detection Using a Composite Neural Network Framework," *IEEE Trans. Cybern.*, vol. 47, no. 6, pp. 1576–1586, Jun. 2017.
51. R. Menchón-Lara and J. Sancho-Gómez, "Ultrasound image processing based on machine learning for the fully automatic evaluation of the Carotid Intima-Media Thickness," in *2014 12th International Workshop on Content-Based Multimedia Indexing (CBMI)*, 2014, pp. 1–4.
52. Z. Yu et al., "A Deep Convolutional Neural Network-Based Framework for Automatic Fetal Facial Standard Plane Recognition," *IEEE J. Biomed. Health Inform.*, vol. 22, no. 3, pp. 874–885, May 2018.
53. J. Hetherington, V. Lessoway, V. Gunka, P. Abolmaesumi, and R. Rohling, "SLIDE: Automatic Spine Level Identification System Using a Deep Convolutional Neural Network," *Int. J. Comput. Assist. Radiol. Surg.*, vol. 12, no. 7, pp. 1189–1198, Jul. 2017.

54. K. Lekadir et al., "A Convolutional Neural Network for Automatic Characterization of Plaque Composition in Carotid Ultrasound," *IEEE J. Biomed. Health Inform.*, vol. 21, no. 1, pp. 48–55, Jan. 2017.
55. P. M. Cheng and H. S. Malhi, "Transfer Learning with Convolutional Neural Networks for Classification of Abdominal Ultrasound Images," *J. Digit. Imaging*, vol. 30, no. 2, pp. 234–243, Apr. 2017.
56. Y. H. Yoon, Yoon, S. Khan, J. Huh, and J. C. Ye, "Efficient B-mode Ultrasound Image Reconstruction from Sub-sampled RF Data using Deep Learning," *IEEE Trans. Med. Imaging*, Aug. 2018, doi: 10.1109/TMI.2018.2864821.
57. S. Wu, Z. Gao, Z. Liu, J. Luo, H. Zhang, and S. Li, "Direct reconstruction of ultrasound elastography using an end-to-end deep neural network: 21st International Conference, Granada, Spain, September 16–20, 2018, Proceedings, Part I," in *Medical Image Computing and Computer Assisted Intervention - MICCAI 2018*, vol. 11070, A. F. Frangi, J. A. Schnabel, C. Davatzikos, C. Alberola-López, and G. Fichtinger, Eds. Cham: Springer International Publishing, 2018, pp. 374-382.
58. A. A. Nair, T. D. Tran, A. Reiter, and M. A. L. Bell, "A deep learning based alternative to beamforming ultrasound images," in *2018 IEEE International Conference on Acoustics, Speech and Signal Processing (ICASSP)*, 2018, pp. 3359–3363.
59. A. C. Luchies and B. C. Byram, "Deep Neural Networks for Ultrasound Beamforming," *IEEE Trans. Med. Imaging*, vol. 37, no. 9, pp. 2010–2021, Sep. 2018.
60. D. Perdios, A. Besson, M. Arditi, and J. Thiran, "A deep learning approach to ultrasound image recovery," in *2017 IEEE International Ultrasonics Symposium (IUS)*, 2017, pp. 1–4.
61. A. H. Abdi et al., "Automatic Quality Assessment of Echocardiograms Using Convolutional Neural Networks: Feasibility on the Apical Four-Chamber View," *IEEE Trans. Med. Imaging*, vol. 36, no. 6, pp. 1221–1230, Jun. 2017.
62. J. Zhang et al., "A web-deployed computer vision pipeline for automated determination of cardiac structure and function and detection of disease by two-dimensional echocardiography," *arXiv preprint arXiv:1706. 07342*, 2017.
63. J. Zhang et al., "Fully Automated Echocardiogram Interpretation in Clinical Practice: Feasibility and Diagnostic Accuracy," *Circulation*, vol. 138, no. 16, pp. 1623–1635, 2018.
64. S. Leclerc et al., "Deep Learning for Segmentation Using an Open Large-Scale Dataset in 2D Echocardiography," *IEEE Trans. Med. Imaging*, Feb. 2019, doi: 10.1109/TMI.2019.2900516.
65. O. Ronneberger, P. Fischer, and T. Brox, "U-Net: Convolutional networks for biomedical image segmentation," in *Medical Image Computing and Computer-Assisted Intervention - MICCAI 2015*, vol. 9351, N. Navab, J. Hornegger, W. M. Wells, and A. F. Frangi, Eds. Cham: Springer International Publishing, 2015, pp. 234–241.

66. G. Carneiro, J. C. Nascimento, and A. Freitas, "The Segmentation of the Left Ventricle of the Heart from Ultrasound Data Using Deep Learning Architectures and Derivative-Based Search Methods," *IEEE Trans. Image Process.*, vol. 21, no. 3, pp. 968–982, Mar. 2012.
67. M. H. Jafari et al., "A unified framework integrating recurrent fully-convolutional networks and optical flow for segmentation of the left ventricle in echocardiography data," in *Deep Learning in Medical Image Analysis and Multimodal Learning for Clinical Decision Support*, 2018, pp. 29–37.
68. M. H. Jafari et al., "Automatic Biplane Left Ventricular Ejection Fraction Estimation with Mobile Point-of-Care Ultrasound Using Multi-Task Learning and Adversarial Training," *Int. J. Comput. Assist. Radiol. Surg.*, vol. 14, no. 6, pp. 1027–1037, Jun. 2019.
69. H. Chen, Y. Zheng, J.-H. Park, P.-A. Heng, and S. K. Zhou, "Iterative multi-domain regularized deep learning for anatomical structure detection and segmentation from ultrasound images," in *Medical Image Computing and Computer-Assisted Intervention – MICCAI 2016*, 2016, pp. 487–495.
70. J. C. Nascimento and G. Carneiro, "Multi-atlas segmentation using manifold learning with deep belief networks," in *2016 IEEE 13th International Symposium on Biomedical Imaging (ISBI)*, 2016, pp. 867–871.
71. O. Oktay et al., "Anatomically Constrained Neural Networks (ACNNs): Application to Cardiac Image Enhancement and Segmentation," *IEEE Trans. Med. Imaging*, vol. 37, no. 2, pp. 384–395, Feb. 2018.
72. A. Madani, R. Arnaout, M. Mofrad, and R. Arnaout, "Fast and Accurate View Classification of Echocardiograms Using Deep Learning," *NPJ Digit. Med.*, vol. 1, Mar. 2018, doi: 10.1038/s41746-017-0013-1.
73. M. D. Zeiler and R. Fergus, "Visualizing and Understanding Convolutional Networks," in *Lecture Notes in Computer Science*, 2014, pp. 818–833.
74. M. D. Zeiler, G. W. Taylor, and R. Fergus, "Adaptive deconvolutional networks for mid and high level feature learning," in *2011 International Conference on Computer Vision*, 2011, doi: 10.1109/iccv.2011.6126474.
75. B. Zhou, A. Khosla, A. Lapedriza, A. Oliva, and A. Torralba, "Learning deep features for discriminative localization," in *2016 IEEE Conference on Computer Vision and Pattern Recognition (CVPR)*, 2016, doi: 10.1109/cvpr.2016.319.
76. K. He, X. Zhang, S. Ren, and J. Sun, "Deep residual learning for image recognition," *arXiv [cs.CV]*, 10-Dec-2015.
77. C. Szegedy, V. Vanhoucke, S. Ioffe, J. Shlens, and Z. Wojna, "Rethinking the inception architecture for computer vision," in *Proceedings of the IEEE Conference on Computer Vision and Pattern Recognition*, 2016, pp. 2818–2826.
78. V. Badrinarayanan, A. Kendall, and R. Cipolla, "SegNet: A Deep Convolutional Encoder-Decoder Architecture for Image Segmentation," *IEEE Trans. Pattern Anal. Mach. Intell.*, vol. 39, no. 12, pp. 2481–2495, Dec. 2017.
79. M. D. Zeiler, D. Krishnan, G. W. Taylor, and R. Fergus, *Deconvolutional Networks*. IEEE Computer Society, 2010, pp. 2528–2535.

80. J. T. Springenberg, A. Dosovitskiy, T. Brox, and M. Riedmiller, "Striving for Simplicity: The All Convolutional Net," *arXiv [cs.LG]*, 21-Dec-2014.
81. B. Zhou, A. Khosla, A. Lapedriza, A. Oliva, and A. Torralba, "Learning deep features for discriminative localization," in *Proceedings of the IEEE Conference on Computer Vision and Pattern Recognition*, 2016, pp. 2921–2929.
82. A. Chattopadhay, A. Sarkar, P. Howlader, and V. N. Balasubramanian, "Grad-CAM++: Generalized gradient-based visual explanations for deep convolutional networks," in *2018 IEEE Winter Conference on Applications of Computer Vision (WACV)*, 2018, pp. 839–847.
83. G. Li and Y. Yu, "Visual Saliency Detection Based on Multiscale Deep CNN Features," *IEEE Trans. Image Process.*, vol. 25, no. 11, pp. 5012–5024, Nov. 2016.
84. K. A. Philbrick et al., "What Does Deep Learning See? Insights From a Classifier Trained to Predict Contrast Enhancement Phase From CT Images," *AJR Am. J. Roentgenol.*, vol. 211, no. 6, pp. 1184–1193, Dec. 2018.

CHAPTER 8

Machine Learning for E/MEG-Based Identification of Alzheimer's Disease

Su Yang

University of West London

London, United Kingdom

Girijesh Prasad, KongFatt Wong-Lin, and Jose Sanchez-Bornot

Ulster University

Londonderry, United Kingdom

CONTENTS

8.1 INTRODUCTION

Electroencephalography (EEG) has been one of the most conventional modalities for diagnosing brain malfunctions. It has been widely used to diagnose diseases such as Alzheimer's disease (AD) and its prodromal stage, mild cognitive impairment (MCI). Due to its portability and relatively low cost, the EEG system receives vast coverage in the hospitals and medical centers. However, it is also well known that due to the relatively small number of electrodes and its nonintrusive nature, using EEG alone has been found difficult to make a definite diagnosis. To alleviate this limitation, magnetoencephalography (MEG) has been introduced for the detection/prediction of AD and MCI. Compared with EEG, MEG collection systems require a much reduced number of contacting electrodes, but effectively increased the quantity of noncontact magnetic sensors. Therefore, MEG is arguably a more powerful modality than EEG. However, due to the entirely different measuring principle between the modalities and much less research devoted, MEG has yet to demonstrate much superior performance to EEG [1].

In this chapter, the recent reports on machine learning (ML)-based MCI/AD diagnosis using E/MEG are reviewed and discussed. In particular, for some of the E/MEG systems with a large number of sensors (100~300), it is possible to perform the source localization to find the accurate spots of the abnormal functions from the cortex/brain. The main content of this chapter is therefore structured in two subsequent sections: sensor-level and source-level. The current issues and limitations in terms of the experimental design for ML-aided MCI/AD detection/prediction, along with a few suggestions for the researchers in this field, are also provided in the Discussion and Conclusion section of the chapter.

8.2 SENSOR-LEVEL ANALYSIS

This section reviews and discusses a few recent works for MCI/AD detection based on sensor space analysis. One of the most intuitive methodologies for feature extraction is to directly explore the signal data in the time domain. In Ref. [2], a new type of entropy namely dispersion entropy (DisEn) was proposed to measure and compare the irregularity of brain signals between AD and Heath Control (HC). A 148-channel MEG system was used to collect the data from 36 AD and 26 HC participants in resting state. The performance was evaluated using boxplots for visual inspection, and the *t*-test was adopted for statistical significance analysis. As a relatively simple approach, it was able to demonstrate that the MEG data from AD have shown more regularity than HC.

A more complex work in Ref. [3] proposed to use EEG-based Event-Related Potential (ERP) as neuromarkers for the classification of AD and MCI, against HC. In total, 61 participants were involved in data collection, which included 15 with AD, 20 with MCI, and 26 with AD. A series of binary classifications (AD vs. HC, MCI vs. HC, and AD vs. MCI) were conducted to study the sensitivity of the working memory task reflected by ERPs. Independent component analysis was used for artifact removal and the spatial relationships of the electrodes were leveraged using the k-means clustering. Here each participant was considered as one cluster in the reported study. The differences in terms of ERP between the classes were compared, and the Kruskal–Wallis statistical tests were adopted to measure the statistical significance of the results. It was reported in comparison to the controlled group that both the AD and MCI groups demonstrated a decreased amplitude in the P450 component. The experiments also indicated that the most significant differences were observed from fronto-centro-parietal electrodes, for HC vs. abnormal groups. These promising results seem to suggest that relatively simple neuromarkers in the time domain could already reflect the abnormal brain state; however, the study has also shown that such markers are not quite effective for the challenging AD vs. MCI classification problem.

Similarly, also through mere visual inspection of the extracted features, researchers have been trying to perform the classification using the frequency domain markers. For example in Ref. [4], a series of the power and the relative power of the signals were used for MCI detection. A 64-channel EEG acquisition system was used to collect data from 22 subjects (11 MCI and 11 HC). The cortex of the brain was divided into 17 regions of interest (ROIs); the statistical analysis of these ROIs was performed by repeated-measures analysis of variance (ANOVA) and *t*-test of an independent sampler. The work claims that the theta band is the main responsible band for MCI detection, and the slowing of EEG rhythms from the left temporal area is significant for MCI.

These recent researches, despite obtaining interesting results and receiving much attention in the community, are still not quite facilitated by ML techniques. These systems could be considered as semi-automated, as the final decisions still need to be made by humans: i.e. visual inspection of the features from different classes. Without incorporating into the ML framework, objective comparison among these systems is therefore quite difficult to make. The existence of such a difficulty is mainly due to that the researchers in the neurological field were traditionally not from the ML field.

With the recent thrive of artificial intelligence applications in various fields, ML-supported detection techniques have been found integrating with the conventional semi-automated diagnosis systems. One typical example in Ref. [5] introduced a pipeline based on a 19-channel EEG system for AD and MCI detections. A series of different features commonly used in the field were extensively explored, including relative power in the conventional frequency bands, median frequency, individual alpha frequency, spectral entropy, Lempel–Ziv complexity, central tendency measure, sample entropy, fuzzy entropy, and auto-mutual information. A feature selection scheme namely fast correlation-based filter was employed, the individual alpha frequency, relative power at the delta frequency band, and sample entropy were eventually kept for classification. Three conventional classifiers, linear discriminant analysis (LDA), quadratic discriminant analysis, and multi-layer perceptron artificial neural network (MLP) were tested, the MLP proved to provide the best recognition performance among the three. With the support of the ML techniques, this fully automated system was evaluated by the standard sensitivity and specificity: On determining whether a subject is not healthy, a sensitivity of 82.35% and a positive predictive value of 84.85% were obtained for HC against AD and MCI; on whether a subject does not suffer from AD, it provided a specificity of 79.41% and a negative predictive value of 84.38% for AD against HC and MCI. It is worth pointing out, despite three classes were involved in the study, effectively the system was still performing two-class classifications: this may indicate currently that it is still quite a challenging task for three-class recognition scenarios. It is well known that MCI is the prodromal phase of AD, and its symptomatic separation with AD and HC is often quite vague.

AD detection using ML techniques has demonstrated much improved performance. Also using a 19-channel EEG system, work reported in Ref. [6] provided more than 10% improvement than the work in Ref. [5]. The subjects (20 AD and 32 HC) were in different states during data collection: hyperventilation, awake, drowsy, and alert, with periods of eyes closed and open. Three types of features, Tsallis entropy (TsEn), Higuchi fractal dimension (HFD), and Lempel–Ziv complexity (LZC), were explored, and the LZC marker showed the best detection performance while an SVM classifier was used: a sensitivity of 100%, a specificity of 92.31%, and a recognition accuracy of 95% were achieved.

Instead of measuring the individual amplitude [3], the functional connectivity between signals attracts more attention in ML-aided AD diagnosing. The method proposed in Ref. [7] demonstrated excellent performance in AD detection using a 16-channel EEG device: a high mean recognition rate of 98.9% was achieved using a nonlinear support vector machine (SVM) classifier. A new biomarker namely permutation disalignment index (PDI) was developed to measure the coupling strength between signals from two electrodes. As a functional connectivity-related marker, PDI is inversely correlational to the coupling strength between the signals. In the experiments, 14 AD and 14 HC participated, and one-way ANOVA was employed for the statistical analysis. It was found by combining the local PDI features and a global complexity measurement namely graph index complexity (GIC), the system performance could receive a considerable boost: more than 6% of the mean accuracy increment was obtained. The reported recognition performance for AD was the average rate of 1,000 random tests. It is worth pointing out, however, that the obtained recognition rates were based on a relatively small pool of 14 participants per class, the robustness of such a newly proposed marker requires further verification across a larger population.

A more challenging task is to predict the conversion from MCI to AD. Such conversions often first occur in only part(s) of the brain, which make the source localization critical. In Ref. [8], researchers proposed an interesting approach to locate the source of interest without performing the conventional source reconstruction algorithms: based on their hypothesis, it is unlikely that a common source generates a simultaneous increase and decrease in power of different frequencies at distant electrode sites, the trial-by-trial negative correlations between the signals. They reported a sensitivity of 95% and a specificity of 80%. It is worth noting particularly that this is a longitudinal study on the conversion from MCI to AD, 15 out of the 25 participants with amnestic MCI developed AD in 3 years. The classification was conducted against 11 elderly controls.

One of the early attempts for ML-aided MCI diagnosis was made in 2015 [9]. The project involved combining a number of MEG databases collected using the same model of 306-channel Vectorview system; in total, the data from 102 MCI and 82 HC were obtained for the study. A series of band-specific mutual information were computed as the markers, which included the theta (4–8 Hz), alpha (8–12 Hz), beta (12–30 Hz), gamma (30–45 Hz), and broadband (2–45 Hz). Multiple classifiers were evaluated and the parameters were optimized for the problem: Random Forest, Bayesian Network, C4.5 induction tree, K-nearest Neighbor, Logistic Regression, and Support Vector Machine. Bootstrapping was selected to validate the diagnosis performances. The optimized results are 100% sensitivity, 69% specificity, and 83% classification accuracy. These pioneer results using MEG are quite promising, especially considering the relatively large number of participants in the study.

As it was discussed, using EEG for AD detection appears to have achieved reasonably good performance [7]; however, EEG for MCI detection is often not effective [8], probably due to the relatively small number of electrodes equipped for EEG systems. MEG, on the other hand, may ease this issue with its larger number of sensors. For example, researchers were able to distinguish the MCI and HC with a success rate of 98.4% using a 148-channel MEG system [10]. Participants (18 MCI and 19 HC) were performing the letter memorizing task during the data collection. The complete ensemble empirical mode decomposition (CEEMD) was used for feature extraction, and the resulting coefficients were used to compute a nonlinear dynamics measure based on permutation entropy analysis. The enhanced probabilistic neural network (EPNN) was adopted to classify the measures. Good performance was obtained, thanks to the CEEMD, which is purposely designed to deal with nonstationary signals such as E/MEG. The related transform has been found quite effective in other EEG applications [11].

Table 8.1 lists a few representative reports on using E/MEG for MCI/AD classifications. For the ML-aided systems, we notice that the SVM and neural network are the two most popular and best-performed classifiers. Researchers tend to instruct the participants in resting state during the data collection. Various biomarkers, across the time and frequency domains, have been developed to capture the informative content from the signals. It appears that the entropy-related features demonstrated good recognition performance [10], which is probably related to the MCI with reduced brain functionality. It is also worth noting that the relatively less popular data transform such as CMMED showed quite promising results, and its original form empirical mode decomposition was purposely designed for analyzing the nonstationary signals such as E/MEG.

8.3 SOURCE-LEVEL ANALYSIS

Due to the complexity and the ill-posed inverse problem in source reconstruction (SR), compared with the sensor-level analysis, relatively fewer attempts were made in this field. However, one of the major appealing factors for source-level analysis, in principle, is the locations of the source points that could be identified in the brain, which is particularly useful for the early diagnosing of MCI/AD.

Early research integrated the SR and ML using a 128-channel EEG system for AD diagnosis [12]. A relatively small number of participants, 17 AD and 17 healthy controls in the resting state with eyes closed, were involved in the data collection. The standardized low-resolution brain electromagnetic tomography (sLORETA) was used for source space reconstruction. The relative logarithmic power spectral density values from four

TABLE 8.1 Recent Reports on MCI/AD Diagnosis at the Sensor Level

State, Modality & Purpose	Method	Participants	Performance & Year
Resting state & 148-channel MEG & AD vs. HC	Dispersion entropy (DisEn) + *t*-test	36 AD, 26 HC	HC shown more irregular MEG than AD. 2016 [2]
Working memory tasks & 32-channel EEG & AD vs. MCI vs. HC classification	Working memory ERP + ICA + k-mean clustering + Kruskal–Wallis statistical tests	15 AD, 20 MCI, 26 HC	Decrease of P450 for abnormal groups. 2017 [3].
Resting, memory and visuospatial tasks & 64-channel EEG & MCI vs. HC	Relative powers + ANOVA + *t*-test	11 MCI, 11 HC	Theta is sensitive. 2017 [4].
Resting state with closed eyes & 19-channel EEG & AD vs. MCI vs. HC	Relative power, alpha frequency, entropy, Lempel–Ziv complexity etc. + FCBF + MLP	37 AD, 37 MCI, 37 HC	HC vs. (MCI & AD): sensitivity of 82.35% and positive predictive value of 84.85%. AD vs. (MCI & HC): specificity of 79.41% and negative predictive value of 84.38%. 2018 [5].
Hyperventilation, awake, drowsy, and alert, with periods of eyes closed and open & 19-channel EEG & AD vs. HC	Tsallis entropy (TsEn), Higuchi Fractal Dimension (HFD), and Lempel–Ziv complexity (LZC) + *P*-value + SVM	20 AD, 32 HC	Using LZC: sensitivity of 100%, specificity of 92.31% and the recognition accuracy of 95%. 2018 [6].
Awake and relaxed state with eyes closed & 16-channel EEG & AD vs. HC	PDI + GIC + ANOVA + SVM	14 AD, 14 HC	98.9% of accuracy. 2018 [7].
Word processing task & 19–32 channels EEG & MCI nonconvertors vs. MCI convertors to AD vs. elderly HC	Trial-by-trial negative correlations + SVM	25 amnestic MCI, 11 elderly HC	Sensitivity 80%, specificity 95%. 2018 [8].

(*Continued*)

TABLE 8.1 (*Continued*) Recent Reports on MCI/AD Diagnosis at the Sensor Level

State, Modality & Purpose	Method	Participants	Performance & Year
Eyes-closed resting state & 306-channel MEG Vectorview system & MCI vs. HC	Mutual information (theta, alpha, beta, gamma and broadband) + multi-classifier bootstrapping	102 MCI, 82 HC	100% sensitivity and 69% specificity, 83% classification accuracy. 2015 [9].
Letters memorizing task & 148-channel MEG & MCI vs. HC	CEEMD + permutation entropy + ANOVA + EPNN HC	18 MCI, 19	98.4% recognition accuracy. 2016 [10].

conventional EEG bands (alpha, beta, delta, and theta) were extracted from 12 selected cortical regions. The results showed that the right temporal region reflected a significant difference between the two groups in all frequency bands; in the left-brain hemisphere, the theta band power increased whereas the alpha band decreased for AD patients. The classification performances using an SVM between AD and HC groups were a sensitivity of 75.0%, a specificity of 93.7%, and an accuracy of 84.4%.

Source-level multi-type MCI detections were also explored [13]. Two types of MCIs, namely single-domain amnestic MCI (sdMCI) and multiple-domain amnestic MCI (mdMCI), were investigated (22 sdMCIs and 30 mdMCIs), which is compared against 29 HCs. Like many conventional studies, the data were collected while subjects were in resting state. A 306-channel MEG system was used to obtain the sensor-level signals, followed by the source space construction using the minimum variance beamformer technique. The time-domain connectivity matrix was computed and used as the marker to distinguish the sdMCI and mdMCI. Three popular classifiers: k-NN, LDA, and SVM were employed to test the recognition performance. Despite that three classes were involved, the study was focusing on the binary classification combinations: HC vs. sdMCI 86.27%, HC vs. mdMCI 81.36%, and sdMCI vs. mdMCI 84.62%. Given the obvious difficulty in MCI detection (compared with AD detection), these results are quite promising, which indicate the great potential of source-level diagnosis.

Later in 2017, a work using weighted minimum norm estimate for source space reconstruction was proposed [14]. Multi-participation PSD coefficients were computed and fed into a Mahalanobis distance classifier, and five-fold cross-validation was used to optimize the results. It was found that the proposed features significantly correlated with memory impairment of AD subjects. It appears that with the number of participants increasing, the classification performance for AD and HC reduced drastically [14]. Compared with the work in Ref. [12] published in 2013, while AD and HC participants (resting state) both increased from 17 to 25, the classification rate reported in Ref. [14] reduced from 84.4% to 78.4%. The work [14] published in 2017 employed an arguably more advanced MEG system with 306-channel (Elekta Neuromag). It may suggest that currently there is a necessity for a standard comparison scheme in the community, in order to justify the meaning of the research.

A recent work proposed in Ref. [15] pointed out an important issue in the current research on ML-aided diagnosis systems. It was reported using five-fold cross-validation, a high classification rate of 98% was achieved, whereas the same biomarkers yielded only about 70% accuracy when leave-one-out cross-validation was used for system evaluation. In detail, MEG data from 24 MCI and 30 HC were collected using a 306-channel Elekta Vectorview system, the subjects remained in a resting state for 4 minutes. The linearly constrained minimum variance (LCMV) beamformer was adopted for the source reconstruction; three connectivity estimators namely phase-locking value (PLV), the imaginary part of PLV (iPLV), and the correlation of the envelope (CorrEnv) were computed and used as the neuromarkers. The classification results were produced using an SVM with RBF kernel. More discussion on this research will be presented in the next section.

A recent work appears to have shown one crucial challenge in the field [16]: the quantity increasing of the data can impact the intra-class variance considerably. The study in Ref. [16] involved 75 MCI and 75 HC, as the relatively new research outcome, with a sensitivity of 73%, a specificity of 64%, and an accuracy of 68.5% were reported. These results were much degraded, compared with the work in Ref. [15] published in the same year. With the number of participants increasing 2~3 times, we can observe a drastic reduction in classification performance. Indeed, in the work in Ref. [16], only a 19-channel EEG system was used for data collection, followed by eLORETA and FFT-based power spectral analysis for source analysis and feature extraction. The SVM and ANOVA were adopted for classification and evaluations.

Table 8.2 provides some reports on the source-level MCI/AD detections. Similar to Table 8.1, it is found the SVM is one of the most popular classifiers. Compared to the sensor-level approaches, source space analysis for the MCI/AD classification appears to be slightly worse. This is not too surprising: the source reconstruction algorithms are designed for the points localization; additional research needs to be done to better facilitate both the classification and localization.

TABLE 8.2 Recent Reports on MCI/AD Diagnosis in the Source Level

State, Modality & Purpose	Method	Participants	Performance & Year
Resting state with eyes closed & 128-channel EEG & AD vs. HC	sLORETA + Band PSDs + SVM	17 AD, 17 HC	Sensitivity 75.0%, specificity of 93.7%, and accuracy of 84.4%. 2013 [12].
Resting state & 306-channel MEG system & HC vs. sdMCIs; HC vs. mdMCIs; mdMCIs vs. sdMCIs	Minimum variance beamformer + time-domain connectivity matrix + k-NN, LDA, SVM	22 sdMCIs, 30 mdMCIs and 29 HC	HC vs. sdMCI 86.27%, HC vs. mdMCI 81.36% and sdMCI vs. mdMCI 84.62%. 2014 [13].
Resting-state with eyes-closed & 306-channel Elekta Neuromag MEG system & AD vs. HC	Weighted minimum norm estimate + multi-participation PSD features + Mahalanobis distance classifier	25 AD, 25 HC	Specificity = 65.68%, sensitivity = 91.11%, the best classification accuracy 78.39%. 2017 [14].
Four minutes of resting state & 306- channel Elekta Vectorview system & MCI vs. HC	LCMV beamformer + PLV + iPLV + CorrEnv + intra and cross-frequency estimators + SVM with RBF kernel	24 MCI, 30 HC	Five-fold cross-validation: 98% accuracy; leave-one-out cross-validation: 70% accuracy. 2018 [15].
Resting-state & 19-channel EEG & MCI vs. HC	eLORETA + FFT-based power spectral analysis + SVM + ANOVA	75 MCI, 75 HC	Sensitivity of 73% and specificity of 64%, an accuracy of 68.5%. 2018 [16].

8.4 DISCUSSION AND CONCLUSION

In this chapter, we discussed a few recent researches on ML-aided MCI/AD diagnosis. It is noted that with the development of ML techniques in other fields, the integration of ML into clinical practice has become increasingly popular. However, it is admitted that currently there is no practically available ML-aided diagnosing system officially used in the actual clinical cases. This is not just an academic matter, but also an issue of trust: patients usually would not risk to solely put their faith on a machine. This is one big obstacle that prevents academic achievements from implementing in the real-world clinical practices.

Traditionally, the computer-aided MCI/AD diagnosis was mainly focusing on the statistical analysis of data; the current new trend aims to combine the statistical analysis with ML algorithms. This completes the pipeline of a typical expert system and makes such diagnosis systems truly automated. With the inclusion of ML modules, it also establishes a standardized framework from a statistical perspective (as opposed to the visual inspection of the plotted performance); within such framework, the evaluation of the systems becomes more objective: the well-recognized metrics in the ML field, such as sensitivity, specificity and recognition accuracy, provide a clearer reflection of the diagnosis performance than the conventional computer-aided systems in the clinical community.

In spite of the promising results for ML-aided MCI/AD diagnosis in recent years, a few issues are noticed in designing the detection systems and need to be carefully addressed for improvement in the future. These important factors are listed as follows:

1. It is noted that with the increasing of the participants involved in the data collection, the classification performance has been found to reduce drastically [9,10,15,16]. This indicates that the within-class difference (i.e. the individual difference between the subjects) is an impacting factor in such clinical scenarios and cannot be just ignored. Given the clinical systems are designed for human users, the existence of such biometric variabilities is well noticed [17]. Theoretically, with the amount of training set increasing, ML systems should be able to provide robustly increasing performance until the curve reaches the plateau stage. One possible way to alleviate such intra-class variance is to introduce the concept of transfer learning: One could purposely extract the useful information from different individuals, which should be commonly shared within the class, yet distinguishable enough between class, we could be expecting a boost in the recognition performance.
2. Most of the state-of-the-art studies are conducted using data from the single session recording for both training and the test of the system. Such design may yield good diagnosis performance in experimental

scenarios if the data are carefully organized, but it is obviously not quite realistic for the clinical scenarios. In real-world practices, such a diagnosis system may be facing different new recordings from the same subjects. The performance of such a case has not been extensively explored. It is recommended to conduct extensive longitudinal studies for E/MEG data, with particular focus on the temple aging effects [17], for example.

3. The various evaluation approaches reported in the literature is another issue that needs to be addressed. It is no secret in the ML community that when using different evaluation approaches, the same system pipeline can demonstrate a huge difference in classification performance. For instance, the work reported in Ref. [14] provided two drastically different accuracies: using a five-fold crossvaldation, the system was able to achieve 98% of the accuracy for MCI detection, whereas using the leave-one-out cross-valiaditon, the same system only provided an accuracy of about 70%. It is suggested that researchers should try to mimic real-life scenarios while doing the experimental design, particularly avoid using the data from same-subject same-session for both training and test.

4. Though the clinical brainwave data (in particular EEG) is quite abundant, according to the literature, a few minutes of recording is enough to provide reasonable accuracy. Additional recording from a single session does not appear to be able to further improve the performance and also it has the liability to introduce redundant data.

5. Most of the current studies are based on using the resting state data. As the early stage baseline study, it is highly recommended. To explore further, in particular the ROIs and their functional responses, different experimental paradigms should be developed. For example, AD affects multiple cognitive areas of the brain, and diverse cognitive stimulation paradigms should be combined to better explore the cognitive changes and their relationships.

Given its minor deployment and relative early developing stage in general, much work could be done in excavating the potential of ML-aided MCI/AD diagnosis. From the perspective of information gain, MEG modality intuitively should to be much more informative than EEG signals, due to its higher sensor density and arguably more information per channel. However, approaches to remove the redundant information should also be carefully designed for MEG-based auto-diagnosis. EEG on the other hand, benefits from its cheap installation and already wide deployment, still playing a supportive role in most of the mainstream clinical practice.

One possible way to boost the prediction performance is to combine the EEG and MEG: a multi-modal recognition system equipped with a well-designed fusion algorithm could synergistically combine complementary information from both modalities. From a broad perspective, using E/MEG-based ML algorithms to classify AD patients and patients with other neurodegenerative diseases (such as Parkinson's disease and Lewy body dementia) may also deserve attention in future investigations.

REFERENCES

1. S. Yang, J. Miguel, S. Bornot, K. Wong-lin, G. Prasad, and S. Member, "M/EEG-based bio-markers to predict the mild cognitive impairment and Alzheimer's disease : A review from the machine learning perspective," *IEEE Trans. Biomed. Eng.*, pp. 1–12.
2. H. Azami, M. Rostaghi, A. Fernandez, and J. Escudero, "Dispersion entropy for the analysis of resting-state MEG regularity in Alzheimer's disease," in *Proceedings of the Annual International Conference of the IEEE Engineering in Medicine and Biology Society, EMBS*, 2016, vol. 2016-Oct, pp. 6417–6420.
3. G. Q. Mamani, F. J. Fraga, G. Tavares, E. Johns, and N. D. Phillips, "EEG-based biomarkers on working memory tasks for early diagnosis of Alzheimer's disease and mild cognitive impairment," *2017 IEEE Healthc. Innov. Point Care Technol.*, pp. 237–240, 2017.
4. J. Ye, Y. Lan, R. Wang, and Y. Yang, "Relative power analysis of electroencephalograph rhythms in elderly with mild cognitive impairment," in *2017 10th International Congress on Image and Signal Processing, BioMedical Engineering and Informatics (CISP-BMEI)*, 2017, no. 91420302, pp. 1–6.
5. S. Ruiz-Gómez et al., "Automated multiclass classification of spontaneous EEG activity in Alzheimer's disease and mild cognitive impairment," *Entropy*, vol. 20, no. 1, p. 35, 2018.
6. A. H. H. Al-Nuaimi, E. Jammeh, L. Sun, and E. Ifeachor, "Complexity measures for quantifying changes in electroencephalogram in Alzheimer's disease," *Complexity*, vol. 2018, pp. 22–24, 2018.
7. H. Yu, X. Lei, Z. Song, J. Wang, X. Wei, and B. Yu, "Functional brain connectivity in Alzheimer's disease: An EEG study based on permutation disalignment index," *Phys. A Stat. Mech. Appl.*, vol. 506, pp. 1093–1103, 2018.
8. A. Mazaheri et al., "EEG oscillations during word processing predict MCI conversion to Alzheimer's disease," *NeuroImage Clin.*, vol. 17, no. October 2017, pp. 188–197, 2018.

9. F. Maestú et al., "A multicenter study of the early detection of synaptic dysfunction in mild cognitive impairment using magnetoencephalography-derived functional connectivity," *NeuroImage Clin.*, vol. 9, pp. 103–109, 2015.
10. J. P. Amezquita-Sanchez, A. Adeli, and H. Adeli, "A new methodology for automated diagnosis of mild cognitive impairment (MCI) using magnetoencephalography (MEG)," *Behav. Brain Res.*, vol. 305, pp. 174–180, 2016.
11. S. Yang and F. Deravi, "Novel HHT-based features for biometric identification using EEG signals," *2014 22nd Int. Conf. Pattern Recognit.*, pp. 1922–1927, Aug. 2014.
12. H. Aghajani, E. Zahedi, M. Jalili, A. Keikhosravi, and B. V. Vahdat, "Diagnosis of early Alzheimer's disease based on EEG source localization and a standardized realistic head model," *IEEE J. Biomed. Heal. Informat.*, vol. 17, no. 6, pp. 1039–1045, 2013.
13. J. A. Pineda-Pardo et al., "Guiding functional connectivity estimation by structural connectivity in MEG: An application to discrimination of conditions of mild cognitive impairment," *Neuroimage*, vol. 101, pp. 765–777, 2014.
14. J. Guillon et al., "Loss of brain inter-frequency hubs in Alzheimer's disease," *Sci. Rep.*, vol. 7, no. 1, pp. 1–14, 2017.
15. S. I. Dimitriadis et al., "How to build a functional connectomic biomarker for mild cognitive impairment from source reconstructed MEG resting-state activity: The combination of ROI representation and connectivity estimator matters," *Front. Neurosci.*, vol. 12, no. JUN, pp. 1–21, 2018.
16. C. Babiloni et al., "Functional cortical source connectivity of resting state electroencephalographic alpha rhythms shows similar abnormalities in patients with mild cognitive impairment due to Alzheimer's and Parkinson's diseases," *Clin. Neurophysiol.*, vol. 129, no. 4, pp. 766–782, 2018.
17. S. Yang and F. Deravi, "On the usability of electroencephalographic signals for biometric recognition: A survey," *IEEE Trans. Human-Machine Syst.*, vol. 47, no. 6, pp. 958–969, 2017.

CHAPTER 9

Some Practical Challenges with Possible Solutions for Machine Learning in Medical Imaging

Naimul Khan, Nabila Abraham, Anika Tabassum, and Marcia Hon

Ryerson University
Toronto, Canada

CONTENTS

9.1 INTRODUCTION

Recent advances in machine learning (ML) have resulted in a flourish of applications in medical imaging and computer-aided diagnosis. Recently, deep learning techniques have gained popularity due to readily available software to deploy state-of-the-art models. Although research results have shown that deep learning models utilizing convolutional neural networks (CNN) have outperformed even human experts in terms of accuracy, there are some practical issues that prevent the widespread deployment of such ML systems in practice. We focus on three such issues in this chapter:

1. **Significant dependence on the size of training data**: Modern ML methods, especially deep learning, is dependent on the amount of training data available. For medical applications, this poses a problem, since acquiring a large amount of labeled training data is expensive in healthcare. Also, dependence on a large amount of training data results in dependence on expensive computational resources, making the technology less accessible for underfunded healthcare centers.
2. **Class imbalance**: Having a significantly reduced number of samples for one of the labeled classes results in class imbalance for supervised learning. Class imbalance happens very frequently for computer-aided diagnosis or segmentation applications. For example, in segmentation, only a few pixels are usually labeled as a foreground (e.g. tumor or lesion), and the rest of the pixels are background. This results in severe class imbalance, which is difficult to deal with by traditional ML algorithms [1].
3. **Confidence tuning**: Most ML methods and their applications in computer-aided diagnosis only report accuracy/F1-score as a performance measure. However, for medical applications, a confidence measure would make the domain expert more comfortable with the system, and a simple tool to tune the confidence-accuracy tradeoff will be useful [2].

In this chapter, we highlight three state-of-the-art research works that we have undertaken at the Ryerson Multimedia Research Laboratory in the past 3 years. These three projects tackle the three aforementioned issues by applying novel methodologies, architectures, and algorithms.

In Section 9.1, we highlight how dependence on a large training set can be reduced by utilizing transfer learning [3,4]. We show that instead of using a large medical training dataset, we can simply utilize natural images from benchmark datasets to learn low-level features, and only train higher layers of deep networks with medical data, selected through an intelligent data filtering mechanism. We present results on the state-of-the-art ADNI dataset [5]. Our results show that transfer learning can help in improving the accuracy of Alzheimer's diagnosis only through a small fraction of training data that is typically required.

In Section 9.2, we show how we can tackle class imbalance through a novel loss function [6], where we achieve a balance between precision and recall using the Tversky index [7]. We incorporate the Tversky index into the focal loss function [1]. Experimental results show that we achieve state-of-the-art results in segmentation of breast ultrasound lesions.

Finally, In Section 9.3, we propose a tunable Bayesian neural network for breast cancer diagnosis, where two tunable parameters can be adjusted to achieve a satisfactory confidence-accuracy tradeoff. We provide an analysis of how the tunable parameters affect the confidence and accuracy.

9.2 UTILIZING TRANSFER LEARNING WITH NATURAL IMAGES

In this section, we show that instead of relying on large training datasets in the medical domain, we can simply use existing large natural image datasets to learn low-level features. Then, through an intelligent data filtering technique based on entropy, we can reduce the dependence on large medical datasets.[1] To show the application of transfer learning, we pick the field of Alzheimer's diagnosis, which has shown promising results recently when applying ML [8].

In the early 2010s, statistical ML approaches have shown promising results with Alzheimer's diagnosis [9]. The recent popularity of deep learning approaches such as CNN and autoencoders has shifted the attention toward deep learning. However, most existing deep learning methods train the architecture from a clean slate. This type of training from scratch has a few issues when applied to a medical application [10]: (1) Deep networks typically have millions of learnable parameters, which require a large amount of labeled data to be properly optimized. Such a large amount of labeled data is expensive to acquire in the medical domain. (2) Having millions of parameters poses another problem, where the model may overfit/underfit that results in very good training performance, but poor performance on unseen data. (3) Training a deep network with such a large amount of data requires a huge number of expensive GPUs, which are not sustainable for underfunded healthcare centers.

Fine-tuning a deep CNN through transfer learning is a recent popular approach that can be utilized instead of training from scratch [11].

Although it is hard to obtain annotated data in the medical domain, plenty of benchmark datasets with annotated objects are available in the natural image domain to solve computer vision problems. One such example is the ImageNet dataset [12]. The basic idea behind transfer learning is to not start training from scratch. Instead, we train a CNN where the parameters are already learned from a natural image dataset such as ImageNet. The network is simply retrained to obtain new knowledge from a different domain (e.g. computer-aided diagnosis of Alzheimer's). It has been shown that CNNs are very good at learning low-level features and can generalize image features given a large training set. If we always train a network from scratch, the extensive research done on natural images and robust architectures created for such problems are not being utilized properly.

In this section, we investigate how we can transfer knowledge learned from natural images to the problem of Alzheimer's diagnosis. The motivation behind reusing knowledge learned from natural images is the reduction of excessive dependency on the size of the training set. Due to the popularity of CNN, there are many established architectures designed with meticulous attention by researchers over the last few years to solve visual classification problems. One of the most popular benchmarks in the visual classification domain is the ImageNet Large Scale Visual Recognition Challenge (ILSVRC). In this challenge, over a million annotated images of 1,000 different objects are provided [12]. Due to the popularity of the challenge, the winning network architectures of this challenge are usually carefully designed and thoroughly tested. For this research, the winners of the aforementioned challenge were carefully explored to pick the architecture most suitable for the problem in hand. We decided to utilize VGG [13]. VGG was picked because of the easy-to-reuse architecture, which consists of multiple convolutional layers, followed by fully connected layers [13]. Typically, the network is trained from a clean slate utilizing natural image datasets such as ImageNet. Then, the convolutional layers are frozen. Only the fully connected layers are retrained for a new problem domain.

However, randomly cutting down the size of the training data will not help in capturing the best possible variation in data, which is required to avoid overfitting/underfitting. To select the best possible training set, we utilize image entropy, which provides us with a relative measurement of the amount of information contained in one image (a slice of the volume MRI image in our case).

In general, for a set of M symbols with probabilities $p_1, p_2, \ldots, p_M$, the entropy can be calculated as follows:

$$H = -\sum_{i=1}^{M} p_i \log p_i \tag{9.1}$$

Image entropy for a 2D slice of a volume image can be calculated through image histograms [14]. The key reason behind using entropy is that it provides a reasonable measure of how much information (or variation of data) a slice of an image contains. Higher entropy typically points to images that have rich information. Instead of using randomly selected images, we can select the most informative slices by utilizing image entropy in this manner, which will result in a more robust dataset.

In Table 9.1, we show that through our proposed entropy-based image filtering combined with transfer learning, we can achieve state-of-the-art classification results for all three classification scenarios in Alzheimer's prediction. The three classification problems are AD vs. normal control (NC), mild cognitive impairment (MCI) vs. AD, and MCI vs. NC on the benchmark ADNI dataset [5]. Although we get a reasonable boost in accuracy, the more important contribution is the reduction in the size of the training set. The closest competitor or proposed method is that of Ref. [16], with a training size of 39,942, while our proposed method has a training size of only 2,560, thus providing a reduction of 16 times. Transfer learning combined with our intelligent training data filtering method can reduce the excessive reliance on a large amount of training data, making deep learning more usable in clinical settings.

We further investigated whether making some convolutional layers trainable results in improved accuracy. In Figure 9.1, we see comparative results for all three classification problems (AD vs. NC, AD vs. MCI, and MCI vs. NC) when groups of convolutional layers are frozen together. The groups correspond to the freezing of VGG16 conv. layers as follows:

1. **All:** None of the convolutional layers are frozen (all of them trainable).

2. **Group 1:** The first four convolutional layers are frozen

TABLE 9.1 Accuracy Results (in %) Compared to State-of-the-Art on the ADNI Dataset.

Architecture	**Training Set (# Images)**	**AD vs. NC**	**AD vs. MCI**	**MCI vs. NC**
Patch-based autoencoder [15]	103,683	94.74	88.1	86.35
3D CNN [16]	39,942	97.6	95	90.8
Inception [17]	46,751	98.84	–	–
Proposed	**2,560**	**99.36**	**99.2**	**99.04**

Note: Best method in Bold

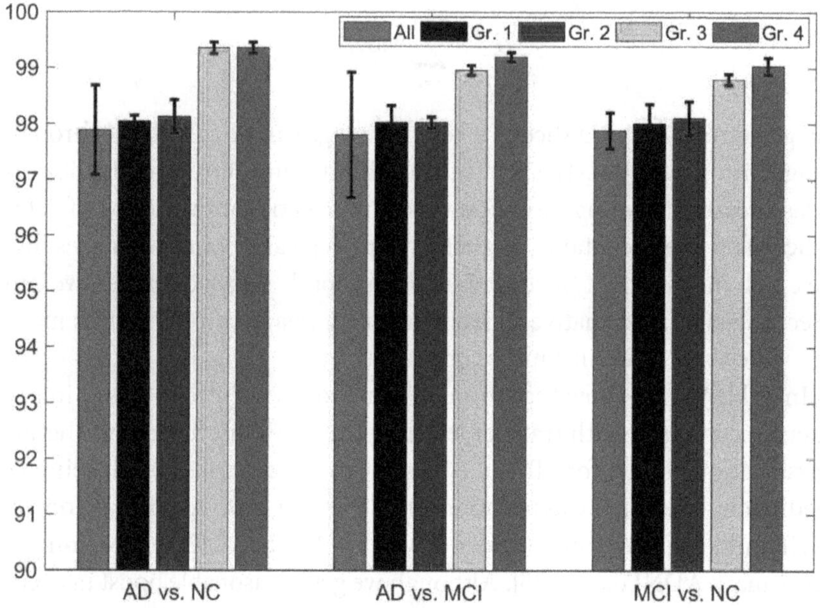

FIGURE 9.1 Results for layer-wise freezing of transfer learning for the three classification problems.

3. **Group 2**: The first eight convolutional layers are frozen.
4. **Group 3**: The first 12 convolutional layers are frozen.
5. **Group 4**: All convolutional layers (1–16) are frozen.

As we can see, for this particular dataset, freezing all convolutional layers (Group 4) resulted in the best accuracy. In general, the early layers of a CNN learn low-level image features that are applicable to most visual problems, but the later layers learn high-level features, which are specific to particular application domains. Therefore, fine-tuning the fully connected layers is usually good enough. However, as discussed in Ref. [10], this behavior can change based on the specific computer-diagnosis problem being worked on. However, the general consensus that we can reach from the results is that transfer learning significantly improves the performance of computer-aided diagnosis problems.

9.3 FOCAL TVERSKY LOSS FUNCTION FOR CLASS IMBALANCE

This section tackles the class imbalance problem, which is common in the biomedical imaging field. Class imbalance is especially common in medical segmentation problems. In segmentation problems such as lesion segmentation, typically the lesion (foreground) only occupies a small portion of the image. Such imbalanced data can result in unstable results in popular segmentation frameworks [18]. In recent literature, CNN have been successful in segmenting lesions in medical imaging data [18]. Instead of typical CNN, segmentation problems employ fully convolutional networks (FCN), where fully connected layers are dropped for efficient pixel-wise segmentation. One of the most popular FCN architectures is U-Net [19]. On top of FCN, U-Net introduces other improvements such as multiple skill connections and up-convolution layers with learnable parameters.

Some recent works propose new loss functions to deal with the class imbalance in medical image segmentation. The focal loss function proposed in Ref. [1], a popular cross-entropy loss function obtained by introducing an exponential factor, emphasizes learning from the class with a smaller number of samples. The focal loss prevents the vast number of easy negative examples from dominating the gradient to alleviate class imbalance. In practice, however, it faces difficulty balancing precision and recall due to very small regions-of-interest (ROI) found in medical images. Research efforts to address small ROI segmentation propose more discriminative models such as attention gated networks [20].

To address the aforementioned issues, we combine attention gated U-Net with a novel variant of the focal loss function, better suited for small lesion segmentation. We propose a novel focal Tversky loss function (FTL) that provides improvement over the focal loss by incorporating the Tversky index into the loss function. We modulate the Tversky index [7] that addresses the imbalance between precision and recall in the focal loss function. Then, we combine this proposed loss function with a deeply supervised attention U-Net [20], improved with a multi-scaled input image pyramid for better intermediate feature representations.[2]

We extend from the Dice loss (DL) function described in Ref. [18], whose limitation is that it equally weighs false positive (FP) and false negative (FN) detections. Failing equally weight FP and FN results in segmentation maps with high precision. However, the recall is lowered because of this issue. Medical segmentation data such as lesion segmentation problems have only a few pixels annotated as ground-truth foreground. Therefore, even a few ground truth foreground pixels being mislabeled will result in a drastic reduction in the recall rate. Therefore, we need to put a higher weight on FN when compared to FP if we want to increase the recall rate.

The Tversky index can help us in achieving a better weighting between FP and FN:

$$TI_c = \frac{\sum_{i=1}^{N} p_{ic} g_{ic} + \epsilon}{\sum_{i=1}^{N} p_{ic} g_{ic} + \alpha \sum_{i=1}^{N} p_{i\bar{c}} g_{ic} + \beta \sum_{i=1}^{N} p_{ic} g_{i\bar{c}} + \epsilon} \tag{9.2}$$

where p_{ic} is the probability that pixel i is of the lesion class c and $p_{i\bar{c}}$ is the probability that pixel i is of the non-lesion class, $\bar{c}$. The same is true for g_{ic} and $g_{i\bar{c}}$, respectively. The total number of pixels in an image is denoted by N. Hyperparameters α and β can be tuned to shift the emphasis to improve recall in the case of large class imbalance. The Tversky index is adapted to a loss function (TL) in Ref. [7] by minimizing $\sum_{c} 1 - TI_c$.

Another issue with the DL is that it struggles to segment small ROIs as they do not contribute to the loss significantly. To address this, we propose the FTL, parametrized by γ, for control between easy background and hard ROI training examples. In Ref. [1], the focal parameter exponentiates the cross-entropy loss to focus on hard classes detected with lower probability. The focal loss has recently been incorporated into the DL function as well [21]. We follow a similar approach to define our FTL:

$$FTL_c = \sum_{c} (1 - TI_c)^{1/\gamma} \tag{9.3}$$

where γ varies in the range $\{1,3\}$. In practice, if a pixel is misclassified with a high Tversky index, the FTL is unaffected. However, if the Tversky index is small and the pixel is misclassified, the FTL will decrease significantly.

When $\gamma > 1$, the loss function focuses more on less accurate predictions that have been misclassified. However, we observe over-suppression of the FTL when the class accuracy is high, usually as the model is close to convergence. To alleviate this issue, we have experimented with higher values of γ. With trial-and-error, we have found that $\gamma = \frac{4}{3}$ achieves the best performance across the board. This is the value we used in all the experiments in this work. To further tackle the over-suppression of FTL, instead of using it for all layers, we only use FTL with the intermediate layers. The very last layer is supervised with the Tversky loss instead to provide

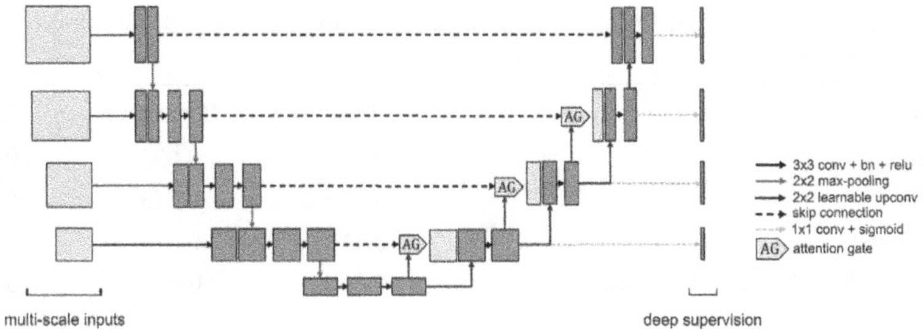

FIGURE 9.2 The proposed attention U-Net architecture.

a strong error signal and mitigate sub-optimal convergence. We hypothesize that using a higher α in our generalized loss function will improve model convergence by shifting the focus to minimize FN predictions. Therefore, we train all models with $\alpha = 0.7$ and $\beta = 0.3$. It is important to note that in the case of $\alpha = \beta = 0.5$, the Tversky index simplifies to the DSC. Moreover, when $\gamma = 1$, the FTL simplifies to the TL.

To obtain an even better precision and recall, we follow the improvements proposed to U-Net in Ref. [20] and combine them with the FTL. However, even after utilizing the attention-based architecture in Ref. [20], we saw that minor spatial details in lesions were getting lost through multiple layers of convolution, since convolution operations tend to blur out minute details. To address this issue, we use soft attention gates to identify relevant spatial information from low-level feature maps and propagate it to the decoding stage. To ease the access of details at different scales even further, we directly feed multi-scale versions of the input image (through forming an image pyramid) to the encoder layers. Combined with deep supervision, this method improves segmentation accuracy for datasets where small ROI features can get lost in multiple stages of convolutions and facilitates the network learning more locality-aware features, which in turn can improve segmentation performance. The proposed network architecture can be seen in Figure 9.2.

To show the effectiveness of the proposed FTL with attention U-Net, we perform experiments on the Breast Ultrasound Lesions 2017 dataset B (BUS) [22],[3] where the lesions occupy 4.84% ± 5.43%. Table 9.2 shows the results. When compared to the baseline U-Net, our method significantly improves Dice scores by 25.7%. This result demonstrates the importance of addressing class imbalance for segmentation and shows that the problem is worth exploring further.

TABLE 9.2 Results on the Bus 2017 Dataset for the Proposed FTL and Attention U-Net Compared to DL

Model	DSC	Precision	Recall
U-Net+DL	0.547	0.653	0.658
U-Net+FTL	0.669	0.775	0.715
Attn U-Net+DL	0.615	0.675	0.658
Proposed (Attn U-Net+multi-input+FTL)	**0.804**	**0.829**	**0.022**

9.4 BAYESIAN NEURAL NETWORKS FOR CONFIDENCE TUNING

While deep neural networks have achieved high accuracy for computer-aided diagnosis problems, for practical consideration, merely an increased accuracy is not enough. Alongside accuracy, a confidence measure will be useful for doctors and healthcare practitioners, to assess how well the system is performing. Bayesian neural networks are a good tool to estimate the confidence of a decision by an ML system [23]. The target of this work is to not only compute such confidence measures efficiently but also provide the doctors with a tool to effectively control the accuracy-coverage tradeoff. The tradeoff can be achieved by using some control parameters for controlling a Bayesian neural network.

In the proposed model, we take a two-stage approach to achieve a tunable confidence measure. The reason for taking a two-stage approach rather than employing an end-to-end Bayesian network is two-fold: (1) employing a traditional CNN for feature extraction, followed by a small Bayesian network, results in a more efficient network architecture, which can result in much faster training and (2) popular CNN architectures such as AlexNet [24], Resnet [25], and VGG [13] are already being deployed at hospitals and clinics. A modular Bayesian architecture can be used simply as an "add-on" to such systems.

The proposed architecture is shown in Figure 9.3. As we can see, a modified ResNet-18 architecture is used as a feature generator, which takes in 224×224 sized images and generates 512-element feature vectors, and a separate small fully connected network that has just three fully connected layers followed by a softmax. Note that this small network only has just over 164 thousand parameters as opposed to the over-11 million parameters in the full network, making the subsequent steps easily executable on commodity hardware. Bayesian inference is performed via a Gaussian process such as stochastic variational inference (SVI) [26], but on the

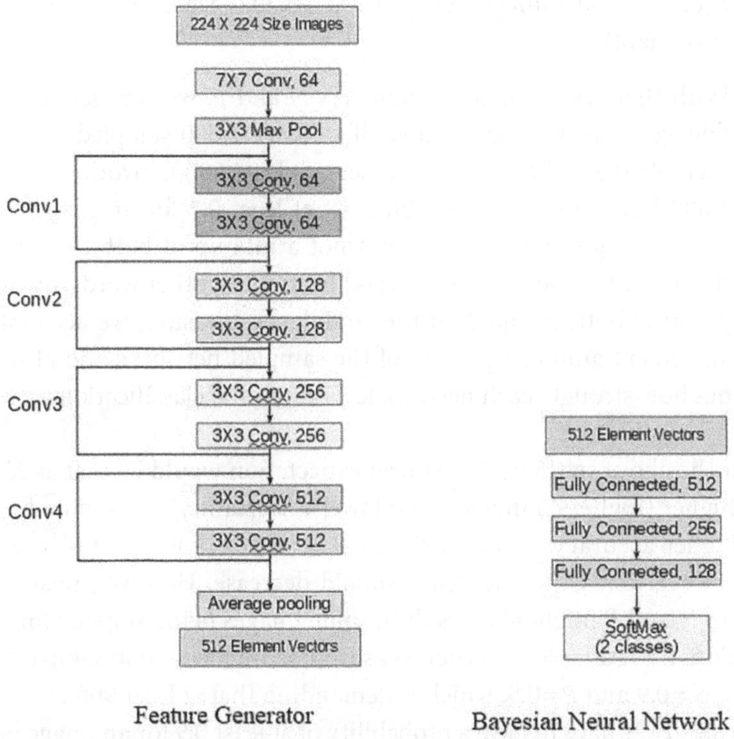

FIGURE 9.3 The proposed two-stage architecture for confidence measurement.

smaller network and with lower-dimensional training data generated from the feature generator, to learn the posterior distribution of the parameters (after having initialized with random normal priors).

Once we have the posterior distributions of the network parameters (weights and biases), the next step is to come up with a confidence measure. Our proposed confidence measure consists of two tunable parameters. The steps to calculate these are described below:

1. Sample a reasonable number (1,000 in our experiments) of networks from the posterior distributions using Monte Carlo sampling. Each of these sampled networks is a deterministic network by itself.
2. Classify each image by each of the sampled networks. Record the probabilities for both classes (benign and malignant) for each image.
3. Use two parameters N and P, where N denotes the fraction of the sampled number of networks that have a minimum probability

P on a certain image being of a particular class (either benign or malignant).

4. With these two tunable parameters N and P, we can define a confidence measure. For example, if we have 1,000 sampled networks, then $N=0.6$ and $P=0.7$ would mean at least 600 networks out of the 1,000 have to have a probability of at least 0.7 for an image being either benign or malignant (but not a mix-up of both); otherwise, the image will be skipped for classification. In other words, by incorporating both N and P in the confidence measure, we account for agreement among a portion of the sampled networks and also find out how strongly each network feels about the classification.

Under the above settings, the natural expectation would be that as N and P go higher (higher confidence and lower uncertainty), we should be getting higher accuracy, while as N and P go lower (lower confidence and higher uncertainty), the accuracy should decrease. However, raising the value of N and P might also result in some images being skipped for classification. For example, consider a case where we have 1,000 sampled networks, $N=0.9$ and $P=0.9$, which is demanding that at least 900 out of the 1,000 networks have to have a probability of at least 0.9 for an image being either benign or malignant – this might result in a number of images being skipped for classification, since we are demanding too high of a confidence. This is the case of lower coverage. At higher values of N and P (higher confidence), we will have lower coverage (many images skipped), but the accuracy on the covered images will be high. On the other hand, at lower values of N and P (lower confidence), we will have higher coverage (not too many images skipped) but the accuracy on the covered images would be lower. In short, tuning the values of N and P gives us a way to decide where in the accuracy-coverage tradeoff we want to settle. Therefore, the N and P values, along with the accuracy and coverage, comprise our new evaluation metric, which can be formalized as a tuple (accuracy, coverage, N, P) where N and P comprise the confidence measure.

Although in this chapter we are using classification accuracy as the primary evaluation criterion, in general, the framework allows any evaluation criterion to be paired with a confidence measure. Other possible candidates include precision, recall, F1-score, ROC AUC score, etc., some of which might make more sense for an imbalanced classification case. However, in this chapter, the goal is not to discuss or compare which evaluation criterion among these is the most appropriate, but to pair a confidence measure with an already chosen evaluation criterion. Ours being a relatively class-balanced classification case, we chose to go with accuracy for our task. The framework is agnostic to the criterion selection.

To evaluate the proposed framework, we performed experiments on the CBIS-DDSM (Curated Breast Imaging Subset of DDSM) [27] dataset. It is an updated and standardized version of the Digital Database for Screening Mammography (DDSM). The original DDSM database consists of 2,620 scanned filmed mammography studies, whereas the CBIS-DDSM includes a subset of the DDSM data curated by a trained mammographer. The ROI-cropped dataset contains 1,696 labeled grayscale images. Of those, 912 are labeled as benign and 784 are labeled as malignant. So, the dataset is reasonably class-balanced. A training to validation ratio of 80:20 was obtained in a stratified manner with regards to the class (benign vs. malignant) distribution. We created five such stratified splits so that each such split can be used for cross-validation to test the generalization of our approach. For each of the five splits, we have 1,357 training images and 339 validation images. All the results we present later show the average of the results on the five validation sets to demonstrate the robustness of our approach.

We sampled 1,000 networks from the posterior distributions using Monte Carlo sampling and performed evaluation by tuning the values of N and P.

We demonstrate the usage of our control parameters N and P and how it affects the classification performance. We have 339 validation images on average. We found that when we set N above 0.9, all test images were skipped and the Bayesian network had no coverage, regardless of the value of P, which is expected because it's unlikely that 95% of the networks would have a minimum probability for a class for any image. In general, if we kept N to a moderate value like 0.5 and then varied P, we noted an upward trend in accuracy and a downward trend in coverage, which is expected. An almost similar trend shows up if we held P at 0.5 and varied N instead, which is also expected. Figure 9.4 shows the accuracy and coverage values and trends for varying N, keeping P at 0.5, while Figure 9.5 shows the accuracy and coverage values and trends for varying P, keeping N constant at 0.5.

We should point out that practically it might make more sense to keep P at a constant value (e.g. 0.5) and tune N, as opposed to keeping N constant and tuning P; this is because tuning N and keeping P constant effectively means varying the degree of polling on the sampled set of networks while

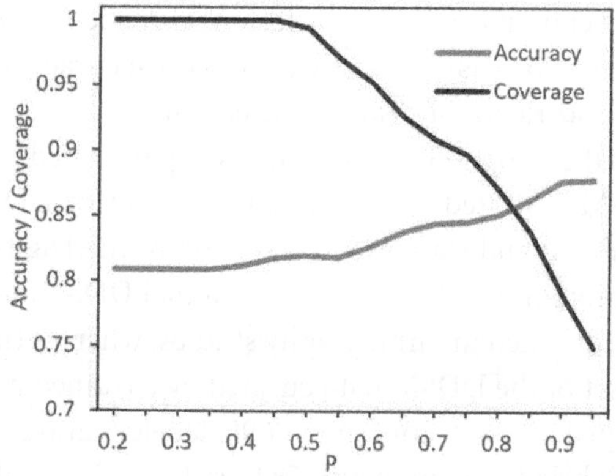

FIGURE 9.4 Accuracy and coverage vs. N (at $P=0.5$).

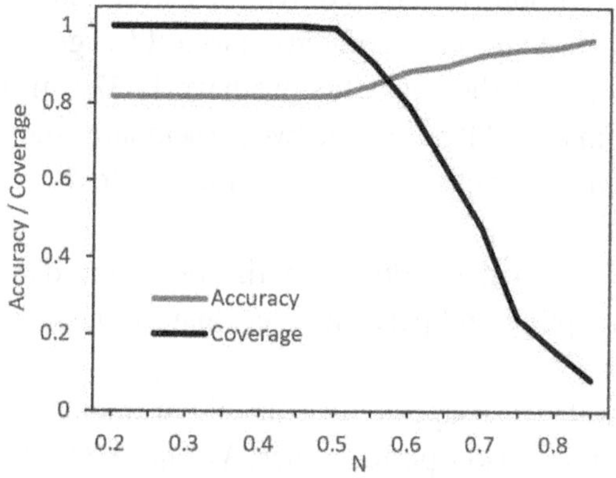

FIGURE 9.5 Accuracy and coverage vs. P (at $N=0.5$).

expecting a fixed minimum classification probability agreement among the polled ones, whereas tuning P keeping N constant means freezing the polling space and varying the value of the minimum classification probability agreement in that frozen network space. In other words, it is N that allows us to choose how much of the sampled network distribution we will cover, and hence it is a better measure of practical uncertainty.

The takeaway from the findings is that the parameters N and P can be tuned to a desirable level and the higher the values of these parameters, the higher the confidence we will have in the predictions/classifications, in exchange for possibly lower coverage. For a domain like medical mammography image classification, it will be up to the mammography experts to determine what value of N and P is reasonable. After setting reasonable values for N and P, previously unseen images that will be classified by the Bayesian network (either as benign or malignant) are more likely to be correctly classified, whereas images that will be skipped and denied classification would need further investigation. The overall framework can be used as a confidence tuning tool for any computer-aided diagnosis problem.

9.5 CONCLUSION

In this chapter, we highlight three practical issues that can arise while deploying an ML model for medical image segmentation or computer-aided diagnosis problems. We tackle the heavy dependence on large training datasets of deep learning models with transfer learning, where we show that utilizing transfer learning from natural images can significantly improve the performance of Alzheimer's diagnosis. To address the issue of class imbalance, which is prevalent for medical image segmentation, we propose a novel FTL, which, combined with Attention U-Net, results in state-of-the-art lesion segmentation performance on a benchmark breast ultrasound dataset. Finally, we propose a confidence tuning tool utilizing a Bayesian neural network, where, through two simple hyperparameters (sampled number of networks and minimum probability), a neural network's accuracy-coverage tradeoff can be tuned to the need of the domain expert.

Although the three sections showed promising results, more work needs to be done to ensure the robustness of the proposed methods before they can be deployed in a clinical setting. For transfer learning, we are investigating whether our solution can be generalized to solve computer-aided diagnosis problems in domains other than Alzheimer's. For our proposed loss function, our next step is to investigate how the solution performs for different types of imbalanced classification problems, especially to investigate how the transfer learning approach can be combined with the proposed loss function. For confidence tuning, an end-to-end Bayesian learning approach on top of transfer learning to keep the computational requirement manageable is something we would be exploring in the future.

NOTES

1 Extended experimental results and analyses on this project was originally published in [3, 4].
2 Extended experimental results and analyses on this project was originally published in [6].
3 Code for this chapter can be found in: https://github.com/nabsabraham/focal-tversky-unet

REFERENCES

1. T.-Y. Lin, P. Goyal, R. Girshick, K. He, and P. Dollár, "Focal loss for dense object detection," *IEEE Transactions on Pattern Analysis and Machine Intelligence*, vol. 42, no. 2, pp 318–327, 2018.
2. B. M. Geller, A. Bogart, P. A. Carney, J. G. Elmore, B. S. Monsees, and D. L. Miglioretti, "Is confidence of mammographic assessment a good predictor of accuracy?" *American Journal of Roentgenology*, vol. 199, no. 1, pp. W134–W141, 2012.
3. N. M. Khan, N. Abraham, and M. Hon, "Transfer learning with intelligent training data selection for prediction of Alzheimer's disease," *IEEE Access*, vol. 7, pp. 72726–72735, 2019.
4. M. Hon and N. M. Khan, "Towards Alzheimer's disease classification through transfer learning," in *IEEE International Conference on Bioinformatics and Biomedicine*, 2017.
5. C. R. Jack et al., "The Alzheimer's disease neuroimaging initiative (ADNI): MRI methods," Journal of *Magnetic Resonance Imaging*, vol. 27, no. 4, pp. 685–691, 2008.
6. N. Abraham and N. M. Khan, "A novel focal Tversky loss function with improved attention U-net for segmentation," in *IEEE Symposium on Biomedical Imaging*, 2019.
7. S. R. Hashemi et al., "Tversky as a loss function for highly unbalanced image segmentation using 3D fully convolutional deep networks," *CoRR*, vol. abs/1803.11078, 2018.
8. S. Klöppel et al., "Accuracy of dementia diagnosis – A direct comparison between radiologists and a computerized method," *Brain*, vol. 131, no. 11, pp. 2969–2974, 2008.
9. C. Plant et al., "Automated detection of brain atrophy patterns based on MRI for the prediction of Alzheimer's disease," Neuroimage, vol. 50, no. 1, pp. 162–174, 2010.
10. N. Tajbakhsh et al., "Convolutional neural networks for medical image analysis: Full training or fine tuning?" *IEEE Transactions on Medical Imaging*, vol. 35, no. 5, pp. 1299–1312, 2016.
11. J. Yosinski, J. Clune, Y. Bengio, and H. Lipson, "How transferable are features in deep neural networks?" in *Advances in Neural Information Processing Systems*, 2014.
12. O. Russakovsky et al., "Imagenet large scale visual recognition challenge," *International Journal of Computer Vision*, vol. 115, no. 3, pp. 211–252, 2015.
13. K. Simonyan and A. Zisserman, "Very deep convolutional networks for large-scale image recognition," *arXiv preprint arXiv:1409*.1556, 2014.
14. C. Studholme, D. L. Hill, and D. J. Hawkes, "An overlap invariant entropy measure of 3D medical image alignment," Pattern *Recognition*, vol. 32, no. 1, pp. 71–86, 1999.
15. A. Gupta, M. Ayhan, and A. Maida, "Natural image bases to represent neuroimaging data," in *International Conference on Machine Learning*, 2013.

16. Hosseini-Asl et al., "Alzheimer's disease diagnostics by adaptation of 3D convolutional network," in *IEEE International Conference Image Processing*, 2016.
17. S. Sarraf et al., "Deepad: Alzheimer's disease classification via deep convolutional neural networks using MRI and fMRI," *bioRxiv*, p. 070441, 2016.
18. C. H. Sudre et al., "Generalised dice overlap as a deep learning loss function for highly unbalanced segmentations," in *Deep Learning in Medical Image Analysis for Clinical Decision Support*. Springer, 2017, pp. 240–248. https://link.springer.com/chapter/10.1007/978-3-319-67558-9_28
19. O. Ronneberger, P. Fischer, and T. Brox, "U-net: Convolutional networks for biomedical image segmentation," in *International Conference on Medical Image Computing and Computer-Assisted Intervention*. Springer, 2015.
20. O. Oktay et al., "Attention U-net: Learning where to look for the pancreas," *arXiv preprint arXiv*:1804.03999, 2018.
21. K. C. Wong et al., "3D segmentation with exponential logarithmic loss for highly unbalanced object sizes," in *International Conference on Medical Image Computing and Computer-Assisted Intervention*. Springer, 2018.
22. M. H. Yap et al., "Automated breast ultrasound lesions detection using convolutional neural networks," *IEEE Journal of Biomedical and Health Informatics*, vol. 22, no. 4, pp. 1218–1226, 2018.
23. C. Leibig, V. Allken, M. S. Ayhan, P. Berens, and S. Wahl, "Leveraging uncertainty information from deep neural networks for disease detection," *Scientific Reports*, vol. 7, no. 1, pp. 1–14, 2017.
24. A. Krizhevsky, I. Sutskever, and G. E. Hinton, "Imagenet classification with deep convolutional neural networks," in *Advances in Neural Information Processing Systems*, 2012, pp. 1097–1105.
25. K. He, X. Zhang, S. Ren, and J. Sun, "Deep residual learning for image recognition," in *Proceedings of the IEEE Conference on Computer Vision and Pattern Recognition*, 2016, pp. 770–778.
26. M. D. Hoffman, D. M. Blei, C. Wang, and J. Paisley, "Stochastic variational inference," *The Journal of Machine Learning Research*, vol. 14, no. 1, pp. 1303–1347, 2013.
27. K. Clark, et al., "The cancer imaging archive (TCIA): Maintaining and operating a public information repository," Journal of *Digital Imaging*, vol. 26, no. 6, pp. 1045–1057, 2013.

CHAPTER 10

Detection of Abnormal Activities Stemming from Cognitive Decline Using Deep Learning

Damla Arifoglu

University College London

London, United Kingdom

Abdelhamid Bouchachia

Bournemouth University

Poole, United Kingdom

CONTENTS

10.1 INTRODUCTION

In recent years, diseases related to cognitive impairment in ageing persons are treated as a major public health concern all over the world. Alzheimer's Disease International estimated the number of people suffering from dementia worldwide in 2018 to be 50 million and it will increase to 82 million by 2030 [1]. These numbers underline a situation that presents a certain level of criticality.

Ageing persons with cognitive impairment have problems with activities that require memory and cognition [2]. They also have difficulties with speaking, writing, distinguishing objects and executing daily life activities such as cleaning, cooking and so on [3]. Elderly people need special care and help from their caregivers leading to a social, psychological, physical and economic challenge to family members, caregivers and the society as a whole.

Most elderly people prefer to lead an independent life. Studies show that it is better for the health of these people to stay in a self-determined private home environment while ageing [7,8].

Changes in daily life activity (preparing food, showering, walking, sleeping, watching television, going to the toilet, having dinner/lunch/breakfast, cleaning the house and so on) patterns and their occurrence time and frequency are key indicators in determining the cognitive status of elderly people. Assessing the cognitive status of elderly people by tracking their daily life activities in a specially designed smart-home would be very useful for caregivers, medical doctors and clinicians so that early treatment would be possible.

Unfortunately, there exists no data assessing the cognitive abilities of ageing persons. Thus, in this study, we tackle the scarcity of the data demonstrating the abnormal behavior of elderly people by generating data. Moreover, we aim to recognise daily life activities by taking their neighbourhood information into account. The spatio-temporal information of activities and their ordering and frequency are important for understanding the cognitive abilities of elderly people. Thus, we emulate activity recognition and abnormal behavior detection problems as a sequence labelling problem. In the present study, we first model activities as a sequence and then detect the abnormal behavior. The rest of the chapter is presented as follows. Section 10.2 provides an overview of dementia indicators. Section 10.3 summarises the literature work, while Section 10.4 describes the datasets used. Section 10.5 describes the methods used and presents the experiments. Lastly, Section 10.6 concludes the chapter.

10.2 INDICATORS OF DEMENTIA

Although the early detection of cognitive impairment would make early treatment possible, studies indicate that 75% of dementia cases are not noticed [9]. Recent research [10] suggests anomalies in the patterns of daily life activities can be clues to detect such cases at an early stage. Moreover, the best indicators could be detected by monitoring the trends and changes of the activities over time such as problems with sleeping or difficulties completing tasks [11]. As an example, forgetting to have dinner, suffering from insomnia, or going to the toilet frequently are signs of cognitive impairment. Moreover, there can be an abnormality in eating habits (for example, having snacks in the middle of the night), waking up frequently in the middle of the night, or dehydration because of not drinking enough water. Sufferers may also have problems that involve risky situations such as forgetting to turn off the heater, the oven, or the stove [11]. Moreover, elderly people with cognitive decline may suffer from the consequences of confusion (for example, not being able to run the dishwasher or confusing names on a phone book).

10.3 LITERATURE OVERVIEW

In this section, we are going to summarise literature work in two parts, namely cognitive assessment and deep learning studies.

10.3.1 Cognitive Status Assessment

Many different studies attack the problem of home-based assessment of the cognitive status of ageing persons automatically [23–30] and different machine learning methods such as Naïve Bayes classifier and Support Vector Machines (SVMs) [31,32,38], Restricted Boltzmann Machines (RBMs) [28,33], Markov Logic Networks [26,27,29], Hidden Markov Models (HMMs) [12,34], Random Forest methods [19], Hidden Conditional Random Fields (CRFs) [35] and Recurrent Neural Networks (RNNs) [36] have been exploited for this purpose.

Current cognitive assessment methods rely on experts testing the elderly persons' ability to answer questionnaires or recall events from the past. This approach requires expert knowledge, which might be biased. In Ref. [23], elderly people are asked to perform a sequence of activities while they are being monitored via a camera to be given scores. Some other studies such as that of Ref. [37] measure the duration of the activities and the number of sensors activated during the execution to assess the cognitive abilities. These types of assessment methodologies cause a distraction as they are not done in the natural flow of daily life activities. On the other hand, rule-based diagnosis methods require the integration of domain knowledge via specific rules and these rules need to be updated for every person as these rules are specific to individuals. For example, the habits of waking up during the night or drinking water in the night might change from person to person. The advantage of our method over these studies is that it doesn't use any expert or domain knowledge. The normal behavior is learnt from training data. Moreover, the assessment is aimed to be done exploiting the daily life routines of elderly people, and thus it provides an unobtrusive way of assessment.

In Ref. [39], movement segments are defined as activity curves and abnormal activities are detected by comparing these curves. In Ref. [40], a probabilistic spatio-temporal model based on location is used to calculate the likelihood of a subject's behavior. Abnormal behavior such as staying in bed for an unusual time or not sleeping in the bedroom is detected using a cross-entropy measure. In Ref. [12], the HMM and fuzzy rules are combined to detect anomalies related to duration, time and frequency.

In Ref. [35], a Hidden State Conditional Random Field (HCRF) method is used to model activities and then abnormal behavior is detected using a threshold-based method, while in Ref. [26], the Markov Logic network is combined with a rule-based and probabilistic reasoning to detect abnormal behavior. One disadvantage of this study is that the steps of activities are defined before the model is constructed. However, the rules change from resident to resident. Moreover, defining the rules is time consuming. In Ref. [27], these rules are automatically detected using a rule induction method and data of normal and abnormal activities. However, our proposed method learns normal activity patterns from the training set and without applying rules. We define abnormal behavior, not activities alone but in the context of sequential information [26,35].

10.3.2 Deep Learning

In recent years, deep learning methods have been used to tackle activity recognition in smart-homes. These methods include Convolutional Neural Networks (CNNs) [41–50,67–69], Deep Belief Networks (DBN) [33], Restricted Boltzman Machines (RBMs) [28,33,51,52] and RNNs [43,44,53]. While RBMs are preferred for feature extraction and selection [51], they perform better than HMMs and NB on the CASAS dataset [52]. CNNs have been popular to recognise activities using wearable sensors [33,41–43,45,48,51]. However, very few studies [52,67–71] use deep learning methods on sensor-based activity recognition, which needs to be further studied.

Auto-encoders are being used for anomaly detection on time-series data [57,58]. In Ref. [56], the authors use Recursive Auto-Encoders for predicting sentiment distributions. Instead of using a bag-of-words model, this model exploits a hierarchical structure and uses compositional semantics to understand the sentiment. In Ref. [59], the authors extract patterns in daily life activities as segments of an activity. This shows that the extracted movement vector can be used to differentiate high-level activities. The idea behind this is residents at a smart-home follow the same routine during the performance of the same activities such as moving around the kitchen sink while washing the dishes.

10.4 DATASETS AND DATA GENERATION

Elderly people suffering from dementia may have difficulties performing activities such as managing medication, cooking and housekeeping. In this research, we analyse sequential daily life activities (performed in a sequential order without any interruption) to detect the abnormal behavior. We also assume that there is only one occupant living in a smart house. Cooking, sleeping, going to the toilet, working, cleaning, washing dishes and so on are examples of daily life activities. We focus on these types of activities since they are promising to reflect on dementia cases in a scenario of daily life. Inspired by data simulation techniques to generate activity instances [17–19], we generate abnormal behavior.

We will first describe the datasets used and then the abnormal behavior generation method will be presented.

10.4.1 Datasets

In this research, we used three datasets:

- **Van Kastereren [60] dataset**: In this dataset, there are daily life activities such as sleeping, cooking, leaving home and so on and the data were collected in three different households in durations less than a month.
- **Aruba testbed of CASAS [16] dataset**: In this dataset, sensors such as motion, door and temperature are used. However, we use motion and door sensors in our study. In total, there are 11 activities in this dataset and the collection was done in 224 days.
- **WSU testbeds of CASAS [16] dataset**: In this dataset, there are five activities, which are making a phone call, hand washing, meal preparation, eating and cleaning. Twenty instances of each activity were performed by 20 students in (1) adlerror and (2) adlnormal versions. While normal behavior is reflected in the adlnormal version, residents were told to include errors in adlerror to simulate the difficulties of elderly people.

10.4.2 Data Generation

Abnormal behavior in the daily life activities of elderly people is divided into two parts: (1) activity-related anomalies and (2) sub-activity–related anomalies. In activity-related anomalies, an activity itself is totally normal while there is an anomaly related to its frequency or its timing in a day. On the other hand, the sub-activity–related anomaly is related to the context and the quality of activity performed such as frequency of sensor activations involved as well as their order and correlation. In the first one, activities as a whole are repeated or forgotten (e.g. having dinner); while in the second one, some steps (sensor activations) of activities are forgotten or repeated (e.g. adding salt to the dish).

10.4.2.1 Activity-Related Abnormal Behavior

To simulate these types of indicators, we insert a set of actions into the whole day actions of activities (see Algorithm 10.1), which will give multiple instances of the same type of an activity. Moreover, insertion in some inadequate time of the day will generate time-related abnormalities such as waking up and eating. We insert the following activities: preparing meal, eating, working, washing dishes, leaving home and entering home into the normal activity sequences of the Aruba dataset.

Algorithm 10.1: Simulation of Activity-Related Abnormal Behavior

Input: Sequence S of sensor activations in a day such as $S = <s_1, s_2, \ldots, s_n>$ where each s_i is a sensor activation. Likewise, an activity is given as a sequence of sensor readings, a_j: $A = <a_1, a_2, \ldots, a_m>$. Here A, which will be inserted into S, is chosen carefully to reflect a dementia-related abnormal behavior (e.g. nutrition problem).

Output: $S = <s_1, s_2, \ldots, s_l, a_1, a_2, \ldots, a_m, s_{p+1}, \ldots, s_n>$

while true do

Choose a random position p in S;

Insert A into S at position p;

end

In all, we manually generate 77 abnormal activity instances on the Aruba dataset. A set of modified abnormal behavior is depicted in Table 10.1. The following abbreviations are used for the activities. S: Sleeping, P: Meal preparation, E: Eating, R: Respirate, W: Working, B: Bed to the toilet and H: Housekeeping. The inserted activities are shown in bold.

Moreover, abnormal activity instances are generated on dataset A of the Van Kasteren dataset, which has the activities. In all, we manually synthesised 135 abnormal activity slices in this dataset.

10.4.2.2 Sub-Activity–Related Abnormal Behavior

This kind of abnormal behavior is generated by repeating specific sensor activations in a given activity. For this purpose, given random instances of working, eating, meal preparation and walking from bed to the toilet, we randomly insert specific sensors (M_{26}, M_{14}, M_{18} and M_4 respectively) involved in these activities (see Algorithm 10.2). For example, for working

TABLE 10.1 Examples of Abnormal Behavior

Original	**Modified**	**Abnormality**
S-P-E	S-**B**-**S**-P-E	Sleep disorder
S-P-E	S-**R**-**S**-P-E	Sleep disorder
S-P-E	S-**R**-**S**-P-E	Sleep disorder
S-P-E	S-**P**-**S**-P-E	Repetition
S- P-E-H	S-P-E-H-**E**-**E**	Repetition
W: M_{26}, M_{28}, M_{27}	M_{26}, M_{28}, $\mathbf{M_{26}}$, $\mathbf{M_{26}}$, M_{27}	Confusion
B: M_4, M_5, M_7	M_4, M_5, $\mathbf{M_5}$, M_7, $\mathbf{M_5}$	Confusion
W: M_{18}, M_{20}, M_{15}	M_{18}, $\mathbf{M_{15}}$, $\mathbf{M_{15}}$, M_{20}, M_{15}	Confusion
E: M_{14}, M_{19}, M_{18}	M_{14}, $\mathbf{M_{14}}$, $\mathbf{M_{14}}$, M_{19}, M_{18}, $\mathbf{M_{14}}$	Confusion
M: M_{18}, M_{19}, M_{15}	M_{18}, $\mathbf{M_{18}}$, $\mathbf{M_{18}}$, M_{19}, M_{15}, $\mathbf{M_{18}}$	Confusion

```
2011-04-01 08:42:35.982779  M026    ON  Work
2011-04-01 08:42:37.732557  M028    OFF
2011-04-01 08:42:37.732557 M26 ONabn
2011-04-01 08:42:41.771143  M027    ON
2011-04-01 08:42:44.654344  M027    OFF
2011-04-01 08:42:49.308347  M026    OFF
2011-04-01 08:42:49.308347 M26 ONabn
2011-04-01 08:42:49.686528  M026    ON
2011-04-01 08:42:49.686528 M26 ONabn
2011-04-01 08:42:56.781314  M026    OFF
2011-04-01 08:42:56.781314 M26 ONabn
2011-04-01 08:42:59.231909  M026    ON
```

FIGURE 10.1 Sensor data after sub-activity–related abnormal behavior is generated.

activity, the sensor M_{26} is repeated more than usual, which can be used to emulate the usage of a computer. A snapshot for sub-activity–related abnormal behavior synthesis is depicted in Figure 10.1, where ONabn shows the inserted sensor activations.

Moreover, an adlerror set of WSU dataset is used because it reflects the confusion and forgetting anomaly types such as forgetting to turn water tap off.

Algorithm 10.2: Simulation of Sub-Activity–Related Abnormal Behavior

Input: Sequence of S of sensor activations of an activity A such as $S = <a_1, a_2, \ldots, a_n>$. A sensor type M that is involved in activity A. A and M are carefully chosen to reflect a dementia-related abnormal behavior (e.g. sensor M_6 in activity *working*).

Output: $S = <a_1, M, a_2, M, a_3, \ldots, M, a_n>$
while true do
Choose a random position p in S
Insert M into S at position p
end

10.5 SPATIO-TEMPORAL ACTIVITY RECOGNITION AND ABNORMAL BEHAVIOR DETECTION

RNNs have shown promising results in some sequence modeling problems such as speech recognition [61], machine translation [62,63], handwriting recognition and generation or translation, language modeling and protein secondary structure prediction [64]. Daily life activities can be modelled as sequences where sensor activations form time-series data. Thus, modeling activity recognition as a sequence labelling problem makes RNNs an appealing approach. In the present study, we exploit RNNs to model activities using their temporal information and then detect abnormal behavior deviating from normal patterns. Also, CNNs are good at encoding spatial information into account and extracting their own features. Thus, in this research, CNNs are used to encode the neighbourhood information of the sensors to recognise daily life activities and then detect abnormal behavior.

The following steps are applied (1) A sliding-window approach inspired by Ref. [20] is applied to segment daily life sequences into time-slice chunks. (2) Time-slices are mapped onto features as described in Ref. [20]. (3) Then, three variations of RNNs, namely Vanilla, GRU and LSTM and CNNs are used to model and classify activities. (4) Lastly, these classifiers are used to flag abnormal behavior based on the classification confusion probability.

The order of sensor readings is important to take the spatial information into account. We use a sliding window approach to segment data into activity instances. We applied the same sliding window approach as in Ref. [20] to extract the sensor reading chunks, which are used as input to RNNs and CNNs. The window size is based on time rather than the number of sensor events (one sensor reading tuple is named as the sensor event). Different time windows can be used such as 1-minute slices, 60-second slices and so on. If 1-minute windows are used, all sensor readings which are in that minute are extracted in a window. These windows are mapped into specific representations as described in the following.

10.5.1 Sensor Data Representation

Raw sensor readings are mapped to the following three representations using a sliding window.

- **Binary**: In this feature, sensors activated in a time-window are assigned to 1, while the ones not activated are assigned to 0.
- **Change-point:** In this feature, in a time-window, if a sensor changes from ON to OFF, or from OFF to On, it is assigned to 1, while it is assigned to 0 if its state remains the same.
- **Last-fired:** In this feature, only one sensor is assigned to 1, indicating the last sensor which is fired last in a time-window.

10.5.2 Abnormal Behavior Detection

Abnormal behavior is detected as follows: The RNNs and CNNs are trained using the train set and then test instances are fed into these models to be classified. The classification confidence scores are used to decide if the test instances are normal or abnormal activities. For this purpose, a threshold, which is the mean of the confidence scores of training instances for each class, is used to decide the abnormality.

In the next section, the Kasteren dataset will be used to evaluate RNNs and Aruba dataset will be used to test the ability of CNNs as well as their combination with LSTM RNNs.

10.5.3 Experiments

In this study, RNN and CNN implementations from Theano [66] and Keras libraries [65] are used. The train and test instances with a batch size of 20 are used and an Adam optimiser is chosen. RNNs and CNNs are compared with the traditional machine learning methods such as SVM (WEKA implementation with default parameters), NB, HMM, HSMM and CRF (implementations of Ref. [20]).

The evaluation metrics, precision, recall, F-measure and accuracy (see Eqs. 10.1–10.4) are chosen to test the success of the proposed methods on activity recognition. Here, the following abbreviations are used: TP: True Positive, TT: Total True labels, TI: Inferred Labels, N: the number classes in the dataset and Total: total number of instances in the dataset.

$$\text{Precision} = 1/N\left(\sum_{i=1}^{N} TPi/TIi\right) \tag{10.1}$$

$$\text{Recall} = 1/N\left(\sum_{i=1}^{N} TPi/TTi\right) \tag{10.2}$$

$$\text{F-measure} = 2 \times \text{Precision} \times \text{Recall}/(\text{Precision} + \text{Recall}) \tag{10.3}$$

$$\text{Accuracy} = \sum_{i=1}^{N} TPi/\text{Total} \tag{10.4}$$

Sensitivity (True Positive Rate) and Specificity (True Negative Rate) metrics (Eqs. 10.5 and 10.6) are used to evaluate the proposed method's success in abnormal behavior detection. A True Positive Rate (TPR) reflects the ability to detect true abnormal behavior, while a True Negative Rate (TNR) measures the ability to identify normal behavior.

$$\text{Sensitivity} = \text{TP}/(\text{TP} + \text{FN}) \tag{10.5}$$

$$\text{Specificity} = \text{TN}/(\text{TN} + \text{FP}) \tag{10.6}$$

10.5.4 Results with Recurrent Neural Networks

For the RNN experiments, Kasteren datasets are divided into train and test sets following a cross-validation approach on a daily basis so that one day data are used for testing while the remaining days are used for training and validation (10% of them are used for validation). The success rate is reported by averaging over the days. Train data are fed into the classifier using batches of 10 in 500 epochs. The RNN network has two layers of 30 and 50 hidden neurons and each time, 25 time-slices are given as an instance. These parameters are set empirically. The results are compared with HMM, HSMM, CRF and NB results of Ref. [20] as depicted in Tables 10.2–10.4.

TABLE 10.2 Activity Recognition Results for Household A of the Van Kasteren Dataset

Model	Feature	Precision	Recall	F-Measure	Accuracy
NB	Binary	48.3 ± 17.7	42.6 ± 16.6	45.1 ± 16.9	77.1 ± 20.8
	Change-point	52.7 ± 17.5	43.2 ± 18.0	47.1 ± 17.2	55.9 ± 18.8
	Last-fired	67.3 ± 17.2	64.8 ± 14.6	65.8 ± 15.5	95.3 ± 2.8
HMM	Binary	37.9 ± 19.8	45.5 ± 19.5	41.0 ± 19.5	59.1 ± 28.7
	Change-point	70.3 ± 16.0	74.3 ± 13.3	72.0 ± 14.2	92.3 ± 5.8
	Last-fired	54.6 ± 17.0	69.5 ± 12.7	60.8 ± 14.9	89.5 ± 8.4
HSMM	Binary	39.5 ± 18.9	48.5 ± 19.5	43.2 ± 19.1	59.5 ± 29.0
	Change-point	70.5 ± 16.0	75.0 ± 12.1	72.4 ± 13.7	91.8 ± 5.9
	Last-fired	60.2 ± 15.4	73.8 ± 12.5	66.0 ± 13.7	91.0 ± 7.2
CRF	Binary	59.2 ± 18.3	56.1 ± 17.3	57.2 ± 17.3	89.8 ± 8.5
	Change-point	73.5 ± 16.6	68.0 ± 16.0	70.4 ± 15.9	91.4 ± 5.6
	Last-fired	66.2 ± 15.8	65.8 ± 14.0	65.9 ± 14.6	96.4 ± 2.4
Vanilla	Binary	46.5 ± 17.7	64.8 ± 16.2	53.5 ± 16.3	86.8 ± 10.6
	Change-point	46.3 ± 19.5	63.8 ± 16.4	53.2 ± 17.9	61.4 ± 16.4
	Last-fired	61.9 ± 19.1	74.3 ± 12.8	67.2 ± 16.4	95.5 ± 3.4

(*Continued*)

TABLE 10.2 (*Continued*) Activity Recognition Results for Household A of the Van Kasteren Dataset

Model	Feature	Precision	Recall	F-Measure	Accuracy
LSTM	Binary	50.8 ± 18.4	63.9 ± 16.5	56.2 ± 17.1	86.7 ± 10.5
	Change-point	46.8 ± 18.7	63.6 ± 14	53.5 ± 16.7	61.4 ± 16.4
	Last-fired	63.7 ± 19.9	73.9 ± 16.8	68.1 ± 18.2	96.7 ± 2.6
GRU	Binary	47.3 ± 18.7	69.1 ± 14.9	55.4 ± 16.5	86.6 ± 10.7
	Change-point	42.9 ± 19	65.0 ± 15.3	51.0 ± 17.1	61.4 ± 16.4
	Last-fired	61.8 ± 16.3	80.6 ± 11.5	69.5 ± 14.0	96.1 ± 2.5
SVM	Binary	45.6 ± 17.9	69.1 ± 15.9	54.2 ± 15.9	85.4 ± 10.4
	Change-point	40.3 ± 19.1	63.4 ± 14.6	48.6 ± 17.0	55.9 ± 18.7
	Last-fired	58.6 ± 16.2	77.2 ± 14.0	66.3 ± 14.9	96.1 ± 2.4

TABLE 10.3 Activity Recognition Results for Household B of the Van Kasteren Dataset

Model	Feature	Precision	Recall	F-Measure	Accuracy
NB	Binary	33.6 ± 10.9	32.5 ± 8.4	32.4 ± 8.9	80.4 ± 18.9
	Change-point	40.9 ± 7.2	38.9 ± 5.7	39.5 ± 5.9	67.8± 18.6
	Last-fired	43.7 ± 8.7	44.6 ± 7.2	43.3 ± 4.8	86.2 ± 13.8
HMM	Binary	38.8 ± 14.7	44.7 ± 13.4	40.7 ± 12.4	63.2 ± 24.7
	Change-point	48.2 ± 17.2	63.1 ± 14.1	53.6 ± 16.5	81.0 ± 14.2
	Last-fired	38.5 ± 15.8	46.6 ± 19.5	41.8 ± 17.1	48.4± 26.9
HSMM	Binary	37.4 ± 16.9	44.6 ± 14.3	39.9 ± 14.3	63.8± 24.2
	Change-point	49.8 ± 15.8	65.2 ± 13.4	55.7 ± 14.6	82.3 ± 13.5
	Last-fired	40.8 ± 11.6	53.3 ± 10.9	45.8 ± 11.2	67.1 ± 24.8
CRF	Binary	35.7 ± 15.2	40.6 ± 12.0	37.5 ± 13.7	78.0 ± 25.9
	Change-point	48.3 ± 8.3	51.5 ± 8.5	49.7 ± 7.9	92.9 ± 6.2
	Last-fired	46.9 ± 12.5	47.8 ± 12.1	46.6 ± 12.9	89.2 ± 13.9
Vanilla	Binary	26.7 ± 13.5	46.9 ± 24.8	32.5 ± 17.9	65.2 ± 34.7
	Change-point	39.6 ± 8	62.4± 15.3	48.3± 10.2	76.9± 13.9
	Last-fired	41.2 ± 12.3	64.4 ± 17.8	49.7 ± 13.6	87.9 ± 13.1
LSTM	Binary	29.1 ± 12.0	44.0 ± 22.0	33.9 ± 16.2	63.5 ± 32.7
	Change-point	40.0 ± 11.2	59.0 ± 16.4	47.5 ± 12.9	76.8± 14.2
	Last-fired	40.8 ± 10.7	60.1 1 16.3	48.2 ± 12.3	87.2 ± 13.2
GRU	Binary	28.5 ± 15.9	36.3 ± 17.2	31.4 ± 16.2	64.5 ± 32.1
	Change-point	37.7 ± 7.6	53.5 ± 9.2	44.9 ± 7.1	76.4 ± 11.5
	Last-fired	41.7 ± 13.2	50.9 ± 17.9	47.5 ± 14.6	87.0 ± 12.9
SVM	Binary	39.6± 10.9	58.5± 17.4	46.7± 12.9	81.6 ± 18.5
	Change-point	32.3 ± 6.5	53.6 ± 7.5	40.0 ± 6.2	67.9± 28.5
	Last-fired	36.4 ± 5.4	54.0 ± 10.4	43.5 ± 6.6	86.2 ± 14.9

TABLE 10.4 Activity Recognition Results for Household C of the Van Kasteren dataset.

Model	Feature	Precision	Recall	F-Measure	Accuracy
NH	Binary	19.61 ± 11.4	16.8 ± 7.5	17.8 ± 9.1	46.5 ± 22.6
	Change-point	39.9 ± 6.9	30.8 ± 4.8	34.5 ± 4.6	57.6 ± 15.4
	Last-fired	40.5 ± 7.4	46.4 ± 14.8	42.3 ± 6.8	87.0 ± 12.2
HMM	Binary	15.2 ± 9.2	17.2 ± 9.3	15.7± 8.8	26.5 ± 22.7
	Change-point	41.4 ± 8.8	50.0 ± 11.4	44.9 ± 8.8	77.2 ± 14.6
	Last-fired	40.7 ± 9.7	53.7 ± 16.2	45.9 ± 11.2	83.9 ± 13.9
HSMM	Binary	15.6 ± 9.2	20.4 ± 10.9	17.3 ± 9.6	31.2 ± 24.6
	Change-point	43.8 ± 10.0	52.3 ± 12.8	47.4 ± 10.5	77.5 ± 15.3
	Last-fired	42.5 ± 10.8	56.0 ± 15.4	47.9 ± 11.3	84.5 ± 13.2
CRF	Binary	17.8 ± 22.1	I 21.8 ± 20.9	19.0 ± 21.8	46.3 ± 25.5'
	Change-point	36.7 ± 18.0	39.6 ± 17.4	38.0 ± 17.6	82.2 ± 13.9
	Last-fired	37.7 ± 17.1	40.41 ± 16.0	38.9 ± 16.5	89.7 ± 8.4
Vanilla	Binary	15.4 ± 5.3	43.1 ± 18.1	22.2 ± 7.3	50.2 ± 22.4
	Change-point	31.3 ± 7.1	54.9 ± 11.3	39.5 ± 8.3	72.2 ± 13.0
	Last-fired	38.3± 16.3	59.6± 15.1	45.8± 14.8	86.7± 12.5
LSTM	Binary	16.8± 6.2	34.8 ± 12.5	22.1 ± 7.4	45.3 ± 21.2
	Change-point	31.0 ± 5.1	53.3 ± 6.5	38.9 ± 5.0	72.0 ± 13.0
	Last-fired	41.3 ± 17.2	57.3 ± 15.9	47.5 ± 16.1	87.4 ± 12.4
CRU	Binary	18.7 ± 8.3	33.2 ± 12.7	23.9 ± 9.6	46.7 ± 23.4
	Change-point	31.2 ± 8.3	47. ± 10.9	31.2 ± 8.5	71.6 ± 12.6
	Last-fired	40.4 ± 16.5	52.7 ± 16.4	45.4 ± 16.9	86.6 ± 12.3
SVM	Binary	19.4 ± 9.0	35.2 ± 12.7	24.0 ± 9.2	37.4 ± 19.0
	Change-point	25.6 ± 6.2	51.4 ± 9.5	34.0 ± 7.2	57.8 ± 15.5
	Last-fired	37.0 ± 7.9	55.5 ± 11.6	44.1 ± 8.5	87.5 ± 12.1

The results on dataset A as depicted in Table 10.2 present that the results with feature representation are mixed and there is not a clear best one. With an accuracy of 96.7%, LSTM is the best method with the last-fired feature and HMM is the worst one, while with a change-point feature, HMM is the best performing method. CRF gives the best accuracy (89.8%) when a binary feature is used, whereas RNNs, NB and SVM do not perform well with change-point representation and HMM and HSMM perform bad with a binary feature. In a nutshell, for the majority of the methods, except HMM and HSMM, last-fired representation is the best one. In terms of recall which reflects better on performance in the presence of imbalanced data, the highest value is obtained by GRU (80.6%). This means that RNNs are good at finding relevant class instances. CRF performs higher precision since it favours the most frequent-class instances while it is not good enough to detect infrequent classes. In general, RNNs outperform better than HMM, NB and HSMM for most of the cases, while CRF is slightly better than these recurrent architectures on dataset A.

Table 10.3 refers to the results obtained on the dataset best method when adopting a binary representation achieving an accuracy of 81.6%. On the other hand, CRF is the best when using the change-point feature and last-fired representations with accuracies of 92.9% and 89.2% respectively. It can be noted that HMM is not as good as the other methods achieving the best case 81.0% with the change-point representation. The closest successful model to CRF is Vanilla RNN and again overall RNNs deliver high recall rates compared to the other methods. Change-point and last-fired representations give the highest recall results except for CRF.

Table 10.4 reports the results on dataset C showing that CRF performs best for change-point and binary representations obtaining 82.2% and 89.7% respectively. Overall, none of the methods performs well when adopting a binary representation. The results are slightly better with change-point but clearly better when applying the last-fired representation. RNNs again give the highest recall values for all representations. Overall, the results show that RNNs perform better than HMM, NB and HSMM in all cases, while CRF is slightly better than RNNs. But in terms of recall, RNNs outperform all methods for all feature representations. The reason behind this is that RNNs perform better for imbalanced data compared to CRF. RNN variants generally perform equally well.

Abnormal activity recognition is tested with LSTM since it is the most promising one and it is compared against NB, HSMM, HMM, SVM and CRF (Table 10.5). We used only the last-fired feature in this experiment. The results indicate that LSTM is the best to prune false negatives compared to the other methods. Methods like NB and One-class SVM, which do not capture the data order, perform the worst. The models ignore the frequency of the activity, but apply the temporal and

TABLE 10.5 Abnormal Activity Detection Results for the Synthetic Dataset

Model	Sensitivity (TPR) (%)	Specificity (TNR) (%)
NB	40.40	56.50
HMM	58.36	3.80
HSMM	68.85	67.8
CRF	66.22	59.45
One-class SVM	72.11	66
LSTM	91.43	59.04

contextual information to make decisions. Results show that LSTM is capable of encoding the order of activities. Hence, when an activity is introduced in a different context or in a different order, LSTM can detect such anomalies.

10.5.5 Results with Convolutional Neural Networks

Given the $N \times M$ input matrix where N is the time-window and M is the number of sensor readings, different network architectures as shown in Figure 10.2 have been tested on the Aruba dataset.

1D Convolution: Convolution is applied on one only dimension as seen in Figure 10.2a, where 100 filters (length of 10) are applied to the temporal dimension. Then a max-pooling layer (stride = 2) and another convolutional layer of 50 filters (length = 5) with a max-pooling layer are added. A flattened layer is added to flatten the features, and then three dense layers with hidden neurons of 512, 128 and 50 are added. Lastly, a soft-max layer is added to produce confidence values to class labels.

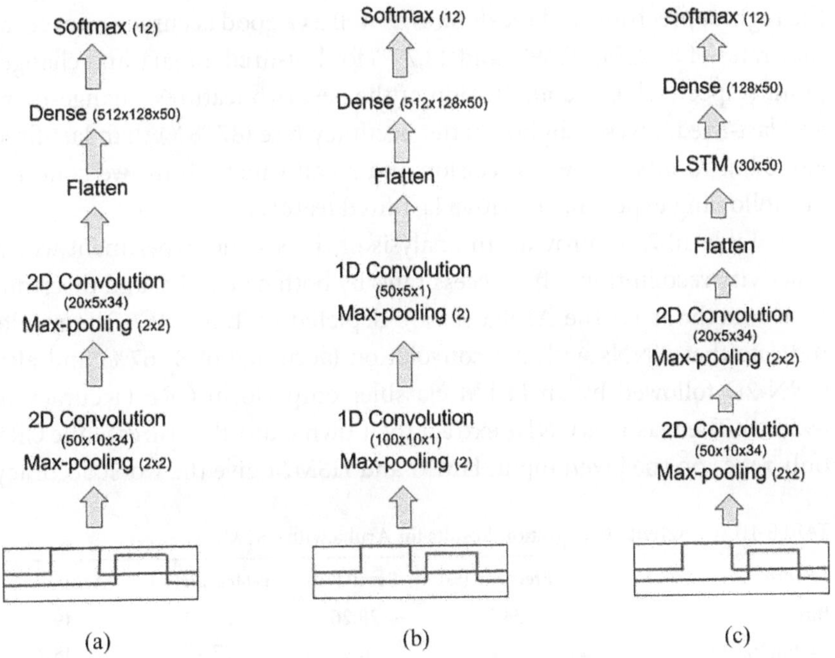

FIGURE 10.2 a) 1D CNN network b) 2D CNN network c) 2D CNN and LSTM network.

2D Convolution: Convolution is applied on both dimensions as seen in Figure 10.2b, where 100 filters (size of 10 × 34) are followed by a max-pooling (2 × 2) layer. The second convolution layer is added (with 20 filters of the size of 5 × 34) and followed by a flattened layer and a soft-max.

CNN and LSTM (2D CNN + LSTM): Because CNNs don't have the ability to encode temporal history, they are combined with LSTM, where the two-layer 2D-CNN mentioned above is merged with two LSTM layers (hidden layers of size 30 × 50). This is followed by two dense layers (128 and 50 hidden units) and a soft-max layer for classification.

Following Ref. [24], the Aruba dataset is divided into train and test sets based on a day in order not to lose the temporal information. For training, 150 days of the Aruba dataset are used, while 15 days are used for validation and the other days are used for testing. The adlnormal set of WSU is used for training while the adlerror version is used for testing.

The first experiment was performed on Aruba to choose the best input representation that gives the highest recognition results. This experiment is performed with the LSTM classifier on 1-minute time slices of sensor readings. Extracted slices are mapped into binary, change-point and last-fired representations. As seen in Table 10.6, last-fired representation gives the highest precision and recall rates as well as a good accuracy rate (accuracy rates of 87.72%, 49.69% and 48.79% for last-fired, binary and change-point respectively). A combination of the best two features: change-point and last-fired, gives a slightly better accuracy rate (87.78%) than last-fired alone but results in lower precision and recall values. Thus, we continue our following experiments with a last-fired feature.

In Table 10.7, we provide an analysis of the second experiment which is activity recognition. The success rates by both generative and discriminative methods on the Aruba set are depicted in Table 10.7. The results indicate that CNNs with 2D convolution (accuracy of 89.67%) and also CNN-2D followed by an LSTM classifier outperform CRF (accuracy of 89.72%). The reason is CNNs extract their own fruitful features while CRF only relies on the given input. HMM and HSMM give the worst accuracy

TABLE 10.6 Activity Recognition Results for Aruba with LSTM

Feature	Precision (%)	Recall (%)	F-Measure(%)	Accuracy(%)
Binary	34.21	28.26	30.95	49.69
Change-point	29.28	26.41	27.77	48.79
Last-fired	43.18	43.37	43.27	87.72
Change-point + Last-fired	37.33	42.42	39.71	87.78

TABLE 10.7 Activity Recognition Results on the Aruba Dataset

Model	Precision (%)	Recall	F-Measure (%)	Accuracy (%)
NB	42.87	61.04%	50.36	84.37
HMM	43.66	72.03%	54.36	77.90
HSMM	43.97	71.56%	54.47	77.98
CRF	50.24	52.83%	51.50	88.58
LSTM	38.65	41.29%	39.92	89.00
CNN-1D	31.42	36.78%	33.89	87.50
CNN-2D	46.84	41.68%	44.11	89.67
CNN-2D + LSTM	51.20	50.55%	50.87	89.72

results (77.90% and 77.98% respectively). NB gives a better accuracy result (84.37%) than HMM and HSMM but it results in lower precision (42.87%) and recall (61.04%) rates. Although HMM and HSMM give the best recall rates (72.03% and 71.56%), they fail in giving good precision rates (43.66% and 43.97% respectively). We see that the CNN-1D network has an accuracy of 87.50% while it fails in high precision (31.42%) and recall (36.78%) values. CNN-1D extracts features on temporal dimension, it takes temporal information within a time-slice chunk into account but on the other hand, it ignores the relationship between sensors since it doesn't do convolution on the feature dimension. Thus, it doesn't learn class-specific feature maps to differentiate between different classes resulting in high accuracy (87.50%) but low precision and recall. When 2D convolution is used, both temporal information and spatial information are considered and the networks learn more informative features. Thus, it gains the ability to learn class-specific features, which results in higher precision and recall values (46.84% and 41.68%) and high accuracy results (89.67%). CNNs cannot remember the previous and the next inputs, but feeding the feature maps into an LSTM layer helps us process the temporal dimension further. As a result, CNN-2D + LSTM networks achieve a precision rate of 51.20%, a recall rate of 50.55% and an accuracy of 89.72%.

The learnt feature patterns are depicted in Figure 10.3. As the features are going to the next layers, it is seen that noise is reduced and features become clearer. The feature dimension is shown on the x-axis and the time axis is depicted on the y-axis while the white pixels show the activations.

Results on the Aruba dataset show that classifiers most successfully detect the instances of leave home and enter home activities since they are the only activities involving door sensors, thus they are not confused with any other activities. Moreover, meal preparation activity is confused with

(a) First layer activations.

(b) Second layer activations.

(c) Flatten layer activations.

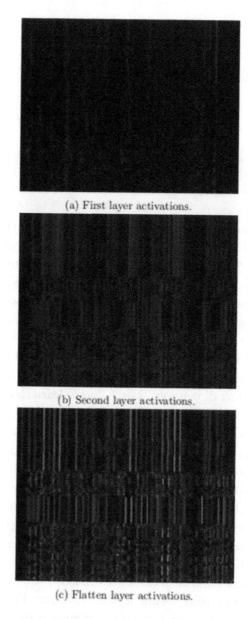

FIGURE 10.3 a) First layer activations b) Second layer activations c) Flatten layer activations.

wash dishes activity most of the time since they involve the same kind of sensors and they both take place in the kitchen. Also, housekeeping activity is generally confused with work activity since they may take place in the same room and may involve the same sensors.

TABLE 10.8 Abnormal Behavior Detection Results on the Modified Aruba Dataset

	Aruba Modified		WSU	
Model	Sensitivity (%)	Specificity (%)	Sensitivity (%)	Specificity (%)
NB	99.33	33.89	46.17	98.42
HMM	45.54	27.71	100	50.55
HSMM	100	35.61	100	42.89
CRF	100	66.03	47.87	72.17
LSTM	98.67	75.48	86.50	77.89
CNN -2D	85.33	33.89	88.70	67.46

In the third experiment, abnormal activity detection is performed firstly on a modified Aruba set. As a representative of CNN networks, we present the result only with the CNN-2D network in order to see the effect of CNNs individually. After training the models with normal behavior, a test set that included abnormal behavior is introduced to the classifier and activity instances that are assigned a label with low confidence values are flagged as abnormal. In Table 10.8, we see that the highest specificity is achieved by LSTM networks giving an accuracy of 75.48% (and a sensitivity rate of 98.67%). Although NB, HMM and HSMM models give higher sensitivity rates (99.33%, 100% and 100% respectively), the specificity rates are smaller (33.89%, 27.71% and 35.61% respectively). HMM gives the worst results (a sensitivity rate of 45.54% and a specificity rate of 27.72%). CNN-2D gives a sensitivity rate of 85.33% and a specificity of 33.89%. This shows that LSTMs are more suitable to detect repetition and order-related abnormal activities since they can relate current input with the upcoming ones what CNN cannot do.

The second part of anomaly detection experiments is performed on the WSU testbed. We extracted 30-second time-slice chunks from sensor readings from WSU. This dataset is not collected in a daily life scenario; thus, sensor readings are not in a sequential order. The sensor readings are available only for activities labelled in the dataset. The adlnormal set is used as a training set and the adlerror set is used as a test dataset. The aim here is to measure how successful the classifiers are to detect the anomalies given the normal dataset. The results in Table 10.8 indicate that the highest sensitivity rate is given by HMM and HSMM (both 100%), while HMM gives a specificity rate of 50.55% and HSMM achieves a specificity of 42.89%. The highest sensitivity rate is achieved by the CNN-2D classifier (86.70%), but LSTM gives a very close sensitivity rate (86.50%) and a higher specificity rate (77.89%) where CNN-2D achieves a specificity rate of 67.47% only. In Ref. [17], the authors present their results as follows. The number of correctly detected activities are 95 for adlnormal and 76 for adlerror, both out of 100 activity instances. We perform experiments on activity slices, on the other hand, they take the whole activity and extract features from that activity and then try to decide if it is normal or abnormal. The problem here is that in a real-life scenario, we cannot know, where an activity starts and ends. Thus, using slice-based detection is more meaningful.

While repetition-related abnormal behavior is detected better by LSTM, abnormal activities stemming from confusion is recognised better by CNN because of its ability to detect variances in feature patterns. The activation order and the relationship between the sensors form steps of activities. When we think about the activity of going to the toilet, it is observed that a person first goes out of bed, walks through the bedroom and then goes to the toilet. As CNN exploits the spatial neighbourhood of the features, it can model this kind of patterns.

The combination of RNNs and CNNs performs the best results since they encode both temporal and spatial information coming from the sensors. However, they fail to understand the intrinsic structure of activities. Thus, we need hierarchical models to understand the sub-activities and their relationships in a given activity and relate them to cognitive decline related to abnormal behavior.

10.6 CONCLUSIONS AND FUTURE WORK

10.6.1 Conclusion

The main goal of this study was to detect abnormal behavior of ageing persons with dementia in the daily routines. Elderly people suffering from dementia tend to confuse things or repeat and skip certain activities in their daily life patterns. Firstly, a method was proposed to synthesise abnormal behavior stemming from dementia. For this purpose, two types of abnormal behavior were generated, which are activity- and sub-activity–related anomalies. Secondly, deep learning methods such as RNNs and CNNs were exploited to detect abnormal behavior. Thirdly, we compared these methods with the traditional machine learning methods such as HMMs, CRFs, Support Vector Machines and Naïve Bayes methods. The results show that the proposed methods are competitive with the state-of-the-art machine learning methods.

First of all, given the scarcity of real-world data available, we proposed a method to manually synthesise abnormal activities to mimic the activity routines of ageing persons. We modified some instances of datasets already available in the literature. The modification was done through injection of abnormal activities in normal daily life activity sequences. We specifically aimed to simulate repetition, sleep disorder and confusion types of abnormal behavior. Repetition and sleep disorder-related abnormal behavior occur at the activity level while confusion-related abnormal behavior occurs at the sub-activity level of activities. However, generating abnormal behavior in this method may fail to reflect user-specific abnormal behavior since people show different habits at different times.

Secondly, the activity recognition problem was emulated as a sequence labelling problem where time-series data of sensor measurements were treated as a sequence. Then, daily life patterns were modelled exploiting RNNs and their variants, namely Long Short Term Memory, Gated Recurrent Units and Vanilla versions, and CNNs. Results with RNNs and CNNs showed that capturing the activity instances and their temporal and spatial relationship was helpful to understand the daily life patterns and their relationships with other activities. With RNNs, we were able to encode the temporal information in daily life in order to model personal environments for dementia support. With CNNs, we tried to extract meaningful and fruitful patterns in the activities and with the help of these patterns, activities were recognised and anomalies were detected. These models were good at detecting anomalies related to repetition of activities and sleep disturbances. However, they are not capable enough to detect anomalies related to confusion since they cannot model sub-activities in an activity. RNNs and CNNs cannot model daily activities at the granular-level, so they cannot understand which sub-activities in these activities are forgotten, repeated and confused. Modeling these sub-activities would give a better understanding of activity recognition.

10.6.2 Future Work

One possible extension of this research would be to take the OFF status of the sensors into account and investigate their impact to detect anomalies. Also, specific features or rules can be considered to understand if a sensor (e.g. item sensors representing medicine or a fridge door sensor to check if it closed or not) is left OFF or not. New features to represent sensor events could be proposed to cover more different types of abnormal behavior (such as forgetting the location of objects at home and confusing how to use kitchen utilities) of the cognitive status of the elderly.

When the disease is progressing slowly, our proposed method might fail to adapt and detect the abnormal behavior. Thus, real-world data can be collected in which gradual deterioration is observed. Moreover, different types of abnormal behavior reflecting dementia-specific habits can be considered. If no real-world data can be collected, simulation methods to artificially generate these kinds of behavior can be proposed.

BIBLIOGRAPHY

1. C. Patterson. The state of the art of dementia research: New frontiers 2018. Tech. rep. Alzheimer's Disease International (ADI), 2018.
2. M. S. Albert et al. "The diagnosis of mild cognitive impairment due to Alzheimer's disease: Recommendations from the National Institute on Aging". In: *Alzheimer's & Dementia* vol. 7, no. 3 (2011), pp. 270–279. doi: 10.1007/ s00406-012-0349-0.
3. W. Thies and L. Bleiler. "2013 Alzheimer's disease facts and figures". In: *Alzheimer's & Dementia: the Journal of the Alzheimer's Association* vol. 9, no. 2 (2013), pp. 208–245.
4. Office for National Statistics. Overview of the UK population: March (2017).
5. Alzhemier. Alzheimer's disease (2017). url: www.alz.org (visited on 08/04/2017).
6. M. Amiribesheli and A. Bouchachia. "Smart homes design for people with dementia". In: *2015 International Conference on Intelligent Environments* (2015), pp. 156–159. doi: 10.1109/IE.2015.33.
7. M. P. Cutchin. "The process of mediated aging-in-place: A theoretically and empirically based model". In: *Social Science and Medicine* vol. 57, no. 6 (2003), pp. 1077–1090. doi: 10.1016/S0277-9536(02)00486-0.
8. A. Wimo, B. Winblad, and L. Jonsson. "The worldwide societal costs of dementia: Estimates for 2009". In: *Alzheimer's & Dementia* vol. 6, no. 2 (2010), pp. 98–103.
9. M. R. Hodges et al. "Automatic assessment of cognitive impairment through electronic observation of object usage". In: *Pervasive Computing.* Berlin, Heidelberg: Springer Berlin Heidelberg (2010), pp. 192–209.
10. K. Wild. "Aging changes". In: *Geraotechnology* vol. 9, no. 2 (2010), pp. 121–125.
11. M. Amiribesheli, A. Benmansour, and A. Bouchachia. "A review of smart homes in healthcare". In: *Journal of Ambient Intelligence and Humanized Computing* vol. 6, no. 4 (2015), pp. 495–517. doi: 10.1007/s12652-015-0270-2.
12. A. R. M. Forkan et al. "A context-aware approach for long- term behavioural change detection and abnormality prediction in ambient assisted living". In: *Pattern Recognition* vol. 48, no. 3 (2015), pp. 628–641. doi: 10.1016/j.patcog.2014.07.007.
13. J. Lundstro zm, E. J'arpe, and A. Verikas. "Detecting and exploring deviating behaviour of smart home residents". In: *Expert Systems with Applications* vol. 55 (2016), pp. 429–440. doi: 10.1016/j.eswa. 2016.02.030. url: http://www.sciencedirect.com/science/article/ pii/S0957417416300616.
14. D. J. Patterson et al. "Fine-grained activity recognition by aggregating abstract object usage". In: *Ninth IEEE International Symposium on Wearable Computers (ISWC'05)* (2005), pp. 44–51. doi: 10.1109/ISWC.2005.22.

15. H. L Chieu, W. S. Lee, and L. P Kaelbling. "Activity recognition from physiological data using conditional random fields". In: *SMA Symposium*. Singapore- MIT Alliance (2006).
16. T. van Kasteren et al. "Accurate activity recognition in a home setting". In: *Proceedings of the 10th International Conference on Ubiquitous Computing*. UbiComp '08 (2008), pp. 1–9. doi: 10.1145/1409635.1409637. url: http: //doi.acm.org/10.1145/1409635.1409637.
17. G. Virone. "Assessing everyday life behavioural rhythms for the older generation". In: *Pervasive and Mobile Computing* vol. 5, no. 5 (2009), pp. 606–622. doi: 10.1016/j.pmcj.2009.06.008.
18. A. R. M. Forkan et al. "A context-aware approach for long- term behavioural change detection and abnormality prediction in ambient assisted living". In: *Pattern Recognition* vol. 48, no. 3 (2015), pp. 628–641. doi: 10.1016/j.patcog.2014.07.007.
19. J. Lundströ̈m, E. J̈arpe, and A. Verikas. "Detecting and exploring deviating behaviour of smart home residents". In: *Expert Systems with Applications* vol. 55 (2016), pp. 429–440. doi: 10.1016/j.eswa. 2016.02.030. url: http://www.sciencedirect.com/science/article/ pii/S0957417416300616.
20. T. Van Kasteren, G. Englebienne, and B. J. A. Krose. "Human activity recognition from wireless sensor network data: Benchmark and software". In: *Activity Recognition in Pervasive Intelligent Environments* (2011), pp. 165–186. doi: 10.2991/978-94-91216-05-3_8.
21. N. Twomey et al. "Unsupervised learning of sensor topologies for improving activity recognition in smart environments". In: *Neurocomputing* vol. 234.C (Apr. 2017), pp. 93–106. ISSN: 0925-2312. doi: 10.1016/j.neucom.2016.12.049. url: https://doi.org/10.1016/j.neucom.2016.12.049.
22. S. S. Akter and L. B. Holder. "Activity recognition using graphical features". In: *2014 13th International Conference on Machine Learning and Applications*. Springer International Publishing (2014), pp. 165–170.
23. M. Seelye Adriana, M. Schmitter-Edgecombe, A. Crandall, and D. J. Cook. "Naturalistic assessment of everyday activities and prompting technologies in mild cognitive impairment". In: *Journal of the International Neuropsychological Society* vol. 2013, no. 4 (2013), pp. 442–452. doi: 10.1017/S135561771200149X.
24. N. K. Suryadevara et al. "Forecasting the behavior of an elderly using wireless sensors data in a smart home". In: *Engineering Applications of Artificial Intelligence* vol. 26, no. 10 (2013), pp. 2641–2652. doi: 10.1016/j.engappai.2013.08.004.
25. P. Dawadi, D. J. Cook, and M. Schmitter-Edgecombe. "Smart home-based longitudinal functional assessment". In: *Proceedings of the 2014 ACM International Joint Conference on Pervasive and Ubiquitous Computing: Adjunct Publication*. UbiComp '14 Adjunct. New York, NY: ACM (2014), pp. 1217–1224. doi: 10.1145/2638728.2638813. url: http://doi.acm.org/10.1145/2638728.2638813.

26. D. Riboni et al. "Fine-grained recognition of abnormal behaviors for early detection of mild cognitive impairment". In: *2015 IEEE International Conference on Pervasive Computing and Communications (PerCom)* (2015), pp. 149–154. doi: 10.1109/PERCOM.2015.7146521.
27. Z. H. Janjua, D. Riboni, and C. Bettini. "Towards automatic induction of abnormal behavioral patterns for recognizing mild cognitive impairment". In: *Proceedings of the 31st Annual ACM Symposium on Applied Computing* (2016), pp. 143–148.
28. N. Hammerla et al. *PD Disease State Assessment in Naturalistic Environments Using Deep Learning.* AAAI Press (2015), pp. 1742–1748. url: http://dl. acm. org/citation.cfm?id=2886521.2886562.
29. K. S. Gayathri, S. Elias, and B. Ravindran. "Hierarchical activity recognition for dementia care using Markov Logic Network". In: *Personal and Ubiquitous Computing* vol. 19, no. 2 (2015), pp. 271–285. doi: 10.1007/s00779-014-0827-7. url: https://doi.org/10.1007/s00779-014-0827–7.
30. Vi Jakkula and D. Cook. "Detecting anomalous sensor events in smart home data for enhancing the living experience". In: *Proceedings of the 7th AAAI Conference on Artificial Intelligence and Smarter Living: The Conquest of Complexity* (2011), pp. 33–37.
31. F. J. Ordóñez, P. de Toledo, and A. Sanchis. "Sensor-based Bayesian detection of anomalous living patterns in a home setting". In: *Personal and Ubiquitous Computing* vol. 19, no. 2 (2015), pp. 259–270. doi: 10.1007/s00779-014-0820-1. url: https://doi.org/10.1007/s00779-014-0820–1.
32. M. Cook and D. J. Schmitter-Edgecombe. "Assessing the quality of activities in a smart environment". In: *Methods of Information in Medicine* vol. 48 (2009), pp. 480–485. doi: 10.3414/ME0592.
33. S. Choi, E. Kim, and S. Oh. "Human behavior prediction for smart homes using deep learning". In: *2013 IEEE RO-MAN* (2013), pp. 173–179. doi: 10.1109/ ROMAN.2013.6628440.
34. W. Kang, D. Shin, and D. Shin. "Detecting and predicting of abnormal behavior using hierarchical Markov model in smart home network". In: *2010 IEEE 17th International Conference on Industrial Engineering and Engineering Management* (2010), pp. 410–414. doi: 10.1109/ICIEEM.2010. 5646583.
35. Y. Tong, R. Chen, and J. Gao. "Hidden state conditional random field for abnormal activity recognition in smart homes". In: *Entropy* vol. 17.3 (2015), p. 1358. doi: 10.3390/e17031358.
36. A. Lotfi et al. "Smart homes for the elderly dementia sufferers: Identification and prediction of abnormal behaviour". In: *Journal of Ambient Intelligence and Humanized Computing* vol. 3, no. 3 (2012), pp. 205–218. doi: 10.1007/s12652-010-0043-x. url: https://doi.org/10.1007/s12652-010-0043–x.
37. P. N. Dawadi, D. J. Cook, and M. Schmitter-Edgecombe. "Automated cognitive health assessment using smart home monitoring of complex tasks". In: *IEEE Transactions on Systems, Man, and Cybernetics: Systems* vol. 43, no. 6 (2013), pp. 1302–1313. ISSN: 2168-2216. doi: 10.1109/TSMC.2013.2252338.

38. P. Dawadi et al. "An approach to cognitive assessment in smart home". In: *Proceedings of the 2011 Workshop on Data Mining for Medicine and Health-care*. DMMH '11. San Diego, CA: ACM (2011), pp. 56–59. ISBN: 978-1-4503-0843-4. doi: 10.1145/2023582.2023592. url: http://doi.acm.org/10.1145/2023582.2023592.
39. P. N. Dawadi, D. J. Cook, and M. Schmitter-Edgecombe. "Modeling patterns of activities using activity curves". In: *Pervasive and Mobile Computing* vol. 28 (June 2016), pp. 51–68. doi: 10.1016/j.pmcj.2015. 09.007.
40. O. Aran et al. "Anomaly detection in elderly daily behaviour in ambient sensing environments". In: *Human Behaviour Understanding: 7th International Workshop* (2016). Ed. by M. Chetouani, J. Cohn, and A. Ali Salah, pp. 51–67.
41. J. Yang et al. "Deep convolutional neural networks on multichannel time series for human activity recognition" (2015), pp. 3995–4001.
42. M. Zeng et al. "Convolutional neural networks for human activity recognition using mobile sensors". In: *6th International Conference on Mobile Computing, Applications and Services* (2014), pp. 197–205. doi: 10.4108/icst.mobicase. 2014.257786.
43. F. J. Ordonez and D. Roggen. "Deep convolutional and LSTM recurrent neural networks for multimodal wearable activity recognition". In: *Sensors* vol. 16, no. 1 (2016), p. 115. doi: 10.3390/s16010115.
44. N. Y. Hammerla, S. Halloran, and T. Pl¨otz. "Deep, convolutional, and recurrent models for human activity recognition using wearables". In: *Proceedings of the Twenty-Fifth International Joint Conference on Artificial Intelligence*. IJCAI'16. AAAI Press (2016), pp. 1533–1540. url: http://dl. acm.org/citation.cfm?id=3060832.3060835.
45. S. Ha and S. Choi. "Convolutional neural networks for human activity recognition using multiple accelerometer and gyroscope sensors". In: *2016 International Joint Conference on Neural Networks (IJCNN)* (2016), pp. 381–388. doi: 10.1109/IJCNN.2016.7727224.
46. C. A. Ronao and S.-B. Cho. "Human activity recognition with smartphone sensors using deep learning neural networks". In: *Expert Systems with Applications* vol. 59 (2016), pp. 235–244. ISSN: 0957-4174. doi: 10.1016/j.eswa.2016.04.032. url: http://www.sciencedirect.com/ science/article/pii/S0957417416302056.
47. R. Yao et al. "Efficient dense labeling of human activity sequences from wearables using fully convolutional networks". In: *CoRR abs/1702.06212* (2017). doi: 10.1016/j.patcog.2017.12.024. url: http: //www.sciencedirect.com/science/article/pii/S0031320317305204.
48. A. Charissa and C. Sung-Bae. "Evaluation of deep convolutional neural network architectures for human activity recognition with smartphone sensors". In: *Proceedings of the KIISE Korea Computer Congress* (2015), pp. 858–860.
49. N. M. Rad et al. "Convolutional neural network for stereo- typical motor movement detection in autism". In: CoRR abs/1511.01865 (2015).

50. K. Wang et al. “Research on healthy anomaly detection model based on deep learning from multiple time-series physiological signals”. In: *Scientific Programming* (2016). doi: 10.1155/2016/5642856.
51. T. Plotz, N. Hammerla, and P. Olivier. “Feature learning for activity recognition in ubiquitous computing”. In: *Proceedings of the 22th International Joint Conference on Artificial Intelligence* vol. 2 (2011), pp. 1729–1734.
52. H. Fang and C. Hu. “Recognizing human activity in smart home using deep learning algorithm”. In: *33rd Chinese Control Conference* (2014), pp. 4716–4720. doi: 10.1109/ChiCC.2014.6895735.
53. H. Fang, H. Si, and L. Chen. “Recurrent neural network for human activity recognition in smart home”. In: *Proceedings of 2013 Chinese Intelligent Automation Conference* (2013). Ed. by Z. Sun and Z. Deng, pp. 341–348.
54. D. Arifoglu, H. Nait-Charif, and A. Bouchachia, “Detecting Indicators of cognitive impairment via Graph Convolutional Networks”. In: *Engineering Applications of Artificial Intelligence* vol. 89, p. 103401 (2020).
55. D. Arifoglu, Y. Wang, and A. Bouchachia, “Detection of dementia-related abnormal behaviour using recursive auto-encoders”. In: *Sensors* vol. 21, no. 1 (2021), p. 260, ISNN: 1424-8220.
56. R. Socher et al. (2011). “Semi- Supervised Recursive Autoencoders for Predicting Sentiment Distributions”. In: *EMNLP 2011 - Conference on Empirical Methods in Natural Language Processing*, Proceedings of the Conference. 151–161.
57. C. Zhou and R. C. Paffenroth. “Anomaly detection with robust deep autoencoders”. In: *Proceedings of the 23rd ACM SIGKDD International Conference on Knowledge Discovery and Data Mining*. KDD ’17 (2017), pp. 665–674. doi: 10.1145/3097983.3098052. url: http://doi.acm.org/10.1145/3097983.3098052.
58. M. Schreyer et al. “Detection of anomalies in large scale accounting data using deep autoencoder networks”. In: CoRR abs/1709.05254 (2017). arXiv: 1709.05254. url: http://arxiv.org/abs/1709.05254.
59. T. Zhang et al. “Learning movement patterns of the occupant in smart home environments: An unsupervised learning approach”. In: *Journal of Ambient Intelligence and Humanized Computing* vol. 8, no. 1 (2017), pp. 133–146. doi: 10.1007/s12652-016-0367-2.
60. T. Van Kasteren, G. Englebienne, and B. J. A. Krose. “Human activity recognition from wireless sensor network data: Benchmark and software”. In: *Activity Recognition in Pervasive Intelligent Environments* (2011), pp. 165–186. doi: 10.2991/978-94-91216-05-3_8.
61. A. Graves, A. R. Mohamed, and G. Hinton. “Speech recognition with deep recurrent neural networks”. In: *2013 IEEE International Conference on Acoustics, Speech and Signal Processing* (2013), pp. 6645–6649. doi: 10.1109/ICASSP. 2013.6638947.
62. I. Sutskever, O. Vinyals, and Q. V. Le. “Sequence to sequence learning with neural networks”. In: *CoRR abs/1409.3215* (2014). url: http://arxiv. org/abs/1409.3215.

63. D. Bahdanau, K. Cho, and Y. Bengio. "Neural machine translation by jointly learning to align and translate". In: *CoRR abs/1409.0473* (2014).
64. K. Greff et al. "LSTM: A search space Odyssey". In: *IEEE Transactions on Neural Networks and Learning Systems* vol. 99 (2016), pp. 1–11. url: http://arxiv.org/abs/1503.04069.
65. C. Francois. Keras (2015). url: https://github.com/fchollet/keras.
66. Theano Development Team. "Theano: A Python framework for fast computation of mathematical expressions". In: *arXiv e-prints abs/1605.02688* (2016).
67. D. Arifoglu and A. Bouchachia. "Activity recognition and abnormal behaviour detection with recurrent neural networks". In: *14th International Conference on Mobile Systems and Pervasive Computing*, pp. 86–93, 2017.
68. D. Arifoglu and A. Bouchachia. "Abnormal behaviour detection for dementia sufferers via transfer learning and recursive auto-encoders". In: *2019 IEEE International Conference on Pervasive Computing and Communications Workshops* (2019), pp. 529–534.
69. D. Arifoglu and A. Bouchachia, "Detection of abnormal behavior for dementia sufferers using Convolutional Neural Networks". In: *Artificial Intelligence in Medicine*, pp. 88–95, 2019.

CHAPTER 11

Classification of Left Ventricular Hypertrophy and NAFLD through Decision Tree Algorithm

Arnulfo González-Cantú
and Maria Elena Romero-Ibarguengoitia
Hospital Clínica Nova de Monterrey
Nuevo Leon, Mexico
Universidad de Monterrey
San Pedro Garza Garcia, Mexico

Baidya Nath Saha
Concordia University of Edmonton
Alberta, Canada

CONTENTS

11.1 INTRODUCTION

Nowadays cardiovascular disease is the most common cause of death throughout the globe [1], and this term includes heart attack, stroke, peripheral arterial disease, and so on. Only during 2016 in the US, 17.6 million deaths were attributed to cardiovascular disease, and its treatments cost billions [2]. The background of metabolic alterations associated with cardiovascular disease is related to a low degree of inflammation caused by low physical activity, non-healthy nutritional behaviour, and obesity. Also, the presence of smoke and alcoholism increases the risk of cardiovascular events and liver disease as non-alcoholic fatty liver disease (NAFLD) by increasing the low-grade inflammation [3].

One of the main causes of cardiovascular disease is arterial hypertension [4]. The blood pressure is regulated by a complex mechanism including the kidney, heart, and blood vessels [5]. The kidney regulates the blood pressure by allowing sodium and water excretion to down-regulate the pressure, and by the renin–angiotensin–aldosterone system (shrinking the lumen of vessels) increasing the pressure. The blood vessels can respond to local mediators like nitric oxide (NO) releasing the pressure, or response to a systemic mediator (i.e. catecholamines) to increase the pressure. The heart as a pump can regulate the blood pressure through the beats frequency or the contraction of the myocardium. Chronic hypertension induces left ventricular hypertrophy (LVH), increasing the metabolism and oxygen requirements; if the process is not reversed, it can increase the risk of a heart attack.

Multiple electrocardiographic criteria are used to diagnose LVH [6]. The accuracy of more frequently used criteria is about 52%–63%, but with very low sensitivity (lower than 56%), and very high specificity (upper than 90%). Though these criteria are used and accepted worldwide, it is desirable to improve the accuracy with a balance between sensitivity and specificity. Not less important and difficult to do is the detection of NAFLD by the way of non-invasive evaluation. Patients with risk factors of NAFLD (i.e. diabetes, obesity, hypertriglyceridemia, and so on) in the presence of high levels of alanine transaminase (ALT) can be assessed with an expensive test as a magnetic resonance of the liver, or with a liver biopsy (with the risks it had).

Nowadays, machine learning (ML) has been used more frequently in medical research to improve the ability to classify (or predict) variables of interest as the presence of diabetes [7], cancer [8] or death. Different algorithms were used for different types of data, and more complex algorithms are needed to handle non-linear relationships [9] or data with high dimensionality [10]. Algorithms such as Adaboost or Support Vector Machine (SVM) can accurately classify diabetic retinopathy [11], cancer [12], and so on; but they cannot offer readable results to doctors without deep enough knowledge in ML. Moreover, there are other ML algorithms with an output that could be more easy to understand by doctors, without sacrificing accuracy. Decision tree (DT) algorithms can be used to predict or classify [13] and handle non-linear relationships between variables.

In this research, we developed a DT-based model aiming to improve the accuracy and automating the classification task of LVH and NAFLD. Our contributions are multifold: (1) DT can automatically generate the hidden complex patterns or rules related to LVH and NAFLD from the patients' data which are clinically relevant and justified by medical experts. (2) Some rules excavated by DT are consistent with the state-of-the-art clinical findings and some of them are new but clinically relevant which are very useful in clinical research. (3) Unlike other ML algorithms, rules generated by DT demonstrate high resemblance with the state-of-the-art diagnostic procedure for LVH and NAFLD which makes the DT-based model useful as a routine diagnostic procedure in clinical settings. (4) Proposed model is very easy to implement and very useful specially in urban and rural hospital settings. (5) Using the proposed tool, emergency doctors can get benefitted from an initial interpretation and enhance their own abilities to classify LVH or NAFLD, which is often complicated to detect, and it can be thoroughly verified by experts later, and thus could dramatically shrink wait times. The proposed tool would enable to process noisy and complex information and make it easier to interpret for clinicians in the field, who necessarily have to make decisions with imperfect data, sometimes under extreme duress. It will definitely give doctors a higher level of confidence when choosing a patient's course of treatment without referring to the experts.

11.2 LITERATURE REVIEW

Previous ML-based research efforts in left ventricular hypertrophy (LVH) and NAFLD are described below.

11.2.1 Left Ventricular Hypertrophy (LVH)

LVH is a major risk to heart attack; though it is easily detected with an echocardiogram, it could be expensive or not available in some places. Electrocardiography is used as a gold standard to diagnose arrhythmias, also, there are multiple diagnostic electrocardiographic criteria described to detect the presence of LVH (i.e. Sokolow-Lyon and Cornell criteria among others); furthermore, these criteria are very specific (>90%), with poor sensitivity (<20%) and an accuracy of ≈50% [6].

Recently some studies have been published aimed to improve the classification of patients with LVH. The majority of these studies includes anthropometric variables also and not electrocardiographic variables only. Lin and Liu [14] classified young adults as having or not having LVH through an SVM algorithm. In this study, 28 electrocardiographic features and other clinical features (age, height, weight, BMI, waist circumference, systolic and diastolic blood pressure and body surface area) were evaluated. The SVM model was compared with the traditional ECG voltage criteria (Cornell and Sokolow-Lyon). Although the SVM model had a more balanced relation between sensitivity and specificity (86.7% and 73.3% each), the Cornel voltage criterion had a higher accuracy (93% vs. 74.2%) [14].

Sparapani and colleagues (2019) describe how the Bayesian Additive Regression Trees can classify the presence fo LVH. This effort was nested in MESA (Multi-Ethnic Study of Atherosclerosis), where 3,214 men and 3,600 women were included. This algorithm is defined by a statistical model with a prior and a likelihood and is a tree-based Bayesian non-parametric method. In this study, 552 amplitude and duration electrocardiographic measurements were included. The MRI were the gold standard method to classify LVH. The proposed model had a ROC AUC of 82.9%, a specificity of 94.6%, and a sensitivity of 29%. Compared with the model of Gen-Min Lin, this model had more specificity (similar to the standard criteria), and in relation to the Cornell voltage product and voltage criteria, the Bayesian Additive Regression Tree showed better performance [15].

12.2.2 Non-Alcoholic Fatty Liver Disease

Nowadays, multiple scores are used to predict NAFLD. Poynard et al. [16] published the SteatoTest, a tool to predict NAFLD [16] in an attempt to reduce the need for liver biopsy. The author used logistic regression to model the probability of the presence of NAFLD; variables such as age, gender, body mass index (BMI), glucose, alanine transaminase, alpha 2 microglobulin, A-1 apolipoprotein, haptoglobin, total bilirubin, total cholesterol and triglycerides were evaluated. This model had an accuracy between 0.8 and 0.9 (varying with the sensitivity and specificity cut-offs). An updated model was published holding the accuracy with a simpler model [17].

Further study tried to improve the classification of NAFLD using previously described variables and some others (i.e. diastolic blood pressure and uric acid) [18], but with a dimensionality reduction with a lasso regression combined with a multivariable logistic regression. In this case, the model was structured with eight variables (including gender, age, total cholesterol, BMI, waistline, diastolic blood pressure, serum uric acid, and course of disease on high-density lipoprotein-cholesterol) and had an accuracy in the training and validation set of 0.848 and 0.809 respectively.

ML algorithms also have been used in the edge of the knowledge of metabolic disease, which includes lipidomics and glycomics. These "omics", includes a larger list of variables and could explain more about the phenomenon behind the disease. Perkakis (2019) evaluated 49 healthy subjects and 31 patients with biopsy-proven NAFLD. The author previously measured some hormone variables also: adiponectin, leptin, activin A and follistatin. The "omics" variables were measured by mass spectrometry and liquid chromatography-mass spectrometry. The ML algorithms included in the analysis were SVM, *k* nearest neighbor, and random forest. In this case, the SVM model with a non-linear kernel had the highest accuracy (with lipidomics variables and with other variables) [19]. However, the uniqueness of the DT algorithm is that it often imitates the human-level thinking, which makes it easier to understand the data and makes some reasonable interpretations. Unlike black-box algorithms such as neural network and SVM, the logic behind the DT algorithm is comprehensible and easy to explicate [20].

11.3 METHODOLOGY

DT is one of the most popular ML algorithms used for both classification and regression problems [20]. A DT exploits a tree-like model where each node represents a feature (attribute), each link (branch) exhibits a decision (rule) and each leaf embodies an outcome (categorical or continuous value). The algorithm of the proposed DT-based model aiming to diagnose LVH and NAFLD is mentioned in Algorithm 11.1.

Algorithm 11.1: Decision Tree Algorithm

Input: Set of possible instances X and label Y
Output: A Decision Tree $f : X \rightarrow Y$
function DECISION TREE (X, Y)

1. Assign all training instances to the root of the tree. Set current node to root node.

2.

a Partition all data instances at the node by the value of the attribute.

b Compute the **information gain ratio** from the partitioning.

$$\text{Gain ratio}(S,A) \equiv \frac{\text{Gain}(S,A)}{\text{Split information}(S,A)}$$

$\text{Gain}(S,A)$ = expected reduction in entropy due to sorting on A, $S = \{X\}$ is a collection of training examples.

$$\text{Gain}(S,A) \equiv \text{Entropy}(S) - \sum_{v \in \text{Values}(A)} \frac{|S_v|}{|S|} \text{Entropy}(S_v)$$

where $\text{Values}(A)$ is the set of all possible values for attribute A, and S_v is the subset of S for which attribute A has value v (i.e., $S_v = \{s \in S \mid A(s) = v\}$).

$$\text{Split information}(S,A) \equiv -\sum_{i=1}^{c} \frac{|S_i|}{|S|} \log_2 \frac{|S_i|}{|S|}$$

where S_i is a subset of S for which A has value v_i, and c is the number of class.

end for

3. Identify a feature that generates the highest information gain ratio. Exploit this feature to be the splitting criterion at the current node.
   if the best information gain ratio is 0 **then**
   label the current node as a leaf and return.

   end if
4. Partition all instances according to the attribute value of the best feature.
5. Denote each partition as a child node of the current node.
6.
   a. If the child node is "pure" (has instances from only one class), label it as a leaf and return.
   b. If not set the child node as the current node and repeat Step 2.

end for

end function

A DT represents a list of disjunctive rules that lead to a class or value; they classify instances by sorting them down the tree from the root to some leaf nodes. Once a DT is learned, it can be used to evaluate new instances to determine their class. The instance is traversed through the tree from the root until it arrives at a leaf. The class assigned to the instance is the class for the leaf. The DT is constructed through a recursive partitioning strategy based on a given training sample, it expands a leaf node unless the given stopping criterion is satisfied, the goal is to split the data into disjoint sets by maximizing the "distance" between groups at each split. In the proposed algorithm, the information gain ratio is used for splitting criteria as shown in Algorithm 11.1. One of the bottlenecks of the DT algorithm is that it suffers from overfitting, i.e. each leaf will represent a very specific set of attribute combinations available in the training data, but unable to classify attribute value combinations that are not seen in the training data. In order to prevent overfitting, it is recommended to prune the DT, i.e. the lower ends (the leaves) of the tree are "snipped" until the tree is much smaller. The proposed pruning algorithm is illustrated in Algorithm 11.2.

Algorithm 11.2: Pruning Algorithm

Input: A Decision Tree f: $X \rightarrow Y$
Output: A Decision Tree $f_1 \subseteq f$
function PRUNING(f)

1. Classify all branches in the tree.
2. Count the total number of leaves in the tree.
3.

while the number of leaves in the tree exceeds the desired number **do**

   a. Find the branch with the least Information Gain.
   b. Remove all child nodes of the branch.
   c. Relabel the branch as a leaf.
   d. Update the leaf count.

end while
end function

11.4 EXPERIMENTAL RESULTS AND DISCUSSIONS

11.4.1 Data Acquisition

To show the effectiveness of DTs to classify patients with LVH and NAFLD, we used data published in Ref. [21,22]. LVH data included 432 patients, out of them 202 patients had LVH and 230 did not have LVH. Among them, 240 were men, and all patients were evaluated with a 12 lead electrocardiogram as shown in Figure 11.1, where the most frequently used measures related to LVH (31 variables). In addition, the Romhilt–Estes multilevel score was calculated to have a point of comparison. The presence of LVH was evaluated with an echocardiogram (the gold standard to diagnose LVH).

Left ventricular morphology patterns for the patients were as follows: normal morphology (n = 100, 23.1%), cardiac remodeling (n = 130, 30.1%), concentric LVH (n = 165, 38.2%) and eccentric LVH (n = 37, 8.6%). LVH severity stage was classified as: mild (n = 77, 38.1%), moderate (n = 50, 24.7%) and severe (n = 75, 37.1%). There was no difference in the severity stage of LVH between males and females (P = 0.420). The distributions of LVMI, RWT and different left ventricle morphologies are shown in Figure 11.2.

Conversely, NAFLD was classified with DT algorithms. Previous studies used structural equation models to find a relationship between the presence of NAFLD and several variables including clinical, family history and even multiple inflammatory variables (IL-2, IL-4, IL-6, tumor necrosis factor-alpha, and such others). In these data, 137 subjects were evaluated with an ultrasound to detect the hyperechogenicity in the liver, related to NAFLD. The ultrasound is not the best non-invasive method to classify NAFLD; however, it is the most inexpensive procedure available to date.

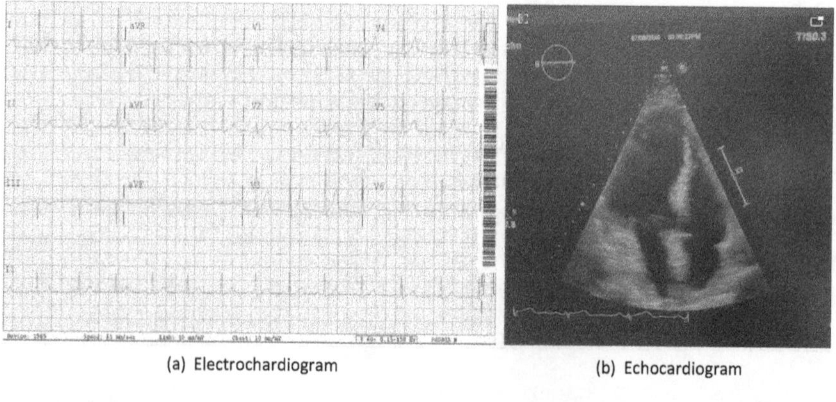

(a) Electrochardiogram

(b) Echocardiogram

FIGURE 11.1 Standard 12-leads electrocardiogram and four-chamber echocardiogram.

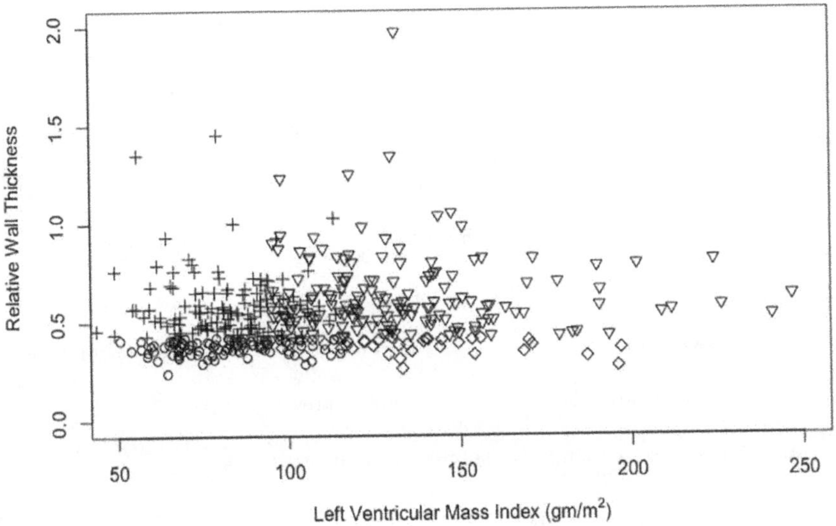

FIGURE 11.2 LVMI distributions and left ventricular morphologies. Morphologies of the left ventricle were defined as: normal (normal LVMI with RWT ≤0.42) (circle), cardiac remodeling (normal LVMI with RWT >0.42) (cross), concentric LVH (elevated LVMI with RWT >0.42) (triangle), and eccentric LVH (elevated LVMI with RWT ≤0.42) (rhomboid). LVH: left ventricular hypertrophy (male: >115 g/m2 and female: >95 g/m2), LVMI: left ventricular mass index, RWT: relative wall thickness.

11.4.2 Decision Tree-Based Model Development for LVH Classification

The proposed model automatically generates a simple, five-level, seven-node DT as shown in Figure 11.3. Each leaf illustrates the probability of having LVH and if its value is greater than 0.5 (50%), the patient will be classified as having LVH and vice-versa. This model was created with 80% of the sample and the remaining 20% was used for internal validation. External validation was conducted in 150 subjects (47.3% LVH positive). The classification performance of the DT model for LVH prediction is illustrated in Table 11.1. Logistic regression was used for dimensionality reduction [20]. Important features estimated by the logistic regression model are illustrated in Table 11.2.

The proposed tree in Figure 11.3 is a particular case, because it was pruned by the algorithm and by an expert in the field (a cardiologist). The algorithm handles the original data and gave a tree, after this "normal" process, the expert evaluated it and made a suggestion about which variable must take it out. These steps were repeated until the expert concludes that the tree had

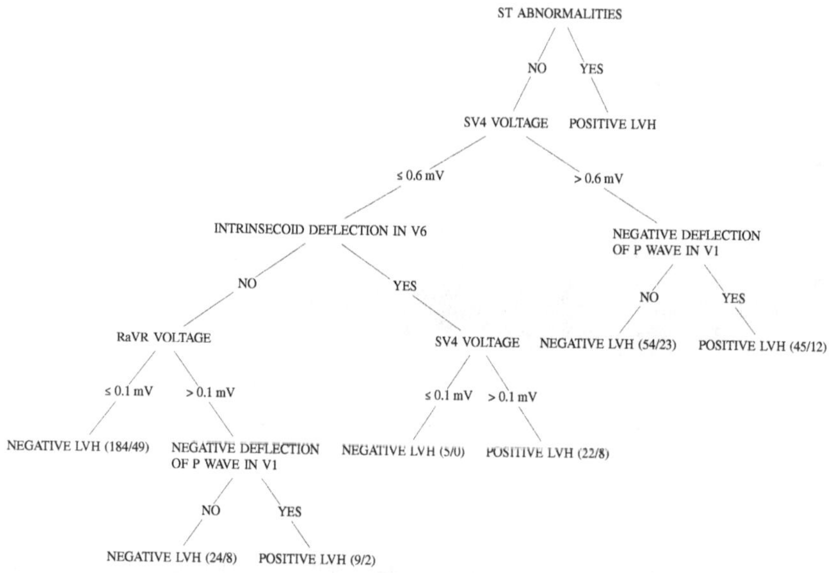

FIGURE 11.3 Decision tree for left ventricular hypertrophy.

TABLE 11.1 Performance of Decision Tree Model for LVH Classification

	Accuracy (%)	Sensitivity (%)	Specificity (%)	PPV (%)	NPV (%)
Internal validation	71.4	79.6	53	66.6	69.3
External validation	73.3	81.6	69.3	56.3	88.6

TABLE 11.2 Logistic Regression Model Used for Dimensionality Reduction in LVH Classification

	Estimate	Std Error	*P*-Value	95% CI
Intercept	−2.7	0.86	0.001	[0.01, 0.34]
ST abnormalities	1.28	0.3	<0.001	[1.98, 6.52]
S V4	0.93	0.36	0.01	[1.24, 5.26]
Intrinsicoid deflection in V6	0.97	0.32	0.002	[1.4, 5.04]
Negative P-wave deflection in V1	0.96	0.24	<0.001	[1.61, 4.22]
R aVR	3.9	1.3	0.002	[4.1, 685.1]
S aVR	0.48	0.34	0.18	[0.83, 3.17]
P-wave duration in V1	−0.009	0.003	0.14	[0.98, 0.99]
S V6	1.91	0.95	0.04	[1.05, 44]
S I	−2.24	1.01	0.27	[0.01, 0.77]
QRS duration	0.01	0.008	0.1	[0.99, 1.03]
R I	0.53	0.37	0.15	[0.81, 3.57]

biological congruency and improved the accuracy of the established LVH criteria. This kind of "modeling" where experts in different fields can work with data scientist is facilitated by the characteristics of DTs.

11.4.3 Decision Tree for NAFLD Classification

The logistic regression model was first applied to NAFLD clinical data discussed in section IV-A to select important features and then a DT was used to classify NAFLD. DT generated as an outcome of the proposed model is demonstrated in Figure 11.4. The classification performance of the proposed DT model for NAFLD prediction in terms of accuracy, sensitivity, specificity, positive predictive value (PPV), and negative predictive value (NPV) is shown in Table 11.3.

Frequently, the variables proposed to be included in a particular model are previously related to the phenomenon of interest, but sometimes these variables had a theoretical association and not a measured relation with the phenomenon. As in the DT in NAFLD, Figure 11.4, the endocrinologist, an expert in the field, supposes a relation of acylcarnitines

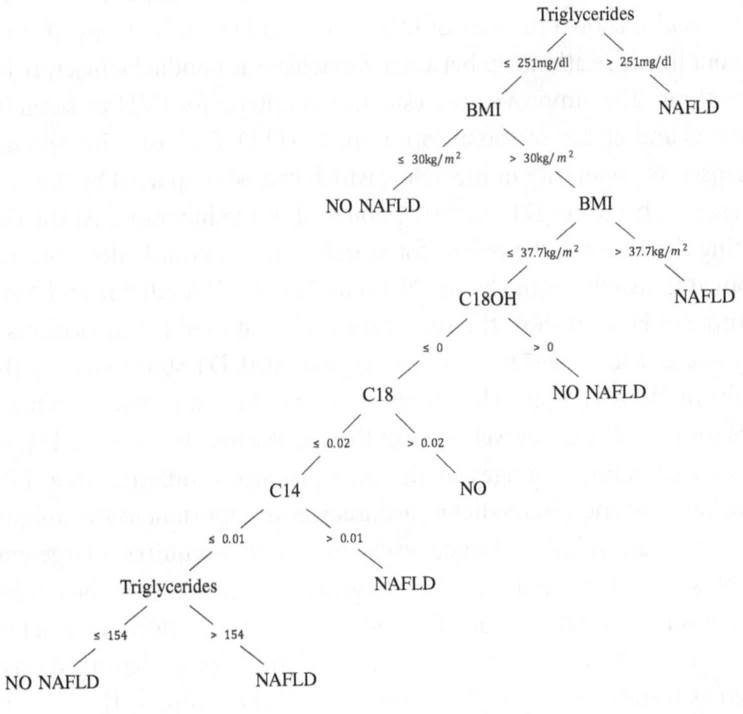

FIGURE 11.4 Proposed decision tree model with logistic regression-based forward selection model.

TABLE 11.3 Performance of Decision Tree to Classify NAFLD

Decision Tree	Accuracy (%)	Sensitivity (%)	Specificity (%)	PPV (%)	NPV (%)
Cross-validation	94.9	80	87.4	66.6	92.2
Confidence interval	78.1–91.7	65.8–94.1	82.4–92.5	54.5–78.7	86.3–98.1

(i.e. C14, C18, C18OH) and other biochemical variables with NAFLD but he does not exactly know how they interact with NAFLD. In this case, the tree proposed by the algorithm can be used as a hypothesis generator (know the relevance between variables) and to classify patients in daily practice (only if the variables are available).

11.5 CONCLUSION AND FUTURE WORKS

We developed a DT-based solution for automating the diagnosis of LVH and NAFLD. The proposed DT-based model is capable of discovering rules to assist in disease diagnosis and they are consistent with the physician's findings. Rules generated by the DT are comprehensible by physicians and is thus more appropriate for using them in clinical settings. The essential characteristics of the DT algorithm have been described in this chapter; the usefulness of it was also shown in cases of LVH and NAFLD. The entropy of this data without linear relationship between variables was handled efficiently by DT algorithms. They improved the established criteria for LVH or suggest new relations and ability of classification for NAFLD. DT's easy interpretability increases its popularity in medicine, which can be supported by the number of research based on DT recently published in the literature. At the time of writing this chapter, the results for search of the keyword "decision tree" in pubmed (a search engine by the National Library of Medicine and National Institute of Health) show the rise of research that used DT algorithms from only one article in 1967 to 1,444 in the year 2020. DT shows state-of-the-art results in many complex classification and prediction problems; however, it faces some challenges as well. One of them is the instability of the DT, which means that subtile changes in the data produce a different tree. Like all branches of science, in medicine, accuracy is as important as the uniqueness of the problem solution. Hence, every experiment requires a large enough sample size and external validation to generalize the utility of the model.

As it was mentioned before, DT had a competitive performance in big and very complex data. Further improvement of the original algorithm was proposed as transfer learning [23], semi-supervised learning [24], and anytime learning [25]. In the future, we aim to develop a more efficient and generalized cost-sensitive and look ahead DT with the help of transfer, semi-supervised, and anytime learning for automating the routine diagnostic procedure.

REFERENCES

1. A. L. Hilliard, D. E. Winchester, T. D. Russell, and R. D. Hilliard, "Myocardial infarction classification and its implications on measures of cardiovascular outcomes, quality, and racial/ethnic disparities," *Clin Cardiol*, vol. 43, no. 10, pp. 1076–1083, Oct 2020.
2. E. J. Benjamin, P. Muntner, A. Alonso, M. S. Bittencourt, C. W. Callaway, A. P. Carson, A. M. Chamberlain, A. R. Chang, S. Cheng, S. R. Das et al., "Heart disease and stroke statistics-2019 update: a report from the American heart association," *Circulation*, vol. 139, no. 10, pp. e56–e528, 2019.
3. M. M. Ruissen, A. L. Mak, U. Beuers, M. E. Tushuizen, and A. G. Holleboom, "Non-alcoholic fatty liver disease: a multidisciplinary approach towards a cardiometabolic liver disease," *Eur J Endocrinol*, vol. 183, no. 3, pp. R57–R73, Sep 2020.
4. U. Goldbourt and E. Grossman, "Blood pressure variability at midlife is associated with all-cause, coronary heart disease and stroke long term mortality," *J Hypert*, vol. 38, no. 9, pp. 1722–1728, Sep 2020.
5. K.-S. Hong, K. Kim, and M. A. Hill, "Regulation of blood flow in small arteries: mechanosensory events underlying myogenic vasoconstriction," *J Exerc Rehabil*, vol. 16, no. 3, pp. 207–215, Jun 2020.
6. F. De la Garza Salazar, E. A. Rodríguez Díaz, A. González Cantú, J. R. Azpiri López, M. Kuri Ayache, and M. E. Romero Ibarguengoitia, "Diagnostic utility of the electrocardiographic left ventricular hypertrophy criteria in specific populations," *Acta Cardiol*, pp. 1–8, Feb 2020.
7. Y. Xiong, L. Lin, Y. Chen, S. Salerno, Y. Li, X. Zeng, and H. Li, "Prediction of gestational diabetes mellitus in the first 19 weeks of pregnancy using machine learning techniques," *J Matern Fetal Neonatal Med*, pp. 1–7, Aug 2020.
8. S. Kweon, J. H. Lee, Y. Lee, and Y. R. Park, "Personal health information inference using machine learning on RNA expression data from patients with cancer: algorithm validation study," *J Med Internet Res*, vol. 22, no. 8, p. e18387, Aug 2020.
9. M. C. Prosperi, A. Altmann, M. Rosen-Zvi, E. Aharoni, G. Borgulya, F. Bazso, A. Sönnerborg, E. Schülter, D. Struck, G. Ulivi et al., "Investigation of expert rule bases, logistic regression, and non-linear machine learning techniques for predicting response to antiretroviral treatment," *Antivir Ther*, vol. 14, no. 3, pp. 433–442, 2009.
10. J. Fan and R. Li, "Statistical challenges with high dimensionality: feature selection in knowledge discovery," *arXiv preprint math/0602133*, 2006.
11. S. Gayathri, V. P. Gopi, and P. Palanisamy, "Automated classification of diabetic retinopathy through reliable feature selection," *Phys Eng Sci Med*, vol. 43. no. 3, pp. 927–945, Sep 2020.
12. Y. Han, Y. Ma, Z. Wu, F. Zhang, D. Zheng, X. Liu, L. Tao, Z. Liang, Z. Yang, X. Li, J. Huang, and X. Guo, "Histologic subtype classification of non-small cell lung cancer using PET/CT images," *Eur J Nucl Med Mol Imaging*, vol. 48, no. 2, pp. 350–360, Feb 2021.
13. Y.-Y. Song and L. Ying, "Decision tree methods: applications for classification and prediction," *Shanghai Arch Psychiatry*, vol. 27, no. 2, p. 130, 2015.

14. G.-M. Lin and K. Liu, "An electrocardiographic system with anthropometrics via machine learning to screen left ventricular hypertrophy among young adults," *IEEE J Transl Eng Health Med*, vol. 8, p. 1800111, 2020.
15. R. Sparapani, N. M. Dabbouseh, D. Gutterman, J. Zhang, H. Chen, D. A. Bluemke, J. A. C. Lima, G. L. Burke, and E. Z. Soliman, "Detection of left ventricular hypertrophy using bayesian additive regression trees: the mesa," *J Am Heart Assoc*, vol. 8, no. 5, p. e009959, 2019.
16. T. Poynard, V. Ratziu, S. Naveau, D. Thabut, F. Charlotte, D. Messous, D. Capron, A. Abella, J. Massard, Y. Ngo, M. Munteanu, A. Mercadier, M. Manns, and J. Albrecht, "The diagnostic value of biomarkers (steatotest) for the prediction of liver steatosis," *Comp Hepatol*, vol. 4, p. 10, Dec 2005.
17. T. Poynard, V. Peta, M. Munteanu, F. Charlotte, Y. Ngo, A. Ngo, H. Perazzo, O. Deckmyn, R. Pais, P. Mathurin, R. Myers, R. Loomba, V. Ratziu, and FLIP consortium, the FibroFrance-CPAM group, the FibroFrance-Obese group, and the Selonsertib group, "The diagnostic performance of a simplified blood test (steatotest-2) for the prediction of liver steatosis," *Eur J Gastroenterol Hepatol*, vol. 31, no. 3, pp. 393–402, 2019.
18. Y. Zhang, R. Shi, L. Yu, L. Ji, M. Li, and F. Hu, "Establishment of a risk prediction model for non-alcoholic fatty liver disease in type 2 diabetes," *Diabetes Ther*, vol. 11, no. 9, pp. 2057–2073, Sep 2020.
19. N. Perakakis, S. A. Polyzos, A. Yazdani, A. Sala-Vila, J. Kountouras, A. D. Anastasilakis, and C. S. Mantzoros, "Non-invasive diagnosis of non-alcoholic steatohepatitis and fibrosis with the use of omics and supervised learning: a proof of concept study," *Metabolism*, vol. 101, p. 154005, 2019.
20. T. M. Mitchell, *Machine Learning*, New York: McGraw-Hill, 1997.
21. F. De la Garza-Salazar, M. E. Romero-Ibarguengoitia, E. A. Rodriguez-Diaz, J. R. Azpiri-Lopez, and A. González-Cantu, "Improvement of electrocardiographic diagnostic accuracy of left ventricular hypertrophy using a machine learning approach," *PLoS One*, vol. 15, no. 5, p. e0232657, 2020.
22. M. E. Romero-Ibarguengoitia, F. Vadillo-Ortega, A. E. Caballero, I. Ibarra-González, A. Herrera-Rosas, M. F. Serratos-Canales, M. León-Hernández, A. González-Chávez, S. Mummidi, R. Duggirala, and J. C. López-Alvarenga, "Family history and obesity in youth, their effect on acylcarnitine/aminoacids metabolomics and non-alcoholic fatty liver disease (nafld). Structural equation modeling approach," *PLoS One*, vol. 13, no. 2, p. e0193138, 2018.
23. J. won Lee and C. Giraud-Carrier, "Transfer learning in decision trees," in *2007 International Joint Conference on Neural Networks*. IEEE, 2007, pp. 726–731.
24. J. Tanha, M. van Someren, and H. Afsarmanesh, "Semi-supervised self-training for decision tree classifiers," *Int J Mach Learn Cybernet*, vol. 8, no. 1, pp. 355–370, 2017.
25. S. Esmeir and S. Markovitch, "Anytime learning of decision trees," *J Mach Learn Res*, vol. 8, no. May, pp. 891–933, 2007.

CHAPTER 12

The Cutting Edge of Surgical Practice: Applications of Machine Learning to Neurosurgery

Omar Khan, Jetan H. Badhiwala,
Muhammad Ali Akbar, and Michael G. Fehlings

University of Toronto
Toronto, Canada

CONTENTS

12.1 INTRODUCTION

As much of this book illustrates, the influence of machine learning (ML) on medicine is quite wide-ranging, as it spans multiple disciplines and affects them in a variety of ways. This applicability is a consequence of

ML's ability to handle large, complex datasets in a manner that circumvents many of the limitations of traditional statistical techniques [1]. Indeed, neurosurgery is certainly not immune to this influence. Recent years have demonstrated a significant rise in the number of articles highlighting the applications of ML to neurosurgical practice [2]. At the same time, diagnostic and epidemiological datasets have burgeoned in size and complexity, making the increase in ML articles one that is born out of both novelty and necessity.

ML is not a monolith; it is more accurate to describe ML as a category of tools that can be subdivided based on the computational tasks that are solved by the algorithm [1,3]. This subdivision breaks down ML into three major categories: supervised learning, unsupervised learning, and reinforcement learning [4,5] (Table 12.1). Of these, reinforcement learning is the most limited with respect to applications within neurosurgery. This is primarily due to its nature as a policy-determining technique that optimizes reward in a specified environment (e.g. a robot playing on a chessboard [environment] that attempts to determine a policy [moves] that maximizes reward and minimizes penalty) [5], which makes it less amenable to being used on epidemiological datasets than the other two categories.

The potential impact of ML on neurosurgical practice is significant. Over the last few years, the literature that has focused on applying ML to

TABLE 12.1 Description of the Three Major Categories of Machine Learning

Attribute	Supervised Learning	Unsupervised Learning	Reinforcement Learning
Labeling	Outcomes are labeled a priori	No labeling of outcomes	No labeling of outcomes
Description	Algorithm uses input variables to predict outcomes with labeled data as a reference	Algorithms separate data into clusters	Algorithms build a policy that maximizes reward and minimizes penalty within an environment
Evaluation metrics	AUC and accuracy relative to actual outcome values	Not applicable, as data are unlabeled	Cumulative reward
Examples	Classification algorithms (e.g. random forest) and regression algorithms (e.g. support vector regression)	k-means clustering, principal component analysis	Q-learning

AUC: area under the receiver operating characteristic curve.

neurosurgery has addressed a large number of clinical practice domains. These domains can be divided into preoperative diagnosis, operative management, and postoperative prognosis. The goal of this chapter is to summarize the role of ML that has thus far been established in these areas. Specifically, Sections 12.2–12.4 of this chapter will respectively discuss the current ML literature relevant to neurosurgical diagnostics, intraoperative care, and neurosurgical prognosis [1,2,6]. Section 12.5 will discuss possible future directions that highlight areas for improvement and potentially exciting research avenues that may be pursued. Finally, Section 12.6 will describe the limitations of ML.

12.2 MACHINE LEARNING AND NEUROSURGICAL DIAGNOSTICS

In imaging applications, ML may serve a promising role in flagging abnormal features or suggesting a list of likely diagnoses, which will undoubtedly assist clinicians with workflow and provide in-depth diagnostic impressions [7]. In recent years, a considerable amount of work has been done around training ML algorithms to read common imaging modalities involving the central nervous system (e.g. magnetic resonance imaging or MRI and computed tomography or CT scans). This work has spanned a host of applications, such as the brain and spinal cord segmentation, stroke imaging, and neuro-oncology.

When a patient presents with a stroke, history is one of the key clinical elements that guide management. In the most recent guidelines for ischemic stroke management, thrombolytic (i.e. 'clot-busting') agents are recommended within 4.5 hours of symptom onset or the patient's last-known baseline state, provided that certain conditions are satisfied [8]. There are additional criteria for the administration of thrombolytic agents for patients presenting between 3 and 4.5 hours of symptom onset (e.g. nonmajor stroke). Thus, it is crucial to identify the onset of symptoms when deciding upon management for a patient with acute ischemic stroke. However, this is frequently not possible, such as when the stroke is severely disabling, when the patient has an additional neurocognitive impairment, or when the neurological deficits are present upon awakening [9,10]. In situations with unclear history, diffusion-weighted and fluid-attenuated inversion recovery (FLAIR) MRI may be done. Patients with diffusion-positive and FLAIR-negative lesions (i.e. DWI-FLAIR mismatch) are deemed to be within the 4.5-hour time window and may be eligible for thrombolytic drugs [10,11].

However, the use of DWI-FLAIR mismatch has low to moderate inter- and intra-rater reliability; in addition, it is not a perfect indicator of ischemic strokes occurring with a 4.5-hour time period [10,12]. Recognizing these limitations, Lee and colleagues developed ML algorithms (logistic regression, support vector machines, and random forest) that utilized MRI features to detect strokes occurring within 4.5 hours [13]. These algorithms were found to be more sensitive than human readers and had no statistically significant difference from human readers with respect to specificity. From these findings, it is possible that the improved performance of ML was due to its detection of additional imaging features in conjunction with the DWI-FLAIR mismatch that may be undetected by human readers. For neurosurgical practice, this has potentially important implications, as patients past the pharmacological thrombolysis window may be eligible for mechanical thrombectomy, which is recommended between 6 and 24 hours of symptom onset or last-known baseline state [8,14]. Thus, accurate identification of patients with the 4.5-hour time window by ML may necessarily change the pool of patients eligible for mechanical thrombectomy by a neurosurgeon.

In neuro-oncology, important strides have been made in the classification, grading, and segmentation of brain tumors. We will summarize these strides here, but a more comprehensive overview can be found in Ref. [15]. Multiple studies have used ML to classify brain tumors as benign or malignant, achieving good to excellent performance, with one study achieving a classification accuracy of 98% [16] and another study achieving an area under the receiver operating characteristic curve (AUC) of 0.911 [17]. Other studies have attempted to use ML for a more granular classification of brain tumors. Zacharaki and colleagues [18], for instance, developed support vector machine (SVM) models to classify different grades of gliomas, meningiomas, and brain metastases based on MRI characteristics. The models generally fared well in most two-class problems (i.e. in distinguishing two different types of tumors) with AUCs between 0.77 and 1. However, their performance was limited in two areas: in distinguishing grade II from grade III gliomas and in multiclass classification (i.e. in distinguishing more than two types of tumors). Later, Wang and colleagues [19] developed ML algorithms to distinguish grade II, III, and IV gliomas via a multiclass approach and achieved significant success (mean accuracy ~90%).

Additional studies of ML in neuro-oncology have focused on tumor segmentation, the process of separating the tumor from the surrounding brain tissue on imaging, which can be indispensable when deciding the treatment approach [20]. Traditionally, manual segmentation of the tumor by physicians is used for treatment planning; however, this process can be inefficient and is subject to imperfect inter-rater reliability [21]. ML is an ideal candidate to address these issues, with current literature comprising multiple articles using either deep learning or k-means clustering to distinguish neoplastic tissue from the regular brain parenchyma. These articles have been able to successfully segment glioblastoma multiforme, low-grade gliomas, meningiomas, and metastatic brain tumors [22,23].

The applications of segmentation algorithms, however, are not solely restricted to an oncologic context. In patients with temporal lobe epilepsy (TLE), a frequent finding is a hippocampal sclerosis [24]. These patients are particularly amenable to surgical treatment (60% seizure-free rate), commonly done via resection of the offending brain areas [25]. However, patients without hippocampal sclerosis are less likely to experience success with surgery, which makes it clinically useful to distinguish between the two subtypes of temporal lobe epilepsy. To this end, Keihaninejad and colleagues [26] have used ML to perform both segmentation and classification of temporal lobe epilepsies on MRI. After segmentation, the authors used SVM algorithms to achieve classification accuracies of 96% and 86% for TLE with and without hippocampal sclerosis respectively. Similar efforts for the segmentation and classification of TLE have been undertaken under slightly different conditions (e.g. detecting TLE based on extrahippocampal findings) [27,28].

Outside the brain, the pool of publications utilizing ML in a diagnostic context for spinal pathology is limited compared to the pool of publications using ML in the setting of intracranial pathology. Nonetheless, the literature for the diagnosis of spinal cord pathology using ML is rapidly expanding and has taken important steps forward thus far. One of these steps was undertaken by Jamaludin and colleagues [29], who developed a model to label vertebrae and intervertebral discs using images from over 12,000 discs. This was followed by the development of a convolutional neural network to predict the extent of disc degeneration according to the Pfirrmann grading scale. Ultimately, the inter-rater agreement between the algorithm and human predictions of 70.1% was similar to the inter-rater agreement of 70.4% between two human radiologists when scoring disc degeneration using the Pfirrmann scale. Other research around spinal deformity, particularly idiopathic scoliosis, has also been undertaken for scoliosis classification and grading [30].

In the realm of spinal cord injury (SCI), Tay and colleagues [31] constructed ML algorithms that used spinal cord imaging obtained from diffusion tensor imaging (DTI) to classify axial images based on whether or not SCI was present. The key feature used to make these predictions was fractional anisotropy, a quantity used as a proxy for the tissue's structural integrity. More specifically, fractional anisotropy is used in DTI to describe the diffusion of water and tissue orientation in the image [32]. After demarcating the spinal cord, the authors used SVM and k-nearest neighbors ML models to classify a spinal cord DTI image as either injured or normal, using fractional anisotropy as a predictor. The algorithms achieved a specificity of 0.952 and a sensitivity of 0.912.

12.3 MACHINE LEARNING AND INTRAOPERATIVE CARE

Neurosurgery is a unique surgical specialty in that it employs a host of organ-specific intraoperative monitoring modalities to ensure surgical success. These modalities include intraoperative imaging, electrophysiological monitoring, and neurophysiological monitoring. Given that neurosurgery relies both on manual skill and quick-thinking diagnostic ability during each operation, the field is a very suitable candidate to additionally employ ML in the intraoperative context.

Parkinson's disease is a movement disorder that arises as a consequence of degeneration of dopaminergic neurons in the substantia nigra of the basal ganglia [33]. Medical management of Parkinson's disease involves boosting dopaminergic activity, bringing about some symptomatic relief [34]. However, in cases that are refractory to medical management, surgical intervention via deep brain stimulation (DBS) of basal ganglia structures (e.g. subthalamic nucleus, STN) is an option [34,35]. In this procedure, a microelectrode recorder is passed through the brain to map out the relevant brain structures and ideally identify the STN. Taghva developed hidden Markov models to detect whether a microelectrode is within the STN during DBS, using simulated brain anatomy involved in the actual procedure [36,37]. The models achieved accuracies between 98% and 99% in classifying the location of the simulated microelectrode, with specificities and sensitivities above 95% when it came to identifying whether the microelectrode was specifically inside the STN. While most seasoned clinicians performing DBS surgery should be able to recognize the STN, this algorithm will be able to augment their recognition and may be generalizable to novel brain targets in Parkinson's.

Intracranial pressure (ICP) monitoring, particularly in patients with traumatic brain injury, is an important tool in the neurosurgeon's arsenal [38]. In the intraoperative context, ICP monitoring has been said to have important therapeutic and prognostic implications [39]. ICP morphology, as a result, can have an important diagnostic value, especially when employed intraoperatively. Nucci and colleagues [40] developed artificial neural networks to detect and classify CSF pressure waveforms. Using the diagnosis of an expert examiner as the 'ground truth', the neural network achieved 88.3% accuracy when it came to classifying CSF pressure waves. Theoretically, these results may be extended to the intraoperative scenario to aid neurosurgeons in the rapid interpretation of ICP.

Spinal surgery frequently carries the risk of cord damage, which means that intraoperative electrophysiological monitoring can be useful in allowing surgeons to recognize and prevent potential neurological deficits. Somatosensory evoked potentials (SEPs) are often used as metrics to gauge the electrophysiological status of the spinal cord [41,42]. However, various surgical and anesthetic factors can hamper the interpretation of the SEP profile; in addition, the use of human experts to interpret SEPs may be subject to inter-rater variations [43]. To rectify these issues, Fan and colleagues [44] created least squares support vector regression models to construct an SEP baseline; the baseline constructed by these models was superior to the nominal baseline as far as allowing successful SEP monitoring and preventing false warnings about spinal cord damage.

12.4 MACHINE LEARNING AND NEUROSURGICAL PROGNOSIS

To date, prognostic ML models have been the most extensively developed in neurosurgery, as they are able to leverage numerical epidemiological data, as opposed to imaging or intraoperative data, which are necessarily more difficult to build models around. Prognostic models can serve a crucial role in clinical practice, by helping to manage expectations, by identifying patients who may potentially require additional intervention, and by even predicting the discharge course of patients. Although these models span a multitude of areas, they generally follow similar principles. They utilize patient data (e.g. age, comorbidities, and preoperative neurological status) to predict postoperative outcomes, which can include functional outcomes, quality-of-life outcomes, and others. ML-based prognostic models have thus far been applied to nearly all areas of neurosurgery, including epilepsy, Parkinson's disease, neurotrauma, neuro-oncology, and spine pathology [45].

A systematic review from 2018 by Senders and colleagues [45] describes in extensive detail how ML-based outcome prediction is used in numerous neurosurgical domains. In the field of epilepsy, the nine articles examined in the review all predicted seizure freedom in patients who underwent surgery for temporal lobe epilepsy using ML algorithms (e.g. SVM, random forest, neural networks, naïve Bayes, and k-nearest neighbor) [46–54]. The nine studies used a multitude of input features, including clinical variables, MRI findings, and EEG findings. Overall, the studies obtained a classification accuracy ranging from 70% to 98% (median: 92%) and an AUC ranging from 0.63 to 0.94. Similarly, four studies used ML to predict survival after either surgical resection, biopsy, or stereotactic radiosurgery on primary or metastatic brain tumors [55–58]. The studies used algorithms such as SVM and neural networks and achieved AUCs between 0.76 and 0.85, indicating good predictive performance. Two other studies additionally predicted cancer recurrence in patients who received either gamma knife radiosurgery for metastatic brain tumors (accuracy: 95% and AUC: 0.88) [59] or gross-total resection for glioblastomas (accuracy: 91%, AUC: 0.84) [60].

In traumatic brain injury, Shi and colleagues [61] used artificial neural networks to predict in-hospital mortality after intracranial decompression (either via craniectomy or hematoma evacuation), achieving an accuracy of 95% and an AUC of 0.89. More recently, Gravesteijn and colleagues [62] developed ML models to predict mortality and unfavorable outcome (defined by a Glasgow Coma Scale < 4) after traumatic brain injury. However, the authors found no difference between ML models (e.g. SVM and random forest) and traditional logistic regression in the discrimination and calibration of predictions. For Parkinson's disease, two studies used ML techniques (e.g. SVM, random forest, and naïve Bayes) to predict motor improvement after DBS of the STN [63,64]. One study achieved an accuracy of 86% when predicting motor improvement 9 months after DBS [64] while the other achieved an accuracy of 95% when predicting motor improvement 2 years after DBS [63].

In the realm of spine disease, ML algorithms have recently begun to be used for outcome prediction in both traumatic and nontraumatic SCI. In traumatic SCI, DeVries and colleagues [65] have developed unsupervised

ML algorithms to predict independence in walking either at discharge or at 1-year follow-up, demonstrating that the ML algorithms were equivalent in performance to their logistic regression counterparts for the same task. Along a similar path of inquiry, Inoue and colleagues [66] recently created an 'xgboost' algorithm to predict recovery in neurological status (judged according to the American Spinal Injury Association Impairment Scale or AIS) 6 months postinjury. Using patient data, MRI findings, and treatment variables among the predictors, the authors demonstrated that the 'xgboost' algorithm was superior in accuracy to a logistic regression model and a decision tree model in making the same predictions (accuracy: 81.1% and AUC: 0.867), although the AUC fell slightly short of the target set by the logistic regression model (0.877).

Nontraumatic SCI can be divided anatomically into cervical spine disease (often termed degenerative cervical myelopathy or DCM) and lumbar spine disease. Hoffman and colleagues [67] published one of the early studies which applied support vector regression to predict the Oswestry Disability Index (ODI, a functional outcome) after surgery for DCM, demonstrating that preoperative ODI and symptom duration were among the most important variables in successful outcome prediction by the ML model. This work was followed up by the works of Merali et al. [68] and Khan et al. [69], who developed multiple ML algorithms to predict functional and health-related quality-of-life outcomes 6 months, 1 year, and 2 years after surgery for DCM. The typical AUC for these models was around 0.7–0.78.

In addition to being used to predict functional and quality-of-life outcomes, ML algorithms have also been developed to predict opioid use after cervical and lumbar spine surgery. In two separate studies, Karhade and colleagues used ML models to predict prolonged opioid use after cervical [70] and lumbar spine surgery [71], using preoperative factors such as insurance status, tobacco use, and history of depression. The authors achieved AUCs of 0.81 for both the cervical spine model (stochastic gradient boosting algorithm) and the lumbar spine model (elastic-net penalized logistic regression). Finally, work has also been done for the prediction of discharge disposition, where Karhade et al. used a large National Surgical Quality Improvement Program database containing 26,000 patients to develop ML algorithms predicting patients with a nonroutine discharge [72]. The developed ML algorithms allowed the authors to achieve good calibration and discrimination (AUC: 0.82).

12.5 FUTURE DIRECTIONS

Table 12.2 summarizes the potential applications of ML to neurosurgery, which span several areas and affect those areas in several ways. Nevertheless, when it comes to being applied to the neurosurgical context, ML is still in a relative state of infancy. While ML in neurosurgery has become a hot-button subject and heavily pursued area of research, there are still numerous gaps that exist that make the present state of the literature far from complete. Therefore, a present-day discussion of ML cannot be complete without discussing the future, which does hold considerable promise. For the diagnosis, treatment, and prognosis of neurological pathologies, we will discuss the future role of ML for neurosurgical practice, including both intracranial and extracranial (e.g. spinal cord) processes.

The core advantages of ML stem from its ability to analyze large and complex datasets with many predictors, its ability to determine important predictors computationally without a priori specification, and its ability to capture nonlinear relationships [73–75]. As described earlier, many studies have been conducted that leverage these ML features to develop powerful diagnostic and prognostic tools. As ML continues to grow in popularity [2], the applications of ML to the areas described in the previous sections will

TABLE 12.2 Summary of the Potential Applications of Machine Learning to Neurosurgical Practice, Sorted by Diagnostic and Intraoperative Applications (Section 12.2) and Prognostication (Section 12.3)

Area of Neurosurgery	Diagnosis and Intraoperative Management	Prognosis
Epilepsy	Segmentation and classification of temporal lobe epilepsy	Prediction of seizure freedom in temporal lobe epilepsy
Neurovascular	Identification of patients within the 4.5-hour time window for acute ischemic stroke	Prediction of outcomes after mechanical thrombectomy [80]
Neuro-oncology	Classification, grading, and segmentation of intracranial neoplasms	Prediction of survival after surgical treatment, prediction of cancer recurrence after gamma knife radiosurgery for metastases
Traumatic brain Injury	Intracranial pressure monitoring	Prediction of mortality and unfavorable outcome after surgery
Spinal cord injury	Spinal cord segmentation, diagnosis of spinal cord injury, intraoperative monitoring of somatosensory evoked potentials	Prediction of functional outcomes, health-related quality-of-life outcomes, prolonged opioid use, and discharge disposition after surgery

become more robust and take a bigger place in clinical practice. Moreover, with the advent of tools such as natural language processing (NLP) and computer vision [6], artificial intelligence tools beyond ML could begin to impact neurosurgical practice in a variety of other ways (e.g. NLP for extracting information from imaging reports [76] and computer vision for analysis of hand function after SCI [77]).

However, in addition to a more broadened scope of ML and artificial intelligence, the path forward requires future studies in ML to achieve greater methodological robustness and reproducibility before ML can be confidently introduced to neurosurgery. To achieve robustness, future literature on ML would benefit from following the 2016 guidelines created by Luo and colleagues [75], which describe a systematic approach to developing ML models. Strategies proposed by the guidelines to ensure robust analysis include using separate training and testing sets to minimize overfitting, using calibration and discrimination metrics, and, when possible, using external datasets for further validation of the model. For reproducibility, ML algorithms by their nature are difficult to express on paper, as they are frequently far too complex to describe via an equation. For this reason, many of the aforementioned ML articles do not include a copy of the model with the paper; however, future studies would benefit from using web-based applications to make their ML models more easily applied. This will inevitably aid the reproducibility and external validation of those studies, allowing those algorithms to eventually become an integral part of future neurosurgical practice.

12.6 LIMITATIONS

Despite its promise, ML carries important limitations that ought to be considered when implementing it into practice. First, compared to logistic regression models, which can be written neatly in equation form, many ML models are more difficult to express in closed form due to their inherent complexity. This makes their interpretation difficult and less intuitive, which is why the development of web-based applications for ML programs developed in future neurosurgical research is crucial to overcome this inherent disadvantage. Second, as a data-driven tool, ML is inherently limited by the quality and quantity of the underlying data [78]. Small, poor-quality datasets will result in worse ML models than larger, high-quality datasets. Additionally, biases within data can make ML algorithms less generalizable. For example, an algorithm making diagnostic predictions based on data from a single hospital site may be more likely to suggest a diagnosis primarily seen at that center, making it less applicable to data from other centers. Third, there are significant medico-legal challenges that can potentially arise from the widespread and unregulated implementation of ML [79]. These challenges can arise from the 'black-box' interpretation of some ML algorithms, which makes it difficult to decipher the parts of the underlying data that the algorithm used to generate an output. For instance, if a user did not have a priori knowledge of the fact that an ML algorithm used the name of the hospital (an otherwise irrelevant variable) as an important predictive variable for a surgical outcome, then that user could be led into utilizing the algorithm inappropriately in multiple contexts. Careful consideration of these issues will also be vital toward properly implementing ML in the future as an adjunct to clinical decision-making in neurosurgery.

REFERENCES

1. O. Khan, J. H. Badhiwala, J. R. F. Wilson, F. Jiang, A. R. Martin, and M. G. Fehlings, "Predictive Modeling of Outcomes after Traumatic and Nontraumatic Spinal Cord Injury Using Machine Learning: Review of Current Progress and Future Directions," (in English), *Neurospine*, vol. 16, no. 4, pp. 678–685, Dec 2019.
2. J. T. Senders et al., "An Introduction and Overview of Machine Learning in Neurosurgical Care," *Acta Neurochirurgica (Wien)*, vol. 160, no. 1, pp. 29–38, Jan 2018.
3. A. V. Karhade et al., "Development of Machine Learning Algorithms for Prediction of 30-Day Mortality after Surgery for Spinal Metastasis," *Neurosurgery*, vol. 85, no. 1, pp. E83–E91, Jul 1, 2019.
4. M. I. Jordan and T. M. Mitchell, "Machine Learning: Trends, Perspectives, and Prospects," (in English), *Science*, vol. 349, no. 6245, pp. 255–260, Jul 17, 2015.
5. M. Wiering and M. van Otterlo, "Reinforcement Learning: State-of-the-Art," (in English), *Reinforcement Learning: State-of-the-Art*, vol. 12, pp. 1–638, 2012.
6. O. Khan, J. H. Badhiwala, G. Grasso, and M. G. Fehlings, "Use of Machine Learning and Artificial Intelligence to Drive Personalized Medicine Approaches for Spine Care," (in English), *World Neurosurgery*, vol. 140, pp. 512–518, Aug 2020.
7. A. S. Lundervold and A. Lundervold, "An Overview of Deep Learning in Medical Imaging Focusing on MRI," (in English), *Zeitschrift Fur Medizinische Physik*, vol. 29, no. 2, pp. 102–127, 2019.
8. W. J. Powers et al., "Guidelines for the Early Management of Patients with Acute Ischemic Stroke: 2019 Update to the 2018 Guidelines for the Early Management of Acute Ischemic Stroke: A Guideline for Healthcare Professionals From the American Heart Association/American Stroke Association," *Stroke*, vol. 50, no. 12, pp. e344–e418, Dec 2019.

9. W. J. Elliott, "Circadian Variation in the Timing of Stroke Onset: A Meta-Analysis," *Stroke*, vol. 29, no. 5, pp. 992–996, May 1998.
10. G. Thomalla et al., "DWI-FLAIR Mismatch for the Identification of Patients with Acute Ischaemic Stroke within 4.5 h of Symptom Onset (PRE-FLAIR): A Multicentre Observational Study," *Lancet Neurology*, vol. 10, no. 11, pp. 978–986, Nov 2011.
11. S. Emeriau, I. Serre, O. Toubas, F. Pombourcq, C. Oppenheim, and L. Pierot, "Can Diffusion-Weighted Imaging-Fluid-Attenuated Inversion Recovery Mismatch (Positive Diffusion-Weighted Imaging/Negative Fluid-Attenuated Inversion Recovery) at 3 Tesla Identify Patients with Stroke at <4.5 hours?," *Stroke*, vol. 44, no. 6, pp. 1647–1651, Jun 2013.
12. B. J. Kim et al., "Color-Coded Fluid-Attenuated Inversion Recovery Images Improve Inter-Rater Reliability of Fluid-Attenuated Inversion Recovery Signal Changes within Acute Diffusion-Weighted Image Lesions," *Stroke*, vol. 45, no. 9, pp. 2801–2804, Sep 2014.
13. H. Lee et al., "Machine Learning Approach to Identify Stroke within 4.5 Hours," *Stroke*, vol. 51, no. 3, pp. 860–866, Mar 2020.
14. M. Mokin et al., "Indications for Thrombectomy in Acute Ischemic Stroke from Emergent Large Vessel Occlusion (ELVO): Report of the SNIS Standards and Guidelines Committee," *Journal of NeuroInterventional Surgery*, vol. 11, no. 3, pp. 215–220, Mar 2019.
15. G. S. Tandel et al., "A Review on a Deep Learning Perspective in Brain Cancer Classification," *Cancers (Basel)*, vol. 11, no. 1, Jan 18, 2019.
16. M. Sasikala and N. Kumaravel, "A Wavelet-Based Optimal Texture Feature Set for Classification of Brain Tumours," *Journal of Medical Engineering & Technology*, vol. 32, no. 3, pp. 198–205, May-Jun 2008.
17. G. Ranjith, R. Parvathy, V. Vikas, K. Chandrasekharan, and S. Nair, "Machine Learning Methods for the Classification of Gliomas: Initial Results Using Features Extracted from MR Spectroscopy," *Neuroradiology Journal*, vol. 28, no. 2, pp. 106–111, Apr 2015.
18. E. I. Zacharaki et al., "Classification of Brain Tumor Type and Grade Using MRI Texture and Shape in a Machine Learning Scheme," *Magnetic Resonance in Medicine*, vol. 62, no. 6, pp. 1609–1618, Dec 2009.
19. X. Wang et al., "Machine Learning Models for Multiparametric Glioma Grading with Quantitative Result Interpretations," (in English), *Frontiers in Neuroscience*, Original Research vol. 12, no. 1046, January 11, 2019.
20. A. Bousselham, O. Bouattane, M. Youssfi, and A. Raihani, "Towards Reinforced Brain Tumor Segmentation on MRI Images Based on Temperature Changes on Pathologic Area," *International Journal of Biomedical Imaging*, vol. 2019, p. 1758948, 2019.
21. C. W. Wee et al., "Evaluation of Variability in Target Volume Delineation for Newly Diagnosed Glioblastoma: A Multi-Institutional Study from the Korean Radiation Oncology Group," (in English), *Radiation Oncology*, vol. 10, Jul 2, 2015.
22. T. L. Jones, T. J. Byrnes, G. Yang, F. A. Howe, B. A. Bell, and T. R. Barrick, "Brain Tumor Classification Using the Diffusion Tensor Image Segmentation (D-SEG) Technique," (in English), *Neuro-Oncology*, vol. 17, no. 3, pp. 466–476, Mar 2015.

23. J. Juan-Albarracin et al., "Automated Glioblastoma Segmentation Based on a Multiparametric Structured Unsupervised Classification," *PLoS One*, vol. 10, no. 5, p. e0125143, 2015.
24. M. Thom, "Review: Hippocampal Sclerosis in Epilepsy: A Neuropathology Review," *Neuropathology and Applied Neurobiology*, vol. 40, no. 5, pp. 520–543, Aug 2014.
25. M. Mohan et al., "The Long-Term Outcomes of Epilepsy Surgery," *PLoS One*, vol. 13, no. 5, p. e0196274, 2018.
26. S. Keihaninejad et al., "Classification and Lateralization of Temporal Lobe Epilepsies with and without Hippocampal Atrophy Based on Whole-Brain Automatic MRI Segmentation," (in English), *PLoS One*, vol. 7, no. 4, Apr 16, 2012.
27. J. Del Gaizo et al., "Using Machine Learning to Classify Temporal Lobe Epilepsy Based on Diffusion MRI," (in English), *Brain and Behavior*, vol. 7, no. 10, Oct 2017.
28. N. K. Focke, M. Yogarajah, M. R. Symms, O. Gruber, W. Paulus, and J. S. Duncan, "Automated MR Image Classification in Temporal Lobe Epilepsy," (in English), *Neuroimage*, vol. 59, no. 1, pp. 356–362, Jan 2, 2012.
29. A. Jamaludin et al., "ISSLS PRIZE IN BIOENGINEERING SCIENCE 2017: Automation of Reading of Radiological Features from Magnetic Resonance Images (MRIs) of the Lumbar Spine without Human Intervention is Comparable with an Expert Radiologist," *European Spine Journal*, vol. 26, no. 5, pp. 1374–1383, May 2017.
30. J. L. Yang et al., "Development and Validation of Deep Learning Algorithms for Scoliosis Screening Using Back Images," (in English), *Communications Biology*, vol. 2, Oct 25, 2019.
31. B. Tay, J. K. Hyun, and S. Oh, "A Machine Learning Approach for Specification of Spinal Cord Injuries Using Fractional Anisotropy Values Obtained from Diffusion Tensor Images," (in English), *Computational and Mathematical Methods in Medicine*, vol. 2014, p. 1–8, 2014.
32. J. M. Soares, P. Marques, V. Alves, and N. Sousa, "A Hitchhiker's Guide to Diffusion Tensor Imaging," *Frontiers in Neuroscience*, vol. 7, p. 31, 2013.
33. F. N. Emamzadeh and A. Surguchov, "Parkinson's Disease: Biomarkers, Treatment, and Risk Factors," *Frontiers in Neuroscience*, vol. 12, p. 612, 2018.
34. P. Rizek, N. Kumar, and M. S. Jog, "An Update on the Diagnosis and Treatment of Parkinson DISEASE," *CMAJ*, vol. 188, no. 16, pp. 1157–1165, Nov 1, 2016.
35. S. J. Groiss, L. Wojtecki, M. Sudmeyer, and A. Schnitzler, "Deep Brain Stimulation in Parkinson's Disease," *Therapeutic Advances in Neurological Disorders*, vol. 2, no. 6, pp. 20–28, Nov 2009.
36. A. Taghva, "An Automated Navigation System for Deep Brain Stimulator Placement Using Hidden Markov Models," (in English), *Neurosurgery*, vol. 66, no. 3, pp. 108–117, Mar 2010.
37. A. Taghva, "Hidden Semi-Markov Models in the Computerized Decoding of Microelectrode Recording Data for Deep Brain Stimulator Placement," *World Neurosurgery*, vol. 75, no. 5–6, pp. 758–763.e4, May–Jun 2011.

38. D. e. Laskowitz and G. e. Grant, *Translational Research in Traumatic Brain Injury*, 1st ed. Boca Raton (FL): CRC Press/Taylor and Francis Group, 2016.
39. T. H. Tsai, T. Y. Huang, S. S. Kung, Y. F. Su, S. L. Hwang, and A. S. Lieu, "Intraoperative Intracranial Pressure and Cerebral Perfusion Pressure for Predicting Surgical Outcome in Severe Traumatic Brain Injury," *Kaohsiung Journal of Medical Sciences*, vol. 29, no. 10, pp. 540–546, Oct 2013.
40. C. G. Nucci et al., "Intracranial Pressure Wave Morphological Classification: Automated Analysis and Clinical Validation," *Acta Neurochirurgica (Wien)*, vol. 158, no. 3, pp. 581–588; discussion 588, Mar 2016.
41. M. R. Nuwer, "Spinal Cord Monitoring with Somatosensory Techniques," *Journal of Clinical Neurophysiology*, vol. 15, no. 3, pp. 183–193, May 1998.
42. T. C. Hammett, B. Boreham, N. A. Quraishi, and S. M. H. Mehdian, "Intraoperative Spinal Cord Monitoring during the Surgical Correction of Scoliosis Due to Cerebral Palsy and Other Neuromuscular Disorders," (in English), *European Spine Journal*, vol. 22, pp. S38–S41, Mar 2013.
43. A. R. Møller, *Intraoperative Neurophysiological Monitoring*, 2nd ed. Totowa, NJ: Humana Press, 2006.
44. B. Fan, H. X. Li, and Y. Hu, "An Intelligent Decision System for Intraoperative Somatosensory Evoked Potential Monitoring," (in English), *IEEE Transactions on Neural Systems and Rehabilitation Engineering*, vol. 24, no. 2, pp. 300–307, Feb 2016.
45. J. T. Senders et al., "Machine Learning and Neurosurgical Outcome Prediction: A Systematic Review," *World Neurosurgery*, vol. 109, pp. 476–486.e1, Jan 2018.
46. A. R. Antony et al., "Functional Connectivity Estimated from Intracranial EEG Predicts Surgical Outcome in Intractable Temporal Lobe Epilepsy," *PLoS One*, vol. 8, no. 10, p. e77916, 2013.
47. J. E. Arle, K. Perrine, O. Devinsky, and W. K. Doyle, "Neural Network Analysis of Preoperative Variables and Outcome in Epilepsy Surgery," *Journal of Neurosurgery*, vol. 90, no. 6, pp. 998–1004, Jun 1999.
48. R. Armananzas et al., "Machine Learning Approach for the Outcome Prediction of Temporal Lobe Epilepsy Surgery," *PLoS One*, vol. 8, no. 4, p. e62819, 2013.
49. B. C. Bernhardt, S. J. Hong, A. Bernasconi, and N. Bernasconi, "Magnetic Resonance Imaging Pattern Learning in Temporal Lobe Epilepsy: Classification and Prognostics," *Annals of Neurology*, vol. 77, no. 3, pp. 436–464, Mar 2015.
50. D. L. Feis, J. C. Schoene-Bake, C. Elger, J. Wagner, M. Tittgemeyer, and B. Weber, "Prediction of Post-Surgical Seizure Outcome in Left Mesial Temporal Lobe Epilepsy," *Neuroimage: Clinical*, vol. 2, pp. 903–911, 2013.
51. J. Grigsby, R. E. Kramer, J. L. Schneiders, J. R. Gates, and W. B. Smith, "Predicting Outcome of Anterior Temporal Lobectomy Using Simulated Neural Networks," (in English), *Epilepsia*, vol. 39, no. 1, pp. 61–66, Jan 1998.
52. N. Memarian, S. Kim, S. Dewar, J. Engel, Jr., and R. J. Staba, "Multimodal Data and Machine Learning for Surgery Outcome Prediction in Complicated Cases of Mesial Temporal Lobe Epilepsy," *Computers in Biology and Medicine*, vol. 64, pp. 67–78, Sep 2015.

53. B. C. Munsell et al., "Evaluation of Machine Learning Algorithms for Treatment Outcome Prediction in Patients with Epilepsy Based on Structural Connectome Data," *Neuroimage*, vol. 118, pp. 219–230, Sep 2015.
54. J. Yankam Njiwa, K. R. Gray, N. Costes, F. Mauguiere, P. Ryvlin, and A. Hammers, "Advanced [(18)F]FDG and [(11)C]flumazenil PET Analysis for Individual Outcome Prediction after Temporal Lobe Epilepsy Surgery for Hippocampal Sclerosis," *Neuroimage: Clinical*, vol. 7, pp. 122–131, 2015.
55. K. E. Emblem, B. Nedregaard, J. K. Hald, T. Nome, P. Due-Tonnessen, and A. Bjornerud, "Automatic Glioma Characterization from Dynamic Susceptibility Contrast Imaging: Brain Tumor Segmentation Using Knowledge-Based Fuzzy Clustering," (in English), *Journal of Magnetic Resonance Imaging*, vol. 30, no. 1, pp. 1–10, Jul 2009.
56. K. E. Emblem et al., "A Generic Support Vector Machine Model for Preoperative Glioma Survival Associations," *Radiology*, vol. 275, no. 1, pp. 228–234, Apr 2015.
57. K. E. Emblem et al., "Machine Learning in Preoperative Glioma MRI: Survival Associations by Perfusion-Based Support Vector Machine Outperforms Traditional MRI," *Journal of Magnetic Resonance Imaging*, vol. 40, no. 1, pp. 47–54, Jul 2014.
58. M. A. Knoll et al., "Survival of Patients with Multiple Intracranial Metastases Treated with Stereotactic Radiosurgery: Does the Number of Tumors Matter?," *American Journal of Clinical Oncology*, vol. 41, no. 5, pp. 425–431, May 2018.
59. P. Azimi, S. Shahzadi, and S. Sadeghi, "Use of Artificial Neural Networks to Predict the Probability of Developing New Cerebral Metastases after Radiosurgery Alone," (in English), *Journal of Neurosurgical Sciences*, vol. 64, no. 1, pp. 52–57, Feb 2020.
60. H. Akbari et al., "Imaging Surrogates of Infiltration Obtained Via Multiparametric Imaging Pattern Analysis Predict Subsequent Location of Recurrence of Glioblastoma," *Neurosurgery*, vol. 78, no. 4, pp. 572–580, Apr 2016.
61. H. Y. Shi, S. L. Hwang, K. T. Lee, and C. L. Lin, "In-Hospital Mortality after Traumatic Brain Injury Surgery: A Nationwide Population-Based Comparison of Mortality Predictors Used in Artificial Neural Network and Logistic Regression Models," *Journal of Neurosurgery*, vol. 118, no. 4, pp. 746–52, Apr 2013.
62. B. Y. Gravesteijn et al., "Machine Learning Algorithms Performed No Better Than Regression Models for Prognostication in Traumatic Brain Injury," (in English), *Journal of Clinical Epidemiology*, vol. 122, pp. 95–107, Jun 2020.
63. K. Kostoglou, K. P. Michmizos, P. Stathis, D. Sakas, K. S. Nikita, and G. D. Mitsis, "Classification and Prediction of Clinical Improvement in Deep Brain Stimulation from Intraoperative Microelectrode Recordings," *IEEE Transactions on Biomedical Engineering*, vol. 64, no. 5, pp. 1123–1130, May 2017.

64. R. R. Shamir, T. Dolber, A. M. Noecker, B. L. Walter, and C. C. McIntyre, "Machine Learning Approach to Optimizing Combined Stimulation and Medication Therapies for Parkinson's Disease," *Brain Stimulation*, vol. 8, no. 6, pp. 1025–1032, Nov–Dec 2015.
65. Z. DeVries et al., "Development of an Unsupervised Machine Learning Algorithm for the Prognostication of Walking Ability in Spinal Cord Injury Patients," *Spine Journal*, vol. 20, no. 2, pp. 213–224, Feb 2020.
66. T. Inoue et al., "XGBoost, a Machine Learning Method, Predicts Neurological Recovery in Patients with Cervical Spinal Cord Injury," *Neurotrauma Reports*, vol. 1, pp. 8–16, Jan 1, 2020.
67. H. Hoffman et al., "Use of Multivariate Linear Regression and Support Vector Regression to Predict Functional Outcome after Surgery for Cervical Spondylotic Myelopathy," (in English), *Journal of Clinical Neuroscience*, vol. 22, no. 9, pp. 1444–1449, Sep 2015.
68. Z. G. Merali, C. D. Witiw, J. H. Badhiwala, J. R. Wilson, and M. G. Fehlings, "Using a Machine Learning Approach to Predict Outcome after Surgery for Degenerative Cervical Myelopathy," *PLoS One*, vol. 14, no. 4, p. e0215133, 2019.
69. O. Khan, J. H. Badhiwala, C. D. Witiw, J. R. Wilson, and M. G. Fehlings, "Machine Learning Algorithms for Prediction of Health-Related Quality-of-Life after Surgery for Mild Degenerative Cervical Myelopathy," *Spine Journal*, Feb 8, 2020.
70. A. V. Karhade et al., "Machine Learning for Prediction of Sustained Opioid Prescription after Anterior Cervical Discectomy and Fusion," *Spine Journal*, vol. 19, no. 6, pp. 976–983, Jun 2019.
71. A. V. Karhade et al., "Development of Machine Learning Algorithms for Prediction of Prolonged Opioid Prescription after Surgery for Lumbar Disc Herniation," *Spine Journal*, vol. 19, no. 11, pp. 1764–1771, Nov 2019.
72. A. V. Karhade et al., "Development of Machine Learning Algorithms for Prediction of Discharge Disposition after Elective Inpatient Surgery for Lumbar Degenerative Disc Disorders," *Neurosurgical Focus*, vol. 45, no. 5, p. E6, Nov 1, 2018.
73. S. Kuhle et al., "Comparison of Logistic Regression with Machine Learning Methods for the Prediction of Fetal Growth Abnormalities: A Retrospective Cohort Study," *BMC Pregnancy Childbirth*, vol. 18, no. 1, p. 333, Aug 15, 2018.
74. J. A. Cruz and D. S. Wishart, "Applications of Machine Learning in Cancer Prediction and Prognosis," *Cancer Informatics*, vol. 2, pp. 59–77, Feb 11, 2007.
75. W. Luo et al., "Guidelines for Developing and Reporting Machine Learning Predictive Models in Biomedical Research: A Multidisciplinary View," *Journal of Medical Internet Research*, vol. 18, no. 12, p. e323, Dec 16, 2016.
76. W. K. Tan et al., "Comparison of Natural Language Processing Rules-based and Machine-learning Systems to Identify Lumbar Spine Imaging Findings Related to Low Back Pain," *Academic Radiology*, vol. 25, no. 11, pp. 1422–1432, Nov 2018.

77. J. Likitlersuang, E. R. Sumitro, T. S. Cao, R. J. Visee, S. Kalsi-Ryan, and J. Zariffa, "Egocentric Video: A New Tool for Capturing Hand Use of Individuals with Spinal Cord Injury at Home," (in English), *Journal of Neuroengineering and Rehabilitation*, vol. 16, Jul 5, 2019.
78. T. S. Toh, F. Dondelinger, and D. Wang, "Looking beyond the Hype: Applied AI and Machine Learning in Translational Medicine," *EBioMedicine*, vol. 47, pp. 607–615, Sep 2019.
79. R. Challen, J. Denny, M. Pitt, L. Gompels, T. Edwards, and K. Tsaneva-Atanasova, "Artificial Intelligence, Bias and Clinical Safety," *BMJ Quality Safety*, vol. 28, no. 3, pp. 231–237, Mar 2019.
80. H. Nishi et al., "Predicting Clinical Outcomes of Large Vessel Occlusion Before Mechanical Thrombectomy Using Machine Learning," (in English), *Stroke*, vol. 50, no. 9, pp. 2379–2388, Sep 2019.

CHAPTER 13

A Novel MRA-Based Framework for the Detection of Cerebrovascular Changes and Correlation to Blood Pressure

Ingy El-Torgoman

Pharos University in Alexandria
Alexandria, Egypt

Ahmed Soliman, Ali Mahmoud, Ahmed Shalaby, and Guruprasad Giridharan

University of Louisville
Louisville, Kentucky

Mohammed Ghazal

Abu Dhabi University
Abu Dhabi, United Arab Emirates

Jasjit S. Suri
AtheroPoint LLC
Roseville, California

Ayman El-Baz
University of Louisville
Louisville, Kentucky
University of Louisville at AlAlamein
International University (UofL-AIU)
New Alamein City, Egypt

CONTENTS

13.1 INTRODUCTION

High blood pressure (HBP) affects approximately 1 in 3 adults in the United States. HBP has been the main reason or has significantly contributed to the mortality rate of 410,000 adults on a yearly basis, with associated healthcare costs of $46 billion [1]. The primary causes for HBP and elevated cerebrovascular perfusion pressure (CPP) vary, but are mainly chronic stress [2], an increasing intake of sodium [3], and problems in kidney functions [4]. CPP is the perfusion pressure in the brain, which is dependent on local vascular impedance and cerebral autoregulation. Blood vessels in the brain are affected by chronically elevated CPP, leading to changes in their structure, as well as disruptions in the mechanisms of cerebral vasoregulation. Significantly, high CPP induces hypertrophic and eutrophic remodeling in cerebral blood vessels [5]. In hypertrophic remodeling, changes in the structure of cerebral blood vessels, caused by elevated CPP, can be seen as the wall of blood vessels becomes thicker and their lumen is reduced. For eutrophic remodeling, cells of smooth muscles undergo a rearrangement that results in maintaining the mass and wall thickness of the totality of the blood vessels, while reducing their lumen. These cerebrovascular changes are hypothesized to be a significant contributor to strokes, brain lesions, cerebral ischemic injury, dementia, and cognitive impairment [5–7].

Currently, HBP is diagnosed and medically managed when systemic BP measurements using a sphygmomanometer are greater than 140/90 mmHg. However, BP measurement via a sphygmomanometer cannot quantify cerebrovascular structural changes that can increase the risk of cerebral adverse events. Many studies have recently concluded that variations in the structure of the cerebrovascular system, as well as those in CPP, may arise before systemic BP becomes elevated, rather than cerebrovascular damage due to sustained exposure to HBP [8–11]. As such, being able to calculate the changes that take place in the cerebrovascular system can lead to the identification and the stratification of those at risk of unfortunate cerebral events. This can lead to treatment well before systemic hypertension sets in, in conjunction with other cognitive tests, and can optimize medical management of HBP patients.

Magnetic Resonance Imaging (MRI) and Magnetic Resonance Angiography (MRA) scans represent imaging techniques, traditionally used to quantify structural changes in organs. In the literature, MRI scanning has been used for volumetric measurement of the ventricular cavities and myocardium [12] and to determine intravascular pressures from magnetic resonance (MR) velocity data in large vessels like the aorta or pulmonary artery [13]. MRA scanning has been used to quantify measurements of the flow in the collateral arteries of patients that have occlusions in the internal carotid artery [14]. To the best of our knowledge, neither MRA nor MRI has been utilized for the estimation of vascular pressure changes in the brain. Detection of cerebrovascular or CPP changes, by analyzing MRAs, has not been successful due to the lack of accurate segmentation algorithms that can mark and separate the small blood vessels within the brain (in comparison to the aorta or pulmonary arteries) from the surrounding soft tissue. Furthermore, there are no methods to measure changes in the cerebrovascular structure and to find the relation between such changes and those in mean arterial pressure, MAP, from MRI/MRA imaging. This manuscript presents novel methodologies to delineate cerebral blood vessels from the surrounding tissue, measure changes in the cerebrovascular structure, and correlate between these changes and MAP.

13.2 METHODS

The aim of the present paper is to develop a new method to detect cerebrovascular structural changes based on the use of MRA and demonstrate the proof-of-concept of correlation between cerebrovascular structural changes to MAP. Patient demographics and details about the proposed methodology and data analysis are presented next.

13.2.1 Patient Demographics

The Institutional Review Board (IRB) at the University of Pittsburgh has granted its approval for the accomplishment of this work. Patients' (n = 15, M = 8, F = 7, and age = 49.2±7.3) data and measurements have been obtained over a period of 700 days. These data and measurements included MRA and systemic BP, respectively. They were all analyzed in retrospect. The selection of the 15 study participants was made so that the changes in their blood pressure (BP) would represent a wide range over the duration of the study. As for MRAs, they were analyzed without identifying BP measurements of the patient whose images were being analyzed. The 3T Trio TIM scanner, employing a 12-channel phased-array head coil, was used to obtain MRA images. The average of four measurements, obtained from readings by a sphygmomanometer, was used to determine BP and MAP. The readings were taken during patient visits right before MRI scanning. Each set of scans consisted of 3D multi-slab high-resolution images, which included 160 slices, whose thickness was 0.5 mm. Image resolution was 384×448. Moreover, the voxel's size was $0.6\times0.6\times1.0\,\text{mm}^3$. The echo time was 3.8 ms, the flip angle was 15°, and the repetition time was 21 ms. The scan took 7 minutes 39 seconds and did not require any contrast.

The subjects had an average day 0 systolic pressure of 122±6.9 mmHg, an average day 0 diastolic pressure of 82±3.8 mmHg, an average day 700 systolic pressure of 118.9±12.4 mmHg, and an average day 700 diastolic pressure of 79.9±11.0 mmHg, i.e. the mean systolic pressure remained comparable over time though some individuals had increased pressure and some had decreased pressure or stayed the same.

13.2.2 Data Analysis

The analysis of patient MRA data consists of five key steps (Figure 13.1) consisting of: (1) manual segmentation of training slices to identify ground

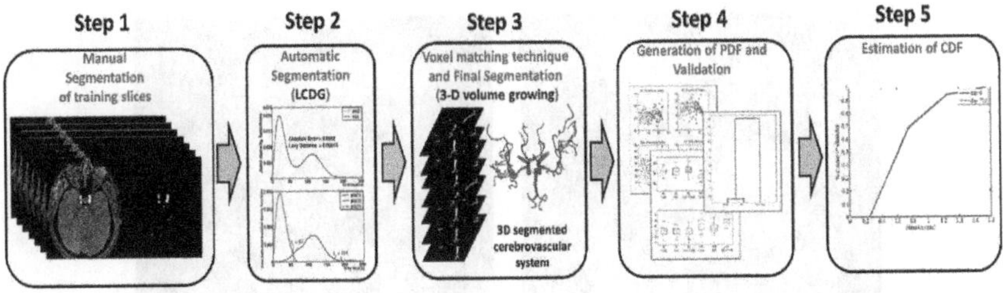

FIGURE 13.1 Framework of the data analysis for quantifying cerebrovascular changes from MRA imaging data.

truth, (2) automatic segmentation for all slices to delineate the blood vessels from the surrounding soft tissue by combining the segmented ground truths with the Linear Combination of Discrete Gaussians (LCDG) models for gray level distribution, (3) voxel matching for obtaining temporal subtraction images to enhance the ability to see cerebrovascular change via a distance map created to quantify the change in patients between day 0 and day 700, (4) generation of a probability distribution function (PDF) which describes the distribution of pixel distances from vascular edges and is used to statistically correlate to BP, and (5) estimation of CDF, otherwise known as the cumulative distribution function, to observe the summated probability of cerebrovascular changes in the same patient from the first day of the trial (day 0) to its very last (day 700).

Manual Segmentation of Training Slices: MRA data from a patient consist of 160 MRA slices. Every tenth slice is manually segmented to extract the blood vessels from surrounding tissue using Adobe Photoshop (Adobe Systems, CA). This methodology allows for delineation of the in-plane blood vessel from the surrounding tissue at a pixel level accuracy where the largest limitation is the resolution of the MRI machine itself. The manually segmented training binary (black for the surrounding tissue and white for the target vasculature) slices are referred to as a ground truth (GT) as the images are correct and free from artifacts or noise (Figure 13.2). The manual segmentation of select slices is used for the initialization and optimization of the segmentation algorithm, which is subsequently used for segmenting all obtained slices.

Automatic Segmentation: One of the most challenging issues relating to common computer-assisted diagnostics is the segmentation of accurate 3D cerebrovascular system information from MRA images. Our approach is to rapidly and accurately extract the blood vessel data by defining the probability models for all regions of interest within the statistical approach and not predefining the probability models [15–17]. For each MRA slice, an

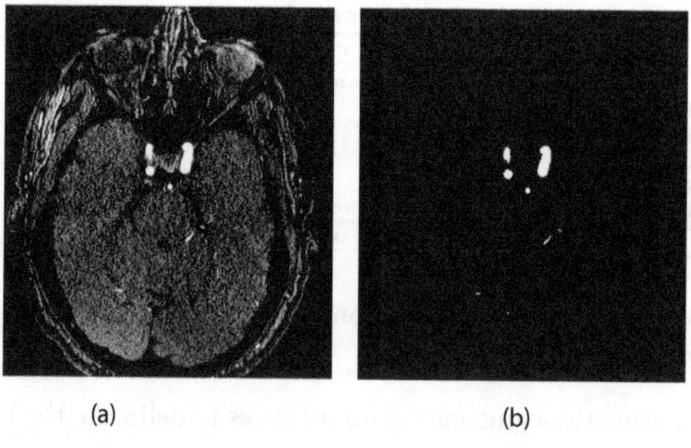

FIGURE 13.2 (a) Original MRA image slice of sample patient at day 0. (b) Manually segmented ground truth (GT) image from the image in (a).

LCDG is used as a close approximation of the empirical gray level distribution. Then, this slice is divided into individualized LCDGs (three per slice). Each of them represents one of the following dominant modes, which are represented by dark gray, light gray, and bright gray, marking bones and fat, brain tissue, and blood vessels, respectively. In order to identify blood vessels in every slice, the determined models mark a certain intensity threshold. The next step is to apply a 3D connectivity filter on the extracted voxels (voxel = volume×element; a representation for a 3D pixel) to select the desired vascular tree. This method results in higher precision region models with higher segmentation accuracy compared to other methods [16].

Adapting the Expectation–Maximization-based technique (EM-based technique) to the LCDG allows to precisely identify the specific model, including its number components (positive and negative) [18], and to identify a continuous LCDG model that contains the probability distribution.

To identify the LCDG model, a criterion, consisting of expected log-likelihoods, is employed [16]. Consider that a 3D MRA image is represented by $\mathbf{X} = (\mathbf{X}_s: s = 1,\ldots, S)$, which contains S co-registered 2D slices $\mathbf{X}_s = (X_s\,(i, j): (i, j) \in R;\, X_s\,(i, j) \in Q)$. On the other hand, a rectangular arithmetic lattice supporting the 3D image is represented by $\mathbf{R}$ and a finite set of gray levels and Q-ary intensities are represented by $\mathbf{Q} = \{0, 1,\ldots, Q{-}1\}$. Consider $\mathbf{F}_s = (f_s\,(q): q \in \mathbf{Q}; \sum_{q\in\mathbf{Q}} f_s\,(q) = 1$; in this equation, q is one of the gray levels, considered to be an empirical marginal probability distribution for gray levels of the slice $\mathbf{X}_s$ within the MRA.

According to Ref. [18], each slice of the MRA image is thought of as a K-modal one, having a determined number K of the main modes of the regions of interest. For the segmentation of the slice by modes separating, it is important to estimate the probability distributions of the signals individually. Said signals associate each mode from $\boldsymbol{F}_s$. $\boldsymbol{F}_s$ is closely approximated with LCDG opposing the conventional mixture of Gaussians, one per region, or slightly more flexible mixtures involving other simple distributions, one per region. Sub-models, each representing a dominant mode, are the result of the division of the LCDG image [19–21].

A discrete Gaussian distribution is defined on the set of integers (gray levels) $\boldsymbol{Q}=\{0,1,\ldots,Q-1\}$ by the probability mass function

$$\psi(q|\theta)=\begin{cases}\Phi(0.5), & q=0\\ \Phi(q+0.5)-\Phi(q-0.5) & 1\le q<Q-1\\ 1-\Phi(q-0.5), & q=Q-1,\end{cases}$$

where the parameter $\theta=(\mu,\sigma)$, and Φ is the CDF of a normal distribution with mean μ and variance σ^2. Then the LCDG with C_p positive components and C_n negative components, such that $C_p \ge K$, has the probability mass function

$$p_{w,\Theta}(q)=\sum_{r=1}^{C_p} w_{p,r}\psi(q|\theta_{p,r})-\sum_{l=1}^{C_n} w_{n,l}\psi(q|\theta_{n,l}) \tag{13.1}$$

The weights $\boldsymbol{w}=(w_{p,1},\ldots,w_{p,C_p},w_{n,1},\ldots,w_{n,C_n})$ are restricted to be all non-negative and to satisfy

$$\sum_{r=1}^{C_p} w_{p,r}-\sum_{l=1}^{C_n} w_{n,l}=1 \tag{13.2}$$

In general, for a probability to be valid, it has to be non-negative: $p_{w,\Theta}(q)\ge 0$ for all $q\in\boldsymbol{Q}$. This implies that a valid subset of all the LCDGs in (13.1) only uses the probability distributions. This subset can however have negative components, $p_{w,\Theta}(q)<0$ for some $q\in\boldsymbol{Q}$.

It is the aim of this study to find a K-modal probability model, which closely approximates the marginal distribution of gray level, which is not known. If $\boldsymbol{F}$ is the Bayesian estimate of $\boldsymbol{F}_s$, the former can be described as follows [22]: $f(q)=(|\mathbf{R}|f_s(q)+1)/(|\mathbf{R}|+Q)$. The model to be devised should work on increasing the expected log-likelihood of the statistically independent empirical data to its maximum limits, along with its other parameters:

$$L(\boldsymbol{w},\Theta)=\sum_{q\in\boldsymbol{Q}} f(q)\log p_{w,\Theta}(q) \tag{13.3}$$

The algorithm used in segmentation in its entirety is as follows [16].

1. For each slice $\boldsymbol{X}_s$, $s = 1, \ldots S$,
   a. The first is to gather the marginal empirical probability distribution F_s, which represents gray levels.
   b. Pinpoint a starting LCDG model, which is close to F_s. This is done with the use of the initialization algorithm, which can approximate the values of C_p–K, C_n, and the parameters $\boldsymbol{w}$, $\boldsymbol{\Theta}$ (marking weights, means, and variances) of both negative and positive discrete Gaussians (DG).
   c. Fix C_p and C_n, use the modified EM algorithm to refine the LCDG-model by manipulating other parameters.
   d. Make K submodels by separating the final LCDG model. There would be a submodel for each dominant mode. This is done by minimizing the misclassification predicted errors and selecting the LCDG-submodel that has the greatest average value (corresponding to the pixels with the highest brightness) to be the model of the wanted vasculature.
   e. Use intensity threshold t to extract the voxels of the blood vessels in the MRA slice, which separates their LCDG-submodel from the background.
2. Remove the artifacts from the extracted voxels whole set with the help of a connection filter, which chooses a system to construct by a 3D growing algorithm, which comes in the form of the greatest connected tree [23]. Algorithm 13.1 summarizes the adopted segmentation approach:

Algorithm 13.1: Main Steps of the Segmentation Approach

For each slice $\boldsymbol{X}_s$, the following steps were completed:

1. LCDG Initialization:

   Find the marginal empirical probability distribution of gray levels ***Fs***.

   - Estimate $C_p - K, C_n, \boldsymbol{W}$, and $\boldsymbol{\Theta}$ of the positive and negative DGs.
   - Find the initial LCDG-model that approximates $\boldsymbol{F}_s$.

2. LCDG Refinement:
    - Fixing C_p and C_n, refine the LCDG-model with the modified EM algorithm by manipulating other parameters.
3. Initial Segmentation:
- Divide the final LCDG-model into K submodels by minimizing the expected errors of misclassification.
    - Select the LCDG-submodel that has the largest mean value to be the model of the wanted vasculature.
    - Use the intensity threshold t to extract the voxels of the blood vessels in the MRA slice, separating their LCDG-submodel from the background.
4. Final Segmentation:
    - Remove the artifacts from the extracted voxels whole set with a connection filter, which chooses the greatest connected tree system built by a 3D growing algorithm.

This procedure aims to decipher each MRA slice's threshold, which will enable the complete extraction of the bright blood vessels while removing the darker unwanted tissue while also separating surrounding non-vasculature tissue that may be of similar brightness and along the same boundaries. When step 1b is initialized, the LCDG with the non-negative beginning probabilities $p_{w,\theta}(q)$ is created. In step 1c, a refinement takes place, increasing the likelihood, but still, probabilities are non-negative. In Ref. [16], experiments showed that the opposite situations never took place.

Automatic segmentation's accuracy is evaluated by calculating total error compared to the ground truths. For evaluation purposes, segmentations are measured, including both true positive (TP) and true negative (TN), as well as false positive (FP) and false negative (FN).

In Figure 13.3, if C is the segmented region, G is the ground truth, and R represents the entire image frame, then the TP = |C∩G|, TN = |R−C∪G|, FP = |C−C∩G|, and FN = |G−C∩G|. The total error ε is given in Ref. [24] as $\varepsilon = (FN + FP)/(TP + FN) = (FN + FP)/G$.

Matching of Voxels: Voxels are defined as an array of volume elements, which constitute a notional 3D space. A 3D affine registration is used to handle the pose, orientation, and the data spacing changes and other scanning parameter changes between day 0 and day 700 [25]. In this step, the determined Euclidian radii are converted into diameter values. The output is then converted into a distance map.

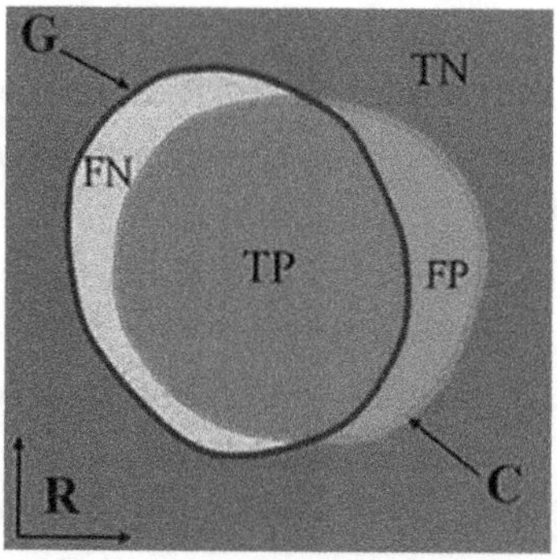

FIGURE 13.3 Illustration of segmentation accuracy and errors of the proposed automatic segmentation (C) by comparing to the ground truth (G) [5].

Generation of Probability Distribution Function and Validation: The EM-based technique is adapted to the LCDG-model. In order to calculate the probability distribution of changes in the cerebrovascular structure, the distance map is used to extract the distribution of pixel distances. The distribution of white pixels is marked by the PDF, as a true value and black pixels being ignored for the data set. The diameters of the blood vessels are determined by estimating Euclidian center point distances from the edge of a vessel. The data points in the generated PDFs are then extracted and compared to the BP data using statistical analysis.

Calculation of Cumulative Distribution Function: The integral of the PDF is used to generate the CDF. (The CDF F_X of a random variable X is calculated from its PDF f_X using $F_X(x)=\int_{-\infty}^{x} f_X(t)dt$.) The CDF shows the total summated probability that a blood vessel will take a value less than or equal to a diameter value that represents an average blood vessel diameter in each slice. It shows the cumulative distribution of the PDF with an upper limit of 1. The more quickly the CDF line approaches 1, the more certain that the diameter of the blood vessel is smaller compared to a CDF that takes longer to approach 1. This is illustrated in the Results section.

13.2.3 Statistical Analysis

Statistical analysis was performed using R software, version 3.3. A mixed effects linear model was used to test the relationship of MRA data with clinical BP measurements. Brain slices were separated into upper (above the circle of Willis) and lower (below the circle of Willis) compartments to determine the correlation with clinical BP readings. The circle of Willis, near the brain base, is where the intracranial cerebral arteries take off from and give rise to progressively smaller vessels [5]. The BP measurements were combined into a single value, the estimated MAP = (2×DBP + SBP)/3, which was a covariate in the model. Also included in the model were patient age, gender, and a random intercept per patient. The dependent variable was the mean of the Euclidean distance map over the entire vascular tree within each compartment. (Two separate models were fit to the upper and lower compartments.) Statistical significance of fixed effects in the fitted models was determined using likelihood ratio chi-squared tests.

13.2.4 3D Reconstruction of the Cerebral Vasculature

A growing tree model that eliminates any unwanted segmented voxels by choosing the greatest connected vascular tree system, coupled with a smoothing algorithm, was used to generate a 3D model based on segmented slices [23]. An example for the resultant vascular system is visualized and illustrated in the Results section.

13.3 RESULTS

Specificity and sensitivity values were obtained from the segmented images as shown below in Table 13.1. The automatically segmented slices for all 15 patients were compared to the manually segmented GTs to determine the accuracy of the algorithm (Figure 13.4). The segmentation algorithm resulted in a cumulative sensitivity of 0.997±0.008 (sensitivity range = 0.969–1) and the cumulative specificity of 0.9998±0.0001 (specificity range = 0.9994–1). The manually segmented training slices (every tenth slice) were excluded in the accuracy calculations of the proposed segmentation approach.

TABLE 13.1 Sensitivity and Specificity Values for Automatically Segmented Images at Day 0, Day 700, and Cumulative Sensitivity and Specificity Values

Time	Sensitivity	Specificity
Day 0	0.997±0.006	0.9998±0.0001
Day 700	0.996±0.008	0.9998±0.0001
Cumulative	0.997±0.008	0.9998±0.0001

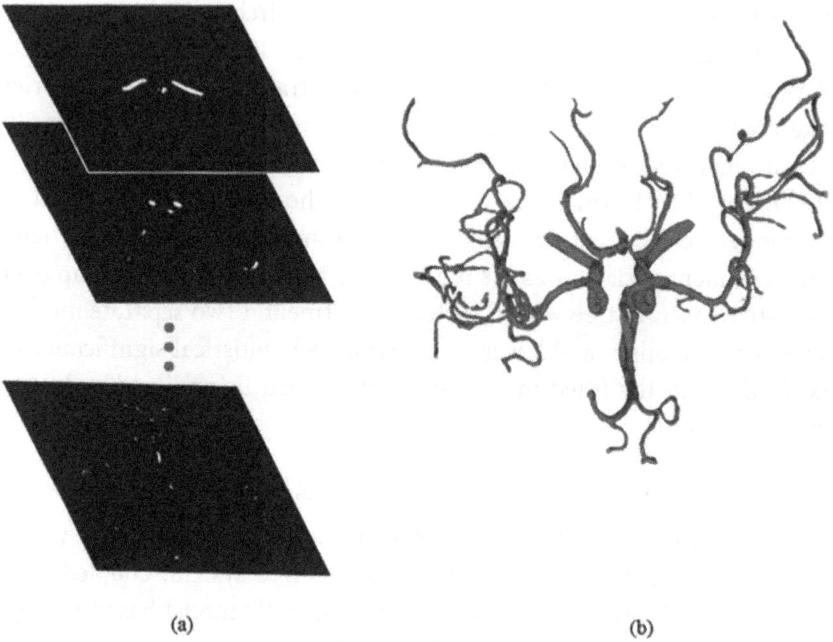

FIGURE 13.4 Example of segmentation algorithm output; (a) sample image slices of a patient at day 0. The automatically segmented slices were compared to the manually segmented ground truths (GT) to determine the accuracy of the segmentation algorithm. (b) Sample 3D reconstruction of the segmented cerebrovascular system using a growing tree model.

The results of the linear mixed effects models analysis (Table 13.2) revealed an inverse relationship between MAP and the mean vessel diameter below the circle of Willis ($P = 0.0007$). The mean diameter of vessels below the circle of Willis was not found to vary significantly with the age of the patient or the gender of the patient. Above the circle of Willis, the mean diameters of vessels showed a statistically significant decrease with age ($P = 0.0005$).

In the analysis, 13 out of 15 patients showed a significant correlation between MAP and the diameters indicated via CDF. Out of the 13 patients that showed CDF correlation with MAP, two example patients (A and B) are shown with the two patients (C and D) where the correlation between CDF and MAP was not found (Figure 13.5). Patient C had a shift in CDF that is in opposition to the MAP change, and patient D had

TABLE 13.2 Mixed Effects Linear Model Statistical Evaluation

	Mean Diameter of Vessels below the Circle of Willis		
	Effect	χ^2	***P*-Value**
Age	3.2 μm/y	0.356	0.551
Gender	F>M by 12.8 μm	0.026	0.872
Mean arterial pressure	−5.3 μm/mmHg	11.63	0.0007
	Mean Diameter of Vessels above the Circle of Willis		
	Effect	χ^2	***P*-Value**
Age	−16.5 μm/y	12.29	0.0005
Gender	F>M by 16.0 μm	0.199	0.655
Mean arterial pressure	1.6 μm/mmHg	0.402	0.525

P-values < 0.05 was considered statistically significant. The diameter denotes the size of vasculature in segmentation images. Age, gender, and timepoints are clinically acquired data.

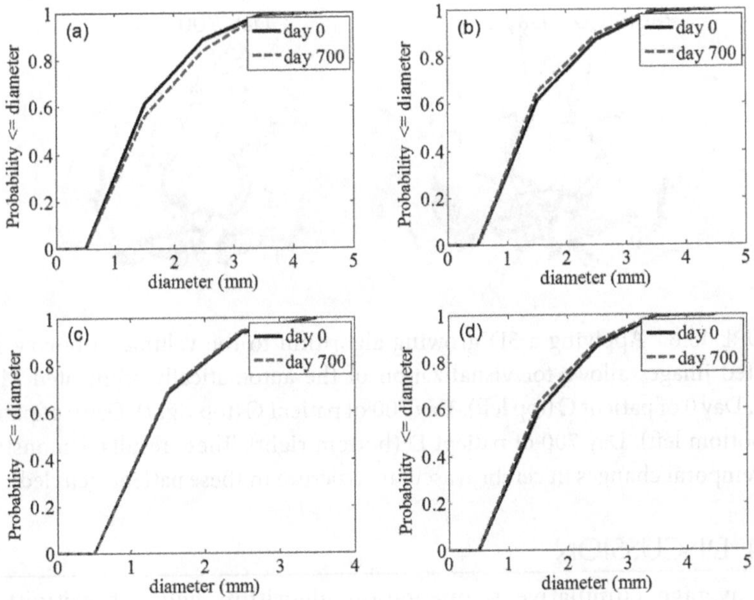

FIGURE 13.5 Sample patient CDFs demonstrating the temporal changes from day 0 to 700. The graphs indicate the probability that blood vessels may be of a certain diameter or less.

a larger shift in CDF compared to the MAP change (Figure 13.5c and d, Table 13.3). The 3D cerebrovascular model reconstruction of patients C and D indicated significant vascular changes between day 0 and day 700 (Figure 13.6).

TABLE 13.3 BP Measurements of Patients A, B, C, and D

	Day 0			Day 700		
Patient	Systolic BP	Diastolic BP	MAP	Systolic BP	Diastolic BP	MAP
A	120	80.5	93.7	103.5	66.5	78.8
B	130.5	83	98.8	143.5	94	110.5
C	118	80.5	93	105.3	69	81.1
D	114	84.5	94.3	120	88	98.7

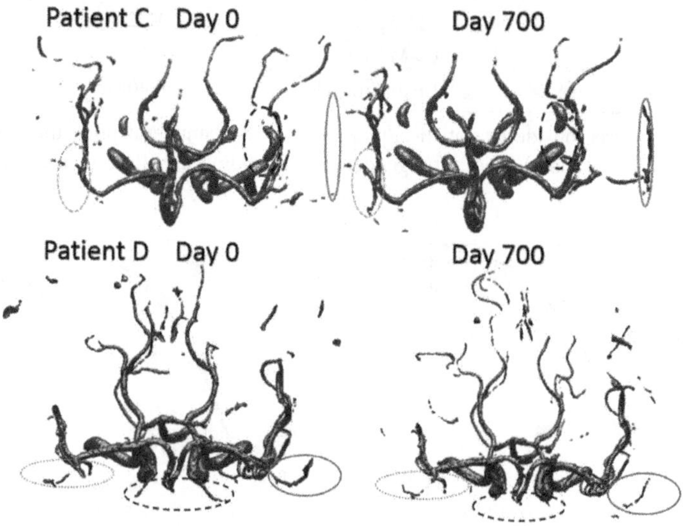

FIGURE 13.6 Applying a 3D growing algorithm to the volume of binary segmented images allows for visualization of the automatically segmented MRA data. Day 0 of patient C (top left). Day 700 of patient C (top right). Day 0 of patient D (bottom left). Day 700 of patient D (bottom right). These results demonstrate the temporal changes in cerebrovascular structure in these patients (circled).

13.4 DISCUSSION

The average cumulative segmentation algorithm had a sensitivity of 0.997±0.008 and a specificity of 0.9998±0.001. This high level of accuracy demonstrates the benefit of using a manual input to initialize automatic segmentation. Using manual segmentation alone would be too time intensive to be used in a practical healthcare setting, while utilizing only an automatic segmentation approach would not provide sufficient segmentation accuracy to delineate and quantify the diameters of the smaller arteriolar (< 10 μm) cerebral blood vessels. The proposed segmentation algorithm combines the accuracy of manual segmentation with the benefit of an automated and less time-intensive approach and provides segmentation with a high degree of accuracy while also minimizing the required time and effort.

The high degree of sensitivity and specificity of our approach in accurately delineating blood vessels from the surrounding brain tissue enables the quantification of cerebrovascular changes. The PDFs indicate the total blood vessel diameter change in time from day 0 to day 700. Below the circle of Willis, there is a statistical correlation between PDFs and systemic BP ($P = 0.0007$), demonstrating that increased MAP and consequently CPP are related to decreased average vessel diameter and PDF. The BP and MAP measurements correlate well with most patients' non-invasive mean PDF diameter measurements below the circle of Willis. Since cerebral changes have been hypothesized to precede systemic hypertension [9,10,26], our methodology may present a tool for potentially initiating early treatment to prevent or optimize management of systemic HBP in conjunction with other approaches including cognitive testing. This finding is important as it suggests that the remodeling of vessels due to increasing BP occurs prior to the onset of diagnosed essential hypertension. Individuals in the current study were explicitly selected to have pre-hypertensive values of BP of equal importance; the methodology can determine the relationship of cerebrovascular remodeling to cortical small vessel disease and lacunar lesions are known to occur with advanced hypertensive disease and with implications for stroke and dementia [27,28]. The correlation of PDF to MAP was independent of patient gender. The difference in PDF of vessels above the circle of Willis was statistically significant with age, which indicates that older patients have constricted cerebral vessels, which may put them at a higher risk of strokes.

In some patients (C and D), the change in CDF did not correlate to changes in MAP, which may indicate impaired autoregulation of cerebral blood flow potentially due to cerebrovascular remodeling [5,26]. The 3D cerebrovascular model reconstruction of these patients demonstrated significant vascular changes between day 0 and day 700. These results may indicate that drug therapies prescribed using systemic BP alone may not provide optimal medical management. Lack of correlation between CDF and MAP may indicate cerebrovascular changes and a higher risk of cerebrovascular adverse events which necessitates more frequent monitoring and/or optimization of medical management, despite having normal systemic BP and MAP. Using a combination of BP and CDF changes may help minimize the occurrence of adverse events.

The proposed approach uses MRA, which directly visualizes the overall cerebrovascular anatomy and provides a higher resolution for small blood vessels compared to Doppler Ultrasound which primarily assesses blood flow or the characteristics of a single or small number of vessels within its field of view. MRA is required for visualization of small cerebral blood vessels to obtain an accurate 3D vascular structure. Routine screening using the proposed MRA-based method would be expensive. The clinical application of importance would be to treatment-resistant hypertension, which is now poorly understood [29]. A recent study presents convincing data suggesting that such patients may have abnormalities of the vasculature, e.g. of the circle of Willis, that could be detected readily with our technique [30]. Other work has suggested that such hypertension may be due to impingement of the cerebral vasculature on brain stem BP regulatory areas [31]. These abnormalities could be detected with our technique. These vascular bases of hypertension, once identified, would guide clinical treatment in these cases which have not been remedied by currently used pharmacological dosing. Additionally, patients at a higher risk of developing hypertension due to familial or clinical history may be screened using the proposed approach despite the higher cost to detect vascular changes and manage high BP before disease onset.

The segmentation algorithm and metrics for vascular and BP changes (CDF and PDF) are not limited to the cerebral vasculature. These methodologies may also be used to quantify vascular changes in other end organs that are sensitive to BP (e.g. Kidneys).

13.5 LIMITATIONS

While our segmentation algorithm significantly improves on automatic segmentation methodologies, it is limited by the resolution limit of the MRI machine performing the MRA scanning. The CDF diameters (Figure 13.5) start at 0.5 mm because the distance map calculations determine the radius from the edge of a blood vessel and a pixel in the MRA imaging represented 0.25 mm. Any value less than 0.5 mm would not be accurately represented due to the resolution limit. Subsequently, the accuracy of the statistical analysis decreases with decreasing blood vessel size (smaller blood vessels $< 10\,\mu m$) above the circle of Willis).

Various over-the-counter medications and supplements were used by the subjects over the time period of this study; however, the BP changes caused by these medications should be minimal. Nonetheless, larger sample sizes are required to establish a definitive relationship with progression to HBP. While elevated CPP is hypothesized to precede systemic hypertension, essential hypertension remains likely due to a mosaic of causes that are not completely understood. Despite these limitations, our method is relevant to understanding brain pathology relevant to hypertension whether such pathology precedes or follows the establishment of clinical hypertension.

13.6 CONCLUSION

Changes in cerebral vasculature can be non-invasively obtained through MRA image analysis. Cerebrovascular changes are correlated to MAP below the circle of Willis. The improved segmentation algorithm coupled with the calculation of CDF and PDF can indicate cerebrovascular and cerebral perfusion pressure changes, which may be a useful tool for clinicians to optimize the medical management of HBP. In addition to the vascular system [32–41], this work could also be applied to various other applications in medical imaging, such as the prostate [42–44], the kidney [45–72], the heart [73–89], the lung [90–137], the brain [138–158], the retina [159–163], the bladder [164], and injury prediction [165] as well as several non-medical applications [166–171].

REFERENCES

1. C. f. D. Control. *About Underlying Cause of Death, 1999-2015*, 2015. Available: http://wonder.cdc.gov/ucd-icd10.html
2. S. Kulkarni, I. O'Farrell, M. Erasi, and M. Kochar, "Stress and hypertension," *WMJ: Official Publication of the State Medical Society of Wisconsin*, vol. 97, no. 11, pp. 34–38, 1998.
3. S. Mohan and N. R. Campbell, "Salt and high blood pressure," *Clinical Science*, vol. 117, no. 1, pp. 1–11, 2009.
4. M. J. Sarnak et al., "Kidney disease as a risk factor for development of cardiovascular disease," *Circulation*, vol. 108, no. 17, pp. 2154–2169, 2003.
5. C. Iadecola and R. L. Davisson, "Hypertension and cerebrovascular dysfunction," *Cell Metabolism*, vol. 7, no. 6, pp. 476–484, 2008.
6. E. J. Van Dijk et al., "The association between blood pressure, hypertension, and cerebral white matter lesions," *Hypertension*, vol. 44, no. 5, pp. 625–630, 2004.
7. M. Willmot, J. Leonardi-Bee, and P. M. Bath, "High blood pressure in acute stroke and subsequent outcome," *Hypertension*, vol. 43, no. 1, pp. 18–24, 2004.

8. J. N. Barnes et al., "Aortic hemodynamics and white matter hyperintensities in normotensive postmenopausal women," *Journal of Neurology*, vol. 264, no. 5, pp. 938–945, 2017.
9. J. R. Jennings et al., "Prehypertensive blood pressures and regional cerebral blood flow independently relate to cognitive performance in midlife," *Journal of the American Heart Association*, vol. 6, no. 3, p. e004856, 2017.
10. J. R. Jennings and Y. Zanstra, "Is the brain the essential in hypertension?," *Neuroimage*, vol. 47, no. 3, pp. 914–921, 2009.
11. L. J. Launer et al., "Vascular factors and multiple measures of early brain health: CARDIA brain MRI study," *PLoS One*, vol. 10, no. 3, p. e0122138, 2015.
12. R. J. Van der Geest and J. H. Reiber, "Quantification in cardiac MRI," *Journal of Magnetic Resonance Imaging*, vol. 10, no. 5, pp. 602–608, 1999.
13. A. A. Amini, J. Chen, and Y. Wang, "Imaging and analysis for determination of cardiovascular mechanics," in *Biomedical Imaging: From Nano to Macro, 2007. ISBI 2007. 4th IEEE International Symposium on*. IEEE, 2007, pp. 692–695.
14. K. Van Everdingen, C. Klijn, L. Kappelle, W. Mali, and J. Van der Grond, "MRA flow quantification in patients with a symptomatic internal carotid artery occlusion," *Stroke*, vol. 28, no. 8, pp. 1595–1600, 1997.
15. A. C. Chung and J. A. Noble, "Statistical 3D vessel segmentation using a Rician distribution," in *International Conference on Medical Image Computing and Computer-Assisted Intervention*. Springer, 1999, pp. 82–89.
16. A. El-Baz et al., "Precise segmentation of 3-D magnetic resonance angiography," *IEEE Transactions on Biomedical Engineering*, vol. 59, no. 7, pp. 2019–2029, 2012.
17. D. L. Wilson and J. A. Noble, "An adaptive segmentation algorithm for time-of-flight MRA data," *IEEE Transactions on Medical Imaging*, vol. 18, no. 10, pp. 938–945, 1999.
18. G. Gimel'farb, A. A. Farag, and A. El-Baz, "Expectation-maximization for a linear combination of Gaussians," in *Pattern Recognition, 2004. ICPR 2004. Proceedings of the 17th International Conference on*. IEEE, 2004, vol. 3, pp. 422–425.
19. N. D. Forkert et al., "Direction-dependent level set segmentation of cerebrovascular structures," in *SPIE Medical Imaging*. International Society for Optics and Photonics, 2011, pp. 79623S–79623S-8.
20. M. Holtzman-Gazit, R. Kimmel, N. Peled, and D. Goldsher, "Segmentation of thin structures in volumetric medical images," *IEEE Transactions on Image Processing*, vol. 15, no. 2, pp. 354–363, 2006.
21. C. Xu and J. L. Prince, "Snakes, shapes, and gradient vector flow," *IEEE Transactions on Image Processing*, vol. 7, no. 3, pp. 359–369, 1998.
22. A. R. Webb, *Statistical Pattern Recognition*, John Wiley & Sons, New York, USA, 2003.
23. M. Sabry, C. B. Sites, A. A. Farag, S. Hushek, and T. Moriarty, "A fast automatic method for 3D volume segmentation of the human cerebrovascular," in *CARS 2002 Computer Assisted Radiology and Surgery*. Springer, 2002, pp. 382–387.

24. K. Suzuki, "Computerized segmentation of organs by means of geodesic active-contour level-set algorithm," in *Multi Modality State-of-the-Art Medical Image Segmentation and Registration Methodologies*. Springer, 2011, pp. 103–128.
25. Y. Itai, H. Kim, S. Ishikawa, S. Katsuragawa, and K. Doi, "Development of a voxel-matching technique for substantial reduction of subtraction artifacts in temporal subtraction images obtained from thoracic MDCT," *Journal of Digital Imaging*, vol. 23, no. 1, pp. 31–38, 2010.
26. J. R. Jennings and A. F. Heim, "From brain to behavior: hypertension's modulation of cognition and affect," *International Journal of Hypertension*, vol. 2012, 2012.
27. P. B. Gorelick et al., "Vascular contributions to cognitive impairment and dementia," *Stroke*, vol. 42, no. 9, pp. 2672–2713, 2011.
28. C. Iadecola et al., "Impact of hypertension on cognitive function: a scientific statement from the American Heart Association," *Hypertension*, vol. 68, no. 6, pp. e67–e94, 2016.
29. P. K. Whelton et al., "2017 ACC/AHA/AAPA/ABC/ACPM/AGS/APhA/ASH/ASPC/NMA/PCNA guideline for the prevention, detection, evaluation, and management of high blood pressure in adults: a report of the American College of Cardiology/American Heart Association Task Force on Clinical Practice Guidelines," *Journal of the American College of Cardiology*, p. 24430, 2017.
30. E. A. Warnert et al., "Is high blood pressure self-protection for the brain?," *Circulation Research*, p. CIRCRESAHA. 116.309493, 2016.
31. E. I. Levy, A. M. Scarrow, and P. J. Jannetta, "Microvascular decompression in the treatment of hypertension: review and update," *World Neurosurgery*, vol. 55, no. 1, pp. 2–10, 2001.
32. A. Mahmoud, A. El-Barkouky, H. Farag, J. Graham, and A. Farag, "A non-invasive method for measuring blood flow rate in superficial veins from a single thermal image," in *Proceedings of the IEEE Conference on Computer Vision and Pattern Recognition Workshops*, 2013, pp. 354–359.
33. A. El-Baz, A. Farag, G. Gimel'farb, M. A. El-Ghar, and T. Eldiasty, "Probabilistic modeling of blood vessels for segmenting MRA images," in *18th International Conference on Pattern Recognition (ICPR'06)*. IEEE, vol. 3, 2006, pp. 917–920.
34. A. El-Baz, A. A. Farag, G. Gimel'farb, M. A. El-Ghar, and T. Eldiasty, "A new adaptive probabilistic model of blood vessels for segmenting MRA images," in *Medical Image Computing and Computer-Assisted Intervention–MICCAI 2006*. Springer, vol. 4191, 2006, pp. 799–806.
35. A. El-baz, A. Shalaby, F. Taher, M. El-Baz, M. Ghazal, M. A. El-Ghar, A. Takieldeen, and J. Suri, "Probabilistic modeling of blood vessels for segmenting magnetic resonance angiography images," in *Medical Research Archives*, 2017, vol. 5, no. 3.
36. A. S. Chowdhury, A. K. Rudra, M. Sen, A. Elnakib, and A. El-Baz, "Cerebral white matter segmentation from MRI using probabilistic graph cuts and geometric shape priors," in *ICIP*, 2010, pp. 3649–3652.

37. Y. Gebru, G. Giridharan, M. Ghazal, A. Mahmoud, A. Shalaby, and A. El-Baz, "Detection of cerebrovascular changes using magnetic resonance angiography," in *Cardiovascular Imaging and Image Analysis*. CRC Press, 2018, pp. 1–22.
38. A. Mahmoud, A. Shalaby, F. Taher, M. El-Baz, J. S. Suri, and A. El-Baz, "Vascular tree segmentation from different image modalities," in *Cardiovascular Imaging and Image Analysis*. CRC Press, 2018, pp. 43–70.
39. F. Taher, A. Mahmoud, A. Shalaby, and A. El-Baz, "A review on the cerebrovascular segmentation methods," in *2018 IEEE International Symposium on Signal Processing and Information Technology (ISSPIT)*. IEEE, 2018, pp. 359–364.
40. H. Kandil, A. Soliman, L. Fraiwan, A. Shalaby, A. Mahmoud, A. ElTanboly, A. Elmaghraby, G. Giridharan, and A. El-Baz, "A novel MRA framework based on integrated global and local analysis for accurate segmentation of the cerebral vascular system," in *2018 IEEE 15th International Symposium on Biomedical Imaging (ISBI 2018)*. IEEE, 2018, pp. 1365–1368.
41. F. Taher, A. Soliman, H. Kandil, A. Mahmoud, A. Shalaby, G. Gimel'farb, and A. El-Baz, "Accurate segmentation of cerebrovasculature from tof-MRA images using appearance descriptors," *IEEE Access*, 2020.
42. I. Reda, M. Ghazal, A. Shalaby, M. Elmogy, A. AbouEl-Fetouh, B. O. Ayinde, M. AbouEl-Ghar, A. Elmaghraby, R. Keynton, and A. El-Baz, "A novel ADCS-based CNN classification system for precise diagnosis of prostate cancer," in *2018 24th International Conference on Pattern Recognition (ICPR)*. IEEE, 2018, pp. 3923–3928.
43. I. Reda, A. Khalil, M. Elmogy, A. Abou El-Fetouh, A. Shalaby, M. Abou El-Ghar, A. Elmaghraby, M. Ghazal, and A. El-Baz, "Deep learning role in early diagnosis of prostate cancer," *Technology in Cancer Research & Treatment*, vol. 17, p. 1533034618775530, 2018.
44. I. Reda, B. O. Ayinde, M. Elmogy, A. Shalaby, M. El-Melegy, M. A. El-Ghar, A. A. El-fetouh, M. Ghazal, and A. El-Baz, "A new CNN-based system for early diagnosis of prostate cancer," in *2018 IEEE 15th International Symposium on Biomedical Imaging (ISBI 2018)*. IEEE, 2018, pp. 207–210.
45. A. S. Chowdhury, R. Roy, S. Bose, F. K. A. Elnakib, and A. El-Baz, "Non-rigid biomedical image registration using graph cuts with a novel data term," in *Proceedings of IEEE International Symposium on Biomedical Imaging: From Nano to Macro, (ISBI'12)*, Barcelona, Spain, May 2–5, 2012, pp. 446–449.
46. A. El-Baz, A. A. Farag, S. E. Yuksel, M. E. El-Ghar, T. A. Eldiasty, and M. A. Ghoneim, "Application of deformable models for the detection of acute renal rejection," in *Deformable Models*, Aly Farag, Ed. Springer, New York, NY, 2007, pp. 293–333.
47. A. El-Baz, A. Farag, R. Fahmi, S. Yuksel, M. A. El-Ghar, and T. Eldiasty, "Image analysis of renal DCE MRI for the detection of acute renal rejection," in *Proceedings of IAPR International Conference on Pattern Recognition (ICPR'06)*, Hong Kong, 2006, pp. 822–825.
48. A. El-Baz, A. Farag, R. Fahmi, S. Yuksel, W. Miller, M. A. El-Ghar, T. El-Diasty, and M. Ghoneim, "A new CAD system for the evaluation of kidney diseases using DCE-MRI," in *Proceedings of International Conference on Medical Image Computing and Computer-Assisted Intervention, (MICCAI'08)*, Copenhagen, Denmark, October 1–6, 2006, pp. 446–453.

49. A. El-Baz, G. Gimel'farb, and M. A. El-Ghar, "A novel image analysis approach for accurate identification of acute renal rejection," in *Proceedings of IEEE International Conference on Image Processing, (ICIP'08)*, San Diego, CA, October 12–15, 2008, pp. 1812–1815.
50. ——, "Image analysis approach for identification of renal transplant rejection," in *Proceedings of IAPR International Conference on Pattern Recognition, (ICPR'08)*, Tampa, Florida, USA, 2008, pp. 1–4.
51. ——, "New motion correction models for automatic identification of renal transplant rejection," in *Proceedings of International Conference on Medical Image Computing and Computer-Assisted Intervention, (MICCAI'07)*, Brisbane, Australia, October 29–November 2, 2007, pp. 235–243.
52. A. Farag, A. El-Baz, S. Yuksel, M. A. El-Ghar, and T. Eldiasty, "A framework for the detection of acute rejection with Dynamic Contrast Enhanced Magnetic Resonance Imaging," in *Proceedings of IEEE International Symposium on Biomedical Imaging: From Nano to Macro, (ISBI'06)*, Arlington, VA, 2006, pp. 418–421.
53. F. Khalifa, G. M. Beache, M. A. El-Ghar, T. El-Diasty, G. Gimel'farb, M. Kong, and A. El-Baz, "Dynamic contrast-enhanced MRI- based early detection of acute renal transplant rejection," *IEEE Transactions on Medical Imaging*, vol. 32, no. 10, pp. 1910–1927, 2013.
54. F. Khalifa, A. El-Baz, G. Gimel'farb, and M. A. El-Ghar, "Non-invasive image-based approach for early detection of acute renal rejection," in *Proceedings of International Conference Medical Image Computing and Computer-Assisted Intervention, (MICCAI'10)*, Beijing, China, September 20–24, 2010, pp. 10–18.
55. F. Khalifa, A. El-Baz, G. Gimel'farb, R. Ouseph, and M. A. El-Ghar, "Shape-appearance guided level-set deformable model for image segmentation," in *Proceedings of IAPR International Conference on Pattern Recognition, (ICPR'10)*, Istanbul, Turkey, August 23–26, 2010, pp. 4581–4584.
56. F. Khalifa, M. A. El-Ghar, B. Abdollahi, H. Frieboes, T. El-Diasty, and A. El-Baz, "A comprehensive non-invasive framework for automated evaluation of acute renal transplant rejection using DCE-MRI," *NMR in Biomedicine*, vol. 26, no. 11, pp. 1460–1470, 2013.
57. F. Khalifa, M. A. El-Ghar, B. Abdollahi, H. B. Frieboes, T. El-Diasty, and A. El-Baz, "Dynamic contrast-enhanced MRI-based early detection of acute renal transplant rejection," in *2014 Annual Scientific Meeting and Educational Course Brochure of the Society of Abdominal Radiology, (SAR'14)*, Boca Raton, FL, March 23–28, 2014, p. CID: 1855912.
58. F. Khalifa, A. Elnakib, G. M. Beache, G. Gimel'farb, M. A. El-Ghar, G. Sokhadze, S. Manning, P. McClure, and A. El-Baz, "3D kidney segmentation from CT images using a level set approach guided by a novel stochastic speed function," in *Proceedings of International Conference Medical Image Computing and Computer-Assisted Intervention, (MICCAI'11)*, Toronto, Canada, September 18–22, 2011, pp. 587–594.
59. F. Khalifa, G. Gimel'farb, M. A. El-Ghar, G. Sokhadze, S. Manning, P. McClure, R. Ouseph, and A. El-Baz, "A new deformable model-based segmentation approach for accurate extraction of the kidney from

abdominal CT images," in *Proceedings of IEEE International Conference on Image Processing, (ICIP'11)*, Brussels, Belgium, September 11–14, 2011, pp. 3393–3396.

60. M. Mostapha, F. Khalifa, A. Alansary, A. Soliman, J. Suri, and A. El-Baz, "Computer-aided diagnosis systems for acute renal transplant rejection: challenges and methodologies," in *Abdomen and Thoracic Imaging*, A. El-Baz and L. S. J. Suri, Eds. Springer, Boston, MA, 2014, pp. 1–35.
61. M. Shehata, F. Khalifa, E. Hollis, A. Soliman, E. Hosseini-Asl, M. A. El-Ghar, M. El-Baz, A. C. Dwyer, A. El-Baz, and R. Keynton, "A new non-invasive approach for early classification of renal rejection types using diffusion-weighted MRI," in *IEEE International Conference on Image Processing (ICIP)*. IEEE, 2016, pp. 136–140.
62. F. Khalifa, A. Soliman, A. Takieldeen, M. Shehata, M. Mostapha, A. Shaffie, R. Ouseph, A. Elmaghraby, and A. El-Baz, "Kidney segmentation from CT images using a 3D NMF-guided active contour model," in *IEEE 13th International Symposium on Biomedical Imaging (ISBI)*. IEEE, 2016, pp. 432–435.
63. M. Shehata, F. Khalifa, A. Soliman, A. Takieldeen, M. A. El-Ghar, A. Shaffie, A. C. Dwyer, R. Ouseph, A. El-Baz, and R. Keynton, "3D diffusion MRI-based cad system for early diagnosis of acute renal rejection," in *Biomedical Imaging (ISBI), 2016 IEEE 13th International Symposium on*. IEEE, 2016, pp. 1177–1180.
64. M. Shehata, F. Khalifa, A. Soliman, R. Alrefai, M. A. El-Ghar, A. C. Dwyer, R. Ouseph, and A. El-Baz, "A level set-based framework for 3D kidney segmentation from diffusion MR images," in *IEEE International Conference on Image Processing (ICIP)*. IEEE, 2015, pp. 4441–4445.
65. M. Shehata, F. Khalifa, A. Soliman, M. A. El-Ghar, A. C. Dwyer, G. Gimel'farb, R. Keynton, and A. El-Baz, "A promising non- invasive cad system for kidney function assessment," in *International Conference on Medical Image Computing and Computer-Assisted Intervention*. Springer, 2016, pp. 613–621.
66. F. Khalifa, A. Soliman, A. Elmaghraby, G. Gimel'farb, and A. El-Baz, "3D kidney segmentation from abdominal images using spatial-appearance models," *Computational and Mathematical Methods in Medicine*, vol. 2017, pp. 1–10, 2017.
67. E. Hollis, M. Shehata, F. Khalifa, M. A. El-Ghar, T. El-Diasty, and A. El-Baz, "Towards non-invasive diagnostic techniques for early detection of acute renal transplant rejection: a review," *The Egyptian Journal of Radiology and Nuclear Medicine*, vol. 48, no. 1, pp. 257–269, 2016.
68. M. Shehata, F. Khalifa, A. Soliman, M. A. El-Ghar, A. C. Dwyer, and A. El-Baz, "Assessment of renal transplant using image and clinical-based biomarkers," in *Proceedings of 13th Annual Scientific Meeting of American Society for Diagnostics and Interventional Nephrology (ASDIN'17)*, New Orleans, LA, February 10–12, 2017.
69. ——, "Early assessment of acute renal rejection," in *Proceedings of 12th Annual Scientific Meeting of American Society for Diagnostics and Interventional Nephrology (ASDIN'16)*, Pheonix, AZ, February 19–21, 2016, 2017.

70. A. Eltanboly, M. Ghazal, H. Hajjdiab, A. Shalaby, A. Switala, A. Mahmoud, P. Sahoo, M. El-Azab, and A. El-Baz, "Level sets-based image segmentation approach using statistical shape priors," *Applied Mathematics and Computation*, vol. 340, pp. 164–179, 2019.
71. M. Shehata, A. Mahmoud, A. Soliman, F. Khalifa, M. Ghazal, M. A. El-Ghar, M. El-Melegy, and A. El-Baz, "3D kidney segmentation from abdominal diffusion MRI using an appearance-guided deformable boundary," *PLoS One*, vol. 13, no. 7, p. e0200082, 2018.
72. H. Abdeltawab et al., "A novel CNN-based cad system for early assessment of transplanted kidney dysfunction," *Scientific Reports*, vol. 9, no. 1, p. 5948, 2019.
73. F. Khalifa, G. Beache, A. El-Baz, and G. Gimel'farb, "Deformable model guided by stochastic speed with application in cine images segmentation," in *Proceedings of IEEE International Conference on Image Processing, (ICIP'10)*, Hong Kong, September 26–29, 2010, pp. 1725–1728.
74. F. Khalifa, G. M. Beache, A. Elnakib, H. Sliman, G. Gimel'farb, K. C. Welch, and A. El-Baz, "A new shape-based framework for the left ventricle wall segmentation from cardiac first-pass perfusion MRI," in *Proceedings of IEEE International Symposium on Biomedical Imaging: From Nano to Macro, (ISBI'13)*, San Francisco, CA, April 7–11, 2013, pp. 41–44.
75. ——, "A new nonrigid registration framework for improved visualization of transmural perfusion gradients on cardiac first–pass perfusion MRI," in *Proceedings of IEEE International Symposium on Biomedical Imaging: From Nano to Macro, (ISBI'12)*, Barcelona, Spain, May 2–5, 2012, pp. 828–831.
76. F. Khalifa, G. M. Beache, A. Firjani, K. C. Welch, G. Gimel'farb, and A. El-Baz, "A new nonrigid registration approach for motion correction of cardiac first-pass perfusion MRI," in *Proceedings of IEEE International Conference on Image Processing, (ICIP'12)*, Lake Buena Vista, FL, September 30–October 3, 2012, pp. 1665–1668.
77. F. Khalifa, G. M. Beache, G. Gimel'farb, and A. El-Baz, "A novel CAD system for analyzing cardiac first-pass MR images," in *Proceedings of IAPR International Conference on Pattern Recognition (ICPR'12)*, Tsukuba Science City, Japan, November 11–15, 2012, pp. 77–80.
78. ——, "A novel approach for accurate estimation of left ventricle global indexes from short-axis cine MRI," in *Proceedings of IEEE International Conference on Image Processing, (ICIP'11)*, Brussels, Belgium, September 11–14, 2011, pp. 2645–2649.
79. F. Khalifa, G. M. Beache, G. Gimel'farb, G. A. Giridharan, and A. El-Baz, "A new image-based framework for analyzing cine images," in *Handbook of Multi Modality State-of-the-Art Medical Image Segmentation and Registration Methodologies*, A. El-Baz, U. R. Acharya, M. Mirmedhdi, and J. S. Suri, Eds. Springer, New York, NY, 2011, vol. 2, Ch. 3, pp. 69–98.
80. ——, "Accurate automatic analysis of cardiac cine images," *IEEE Transactions on Biomedical Engineering*, vol. 59, no. 2, pp. 445–455, 2012.

81. F. Khalifa, G. M. Beache, M. Nitzken, G. Gimel'farb, G. A. Giridharan, and A. El-Baz, "Automatic analysis of left ventricle wall thickness using short-axis cine CMR images," in *Proceedings of IEEE International Symposium on Biomedical Imaging: From Nano to Macro, (ISBI'11)*, Chicago, IL, March 30–April 2, 2011, pp. 1306–1309.
82. M. Nitzken, G. Beache, A. Elnakib, F. Khalifa, G. Gimel'farb, and A. El-Baz, "Accurate modeling of tagged CMR 3D image appearance characteristics to improve cardiac cycle strain estimation," in *Image Processing (ICIP), 2012 19th IEEE International Conference on*. Orlando, FL. IEEE, Sep. 2012, pp. 521–524.
83. ——, "Improving full-cardiac cycle strain estimation from tagged CMR by accurate modeling of 3D image appearance characteristics," in *Biomedical Imaging (ISBI), 2012 9th IEEE International Symposium on*. Barcelona, Spain. IEEE, May 2012, pp. 462–465, (Selected for oral presentation).
84. M. J. Nitzken, A. S. El-Baz, and G. M. Beache, "Markov–Gibbs random field model for improved full-cardiac cycle strain estimation from tagged cmr," *Journal of Cardiovascular Magnetic Resonance*, vol. 14, no. 1, pp. 1–2, 2012.
85. H. Sliman, A. Elnakib, G. Beache, A. Elmaghraby, and A. El-Baz, "Assessment of myocardial function from cine cardiac MRI using a novel 4D tracking approach," *Journal of Computer Science and Systems Biology*, vol. 7, pp. 169–173, 2014.
86. H. Sliman, A. Elnakib, G. M. Beache, A. Soliman, F. Khalifa, G. Gimel'farb, A. Elmaghraby, and A. El-Baz, "A novel 4D PDE-based approach for accurate assessment of myocardium function using cine cardiac magnetic resonance images," in *Proceedings of IEEE International Conference on Image Processing (ICIP'14)*, Paris, France, October 27–30, 2014, pp. 3537–3541.
87. H. Sliman, F. Khalifa, A. Elnakib, G. M. Beache, A. Elmaghraby, and A. El-Baz, "A new segmentation-based tracking framework for extracting the left ventricle cavity from cine cardiac MRI," in *Proceedings of IEEE International Conference on Image Processing, (ICIP'13)*, Melbourne, Australia, September 15–18, 2013, pp. 685–689.
88. H. Sliman, F. Khalifa, A. Elnakib, A. Soliman, G. M. Beache, A. Elmaghraby, G. Gimel'farb, and A. El-Baz, "Myocardial borders segmentation from cine MR images using bi-directional coupled parametric deformable models," *Medical Physics*, vol. 40, no. 9, pp. 1–13, 2013.
89. H. Sliman, F. Khalifa, A. Elnakib, A. Soliman, G. M. Beache, G. Gimel'farb, A. Emam, A. Elmaghraby, and A. El-Baz, "Accurate segmentation framework for the left ventricle wall from cardiac cine MRI," in *Proceedings of International Symposium on Computational Models for Life Science, (CMLS'13)*, vol. 1559, Sydney, Australia, November 27–29, 2013, pp. 287–296.
90. B. Abdollahi, A. C. Civelek, X.-F. Li, J. Suri, and A. El-Baz, "PET/CT nodule segmentation and diagnosis: a survey," in *Multi Detector CT Imaging*, L. Saba and J. S. Suri, Eds. Taylor & Francis, Boca Raton, 2014, Ch. 30, pp. 639–651.

91. B. Abdollahi, A. El-Baz, and A. A. Amini, "A multi-scale non-linear vessel enhancement technique," in *Engineering in Medicine and Biology Society, EMBC, 2011 Annual International Conference of the IEEE*. IEEE, 2011, pp. 3925–3929.
92. B. Abdollahi, A. Soliman, A. Civelek, X.-F. Li, G. Gimel'farb, and A. El-Baz, "A novel gaussian scale space-based joint MGRF framework for precise lung segmentation," in *Proceedings of IEEE International Conference on Image Processing, (ICIP'12)*. IEEE, 2012, pp. 2029–2032.
93. ——, "A novel 3D joint MGRF framework for precise lung segmentation," in *Machine Learning in Medical Imaging*. Springer, 2012, pp. 86–93.
94. A. M. Ali, A. S. El-Baz, and A. A. Farag, "A novel framework for accurate lung segmentation using graph cuts," in *Proceedings of IEEE International Symposium on Biomedical Imaging: From Nano to Macro, (ISBI'07)*. IEEE, 2007, pp. 908–911.
95. A. El-Baz, G. M. Beache, G. Gimel'farb, K. Suzuki, and K. Okada, "Lung imaging data analysis," *International Journal of Biomedical Imaging*, vol. 2013, pp. 1–2, 2013.
96. A. El-Baz, G. M. Beache, G. Gimel'farb, K. Suzuki, K. Okada, A. Elnakib, A. Soliman, and B. Abdollahi, "Computer-aided diagnosis systems for lung cancer: challenges and methodologies," *International Journal of Biomedical Imaging*, vol. 2013, pp. 1–46, 2013.
97. A. El-Baz, A. Elnakib, M. Abou El-Ghar, G. Gimel'farb, R. Falk, and A. Farag, "Automatic detection of 2D and 3D lung nodules in chest spiral CT scans," *International Journal of Biomedical Imaging*, vol. 2013, pp. 1–11, 2013.
98. A. El-Baz, A. A. Farag, R. Falk, and R. La Rocca, "A unified approach for detection, visualization, and identification of lung abnormalities in chest spiral CT scans," in *International Congress Series*. Elsevier, vol. 1256, 2003, pp. 998–1004.
99. ——, "Detection, visualization and identification of lung abnormalities in chest spiral CT scan: Phase-I," in *Proceedings of International conference on Biomedical Engineering*, Cairo, Egypt, vol. 12, no. 1, 2002.
100. A. El-Baz, A. Farag, G. Gimel'farb, R. Falk, M. A. El-Ghar, and T. Eldiasty, "A framework for automatic segmentation of lung nodules from low dose chest CT scans," in *Proceedings of International Conference on Pattern Recognition, (ICPR'06)*. IEEE, vol. 3, 2006, pp. 611–614.
101. A. El-Baz, A. Farag, G. Gimel'farb, R. Falk, and M. A. El-Ghar, "A novel level set-based computer-aided detection system for automatic detection of lung nodules in low dose chest computed tomography scans," *Lung Imaging and Computer Aided Diagnosis*, vol. 10, pp. 221–238, 2011.
102. A. El-Baz, G. Gimel'farb, M. Abou El-Ghar, and R. Falk, "Appearance-based diagnostic system for early assessment of malignant lung nodules," in *Proceedings of IEEE International Conference on Image Processing, (ICIP'12)*. IEEE, 2012, pp. 533–536.

103. A. El-Baz, G. Gimel'farb, and R. Falk, "A novel 3D framework for automatic lung segmentation from low dose CT images," in *Lung Imaging and Computer Aided Diagnosis*, A. El-Baz and J. S. Suri, Eds. Taylor & Francis, Boca Raton, 2011, Ch. 1, pp. 1–16.
104. A. El-Baz, G. Gimel'farb, R. Falk, and M. El-Ghar, "Appearance analysis for diagnosing malignant lung nodules," in *Proceedings of IEEE International Symposium on Biomedical Imaging: From Nano to Macro (ISBI'10)*. IEEE, 2010, pp. 193–196.
105. A. El-Baz, G. Gimel'farb, R. Falk, and M. A. El-Ghar, "A novel level set-based CAD system for automatic detection of lung nodules in low dose chest CT scans," in *Lung Imaging and Computer Aided Diagnosis*, A. El-Baz and J. S. Suri, Eds. Taylor & Francis, Boca Raton, 2011, vol. 1, Ch. 10, pp. 221–238.
106. ——, "A new approach for automatic analysis of 3D low dose CT images for accurate monitoring the detected lung nodules," in *Proceedings of International Conference on Pattern Recognition, (ICPR'08)*. IEEE, 2008, pp. 1–4.
107. ——, "A novel approach for automatic follow-up of detected lung nodules," in *Proceedings of IEEE International Conference on Image Processing, (ICIP'07)*. IEEE, vol. 5, 2007, pp. V–501.
108. ——, "A new CAD system for early diagnosis of detected lung nodules," in *Image Processing, 2007. ICIP 2007. IEEE International Conference on*. IEEE, vol. 2, 2007, pp. II–461.
109. A. El-Baz, G. Gimel'farb, R. Falk, M. A. El-Ghar, and H. Refaie, "Promising results for early diagnosis of lung cancer," in *Proceedings of IEEE International Symposium on Biomedical Imaging: From Nano to Macro, (ISBI'08)*. IEEE, 2008, pp. 1151–1154.
110. A. El-Baz, G. L. Gimel'farb, R. Falk, M. Abou El-Ghar, T. Holland, and T. Shaffer, "A new stochastic framework for accurate lung segmentation," in *Proceedings of Medical Image Computing and Computer-Assisted Intervention, (MICCAI'08)*, 2008, pp. 322–330.
111. A. El-Baz, G. L. Gimel'farb, R. Falk, D. Heredis, and M. Abou El-Ghar, "A novel approach for accurate estimation of the growth rate of the detected lung nodules," in *Proceedings of International Workshop on Pulmonary Image Analysis*, 2008, pp. 33–42.
112. A. El-Baz, G. L. Gimel'farb, R. Falk, T. Holland, and T. Shaffer, "A framework for unsupervised segmentation of lung tissues from low dose computed tomography images," in *Proceedings of British Machine Vision, (BMVC'08)*, 2008, pp. 1–10.
113. A. El-Baz, G. Gimel'farb, R. Falk, and M. A. El-Ghar, "3D MGRF-based appearance modeling for robust segmentation of pulmonary nodules in 3D LDCT chest images," in *Lung Imaging and Computer Aided Diagnosis*, Ayman El-Baz and Jasjit S. Suri, Eds. CRC Press, Boca Raton, 2011, Ch. 3, pp. 51–63.
114. ——, "Automatic analysis of 3D low dose CT images for early diagnosis of lung cancer," *Pattern Recognition*, vol. 42, no. 6, pp. 1041–1051, 2009.

115. A. El-Baz, G. Gimel'farb, R. Falk, M. A. El-Ghar, S. Rainey, D. Heredia, and T. Shaffer, "Toward early diagnosis of lung cancer," in *Proceedings of Medical Image Computing and Computer-Assisted Intervention, (MICCAI'09)*. Springer, 2009, pp. 682–689.
116. A. El-Baz, G. Gimel'farb, R. Falk, M. A. El-Ghar, and J. Suri, "Appearance analysis for the early assessment of detected lung nodules," in *Lung Imaging and Computer Aided Diagnosis*, 2011, Ch. 17, pp. 395–404.
117. A. El-Baz, F. Khalifa, A. Elnakib, M. Nitkzen, A. Soliman, P. McClure, G. Gimel'farb, and M. A. El-Ghar, "A novel approach for global lung registration using 3D Markov Gibbs appearance model," in *Proceedings of International Conference Medical Image Computing and Computer-Assisted Intervention, (MICCAI'12)*, Nice, France, October 1–5, 2012, pp. 114–121.
118. A. El-Baz, M. Nitzken, A. Elnakib, F. Khalifa, G. Gimel'farb, R. Falk, and M. A. El-Ghar, "3D shape analysis for early diagnosis of malignant lung nodules," in *Proceedings of International Conference Medical Image Computing and Computer-Assisted Intervention, (MICCAI'11)*, Toronto, Canada, September 18–22, 2011, pp. 175–182.
119. A. El-Baz, M. Nitzken, G. Gimel'farb, E. Van Bogaert, R. Falk, M. A. El-Ghar, and J. Suri, "Three-dimensional shape analysis using spherical harmonics for early assessment of detected lung nodules," in *Lung Imaging and Computer Aided Diagnosis*, 2011, Ch. 19, pp. 421–438.
120. A. El-Baz, M. Nitzken, F. Khalifa, A. Elnakib, G. Gimel'farb, R. Falk, and M. A. El-Ghar, "3D shape analysis for early diagnosis of malignant lung nodules," in *Proceedings of International Conference on Information Processing in Medical Imaging, (IPMI'11)*, Monastery Irsee, Germany (Bavaria), July 3–8, 2011, pp. 772–783.
121. A. El-Baz, M. Nitzken, E. Vanbogaert, G. Gimel'Farb, R. Falk, and M. Abo El-Ghar, "A novel shape-based diagnostic approach for early diagnosis of lung nodules," in *Biomedical Imaging: From Nano to Macro, 2011 IEEE International Symposium on*. IEEE, 2011, pp. 137–140.
122. A. El-Baz, P. Sethu, G. Gimel'farb, F. Khalifa, A. Elnakib, R. Falk, and M. A. El-Ghar, "Elastic phantoms generated by microfluidics technology: validation of an imaged-based approach for accurate measurement of the growth rate of lung nodules," *Biotechnology Journal*, vol. 6, no. 2, pp. 195–203, 2011.
123. ——, "A new validation approach for the growth rate measurement using elastic phantoms generated by state-of-the-art microfluidics technology," in *Proceedings of IEEE International Conference on Image Processing, (ICIP'10)*, Hong Kong, September 26–29, 2010, pp. 4381–4383.
124. A. El-Baz, P. Sethu, G. Gimel'farb, F. Khalifa, A. Elnakib, R. Falk, and M. A. E.-G. J. Suri, "Validation of a new imaged-based approach for the accurate estimating of the growth rate of detected lung nodules using real CT images and elastic phantoms generated by state-of-the-art microfluidics technology," in *Handbook of Lung Imaging and Computer Aided Diagnosis*, A. El-Baz and J. S. Suri, Eds. Taylor & Francis, New York, NY, 2011, vol. 1, Ch. 18, pp. 405–420.

125. A. El-Baz, A. Soliman, P. McClure, G. Gimel'farb, M. A. El-Ghar, and R. Falk, "Early assessment of malignant lung nodules based on the spatial analysis of detected lung nodules," in *Proceedings of IEEE International Symposium on Biomedical Imaging: From Nano to Macro, (ISBI'12)*. IEEE, 2012, pp. 1463–1466.
126. A. El-Baz, S. E. Yuksel, S. Elshazly, and A. A. Farag, "Non-rigid registration techniques for automatic follow-up of lung nodules," in *Proceedings of Computer Assisted Radiology and Surgery, (CARS'05)*. Elsevier, vol. 1281, 2005, pp. 1115–1120.
127. A. S. El-Baz and J. S. Suri, *Lung Imaging and Computer Aided Diagnosis*. CRC Press, Boca Raton, 2011.
128. A. Soliman, F. Khalifa, N. Dunlap, B. Wang, M. El-Ghar, and A. El-Baz, "An iso-surfaces based local deformation handling framework of lung tissues," in *Biomedical Imaging (ISBI), 2016 IEEE 13th International Symposium on*. IEEE, 2016, pp. 1253–1259.
129. A. Soliman, F. Khalifa, A. Shaffie, N. Dunlap, B. Wang, A. Elmaghraby, and A. El-Baz, "Detection of lung injury using 4D-CT chest images," in *Biomedical Imaging (ISBI), 2016 IEEE 13th International Symposium on*. IEEE, 2016, pp. 1274–1277.
130. A. Soliman, F. Khalifa, A. Shaffie, N. Dunlap, B. Wang, A. Elmaghraby, G. Gimel'farb, M. Ghazal, and A. El-Baz, "A comprehensive framework for early assessment of lung injury," in *Image Processing (ICIP), 2017 IEEE International Conference on*. IEEE, 2017, pp. 3275–3279.
131. A. Shaffie, A. Soliman, M. Ghazal, F. Taher, N. Dunlap, B. Wang, A. Elmaghraby, G. Gimel'farb, and A. El-Baz, "A new framework for incorporating appearance and shape features of lung nodules for precise diagnosis of lung cancer," in *Image Processing (ICIP), 2017 IEEE International Conference on*. IEEE, 2017, pp. 1372–1376.
132. A. Soliman, F. Khalifa, A. Shaffie, N. Liu, N. Dunlap, B. Wang, A. Elmaghraby, G. Gimel'farb, and A. El-Baz, "Image-based cad system for accurate identification of lung injury," in *Image Processing (ICIP), 2016 IEEE International Conference on*. IEEE, 2016, pp. 121–125.
133. A. Soliman, A. Shaffie, M. Ghazal, G. Gimel'farb, R. Keynton, and A. El-Baz, "A novel cnn segmentation framework based on using new shape and appearance features," in *2018 25th IEEE International Conference on Image Processing (ICIP)*. IEEE, 2018, pp. 3488–3492.
134. A. Shaffie, A. Soliman, H. A. Khalifeh, M. Ghazal, F. Taher, R. Keynton, A. Elmaghraby, and A. El-Baz, "On the integration of CT- derived features for accurate detection of lung cancer," in *2018 IEEE International Symposium on Signal Processing and Information Technology (ISSPIT)*. IEEE, 2018, pp. 435–440.
135. A. Shaffie, A. Soliman, H. A. Khalifeh, M. Ghazal, F. Taher, A. Elmaghraby, R. Keynton, and A. El-Baz, "Radiomic-based framework for early diagnosis of lung cancer," in *2019 IEEE 16th International Symposium on Biomedical Imaging (ISBI 2019)*. IEEE, 2019, pp. 1293–1297.

136. A. Shaffie, A. Soliman, M. Ghazal, F. Taher, N. Dunlap, B. Wang, V. Van Berkel, G. Gimelfarb, A. Elmaghraby, and A. El-Baz, "A novel autoencoder-based diagnostic system for early assessment of lung cancer," in *2018 25th IEEE International Conference on Image Processing (ICIP)*. IEEE, 2018, pp. 1393–1397.
137. A. Shaffie et al., "A generalized deep learning-based diagnostic system for early diagnosis of various types of pulmonary nodules," *Technology in Cancer Research & Treatment*, vol. 17, p. 1533033818798800, 2018.
138. Y. ElNakieb et al., "Autism spectrum disorder diagnosis framework using diffusion tensor imaging," in *2019 IEEE International Conference on Imaging Systems and Techniques (IST)*. IEEE, 2019, pp. 1–5.
139. R. Haweel, O. Dekhil, A. Shalaby, A. Mahmoud, M. Ghazal, R. Keynton, G. Barnes, and A. El-Baz, "A machine learning approach for grading autism severity levels using task-based functional MRI," in *2019 IEEE International Conference on Imaging Systems and Techniques (IST)*. IEEE, 2019, pp. 1–5.
140. Dekhil, O., Ali, M., Haweel, R., Elnakib, Y., Ghazal, M., Hajjdiab, H., Fraiwan, L., Shalaby, A., Soliman, A., Mahmoud, A. and Keynton, R., 2020, July. A Comprehensive Framework for Differentiating Autism Spectrum Disorder From Neurotypicals by Fusing Structural MRI and Resting State Functional MRI. In *Seminars in Pediatric Neurology* (Vol. 34, p. 100805). WB Saunders.
141. R. Haweel, O. Dekhil, A. Shalaby, A. Mahmoud, M. Ghazal, A. Khalil, R. Keynton, G. Barnes, and A. El-Baz, "A novel framework for grading autism severity using task-based fMRI," in *2020 IEEE 17th International Symposium on Biomedical Imaging (ISBI)*. IEEE, 2020, pp. 1404–1407.
142. B. Dombroski, M. Nitzken, A. Elnakib, F. Khalifa, A. El-Baz, and M. F. Casanova, "Cortical surface complexity in a population-based normative sample," *Translational Neuroscience*, vol. 5, no. 1, pp. 17–24, 2014.
143. A. El-Baz, M. Casanova, G. Gimel'farb, M. Mott, and A. Switala, "An MRI-based diagnostic framework for early diagnosis of dyslexia," *International Journal of Computer Assisted Radiology and Surgery*, vol. 3, no. 3–4, pp. 181–189, 2008.
144. A. El-Baz, M. Casanova, G. Gimel'farb, M. Mott, A. Switala, E. Vanbogaert, and R. McCracken, "A new CAD system for early diagnosis of dyslexic brains," in *Proceedings on International Conference on Image Processing (ICIP'2008)*. IEEE, 2008, pp. 1820–1823.
145. A. El-Baz, M. F. Casanova, G. Gimel'farb, M. Mott, and A. E. Switwala, "A new image analysis approach for automatic classification of autistic brains," in *Proceedings on IEEE International Symposium on Biomedical Imaging: From Nano to Macro (ISBI'2007)*. IEEE, 2007, pp. 352–355.
146. A. El-Baz, A. A. Farag, G. Gimel'farb, and S. G. Hushek, "Automatic cerebrovascular segmentation by accurate probabilistic modeling of TOF-MRA images," in *Medical Image Computing and Computer-Assisted Intervention–MICCAI 2005*. Springer, 2005, pp. 34–42.

147. A. El-Baz, A. Farag, A. Elnakib, M. F. Casanova, G. Gimel'farb, A. E. Switala, D. Jordan, and S. Rainey, "Accurate automated detection of autism related corpus callosum abnormalities," *Journal of Medical Systems*, vol. 35, no. 5, pp. 929–939, 2011.
148. El-Baz, A., Farag, A. and Gimelfarb, G., 2005, June. Cerebrovascular segmentation by accurate probabilistic modeling of TOF-MRA images. In *Scandinavian Conference on Image Analysis* (pp. 1128–1137). Springer, Berlin, Heidelberg.
149. A. El-Baz, G. Gimel'farb, R. Falk, M. A. El-Ghar, V. Kumar, and D. Heredia, "A novel 3D joint Markov–Gibbs model for extracting blood vessels from PC–MRA images," in *Medical Image Computing and Computer-Assisted Intervention-MICCAI 2009*, vol. 5762. Springer, 2009, pp. 943–950.
150. A. Elnakib, A. El-Baz, M. F. Casanova, G. Gimel'farb, and A. E. Switala, "Image-based detection of corpus callosum variability for more accurate discrimination between dyslexic and normal brains," in *Proceedings on IEEE International Symposium on Biomedical Imaging: From Nano to Macro (ISBI'2010)*. IEEE, 2010, pp. 109–112.
151. A. Elnakib, M. F. Casanova, G. Gimel'farb, A. E. Switala, and A. El-Baz, "Autism diagnostics by centerline-based shape analysis of the corpus callosum," in *Proceedings on IEEE International Symposium on Biomedical Imaging: From Nano to Macro (ISBI'2011)*. IEEE, 2011, pp. 1843–1846.
152. A. Elnakib, M. Nitzken, M. Casanova, H. Park, G. Gimel'farb, and A. El-Baz, "Quantification of age-related brain cortex change using 3D shape analysis," in *Pattern Recognition (ICPR), 2012 21st International Conference on*. IEEE, 2012, pp. 41–44.
153. M. Nitzken, M. Casanova, G. Gimel'farb, A. Elnakib, F. Khalifa, A. Switala, and A. El-Baz, "3D shape analysis of the brain cortex with application to dyslexia," in *Image Processing (ICIP), 2011 18th IEEE International Conference on*. Brussels, Belgium: IEEE, Sep. 2011, pp. 2657–2660, (Selected for oral presentation. Oral acceptance rate is 10% and the overall acceptance rate is 35%).
154. F. E.-Z. A. El-Gamal, M. M. Elmogy, M. Ghazal, A. Atwan, G. N. Barnes, M. F. Casanova, R. Keynton, and A. S. El-Baz, "A novel cad system for local and global early diagnosis of Alzheimer's disease based on pib-pet scans," in *2017 IEEE International Conference on Image Processing (ICIP)*. IEEE, 2017, pp. 3270–3274.
155. M. M. Ismail, R. S. Keynton, M. M. Mostapha, A. H. ElTanboly, M. F. Casanova, G. L. Gimel'farb, and A. El-Baz, "Studying autism spectrum disorder with structural and diffusion magnetic resonance imaging: a survey," *Frontiers in Human Neuroscience*, vol. 10, p. 211, 2016.
156. A. Alansary et al., "Infant brain extraction in t1-weighted MR images using bet and refinement using LCDG and MGRF models," *IEEE Journal of Biomedical and Health Informatics*, vol. 20, no. 3, pp. 925–935, 2016.
157. E. H. Asl, M. Ghazal, A. Mahmoud, A. Aslantas, A. Shalaby, M. Casanova, G. Barnes, G. Gimel'farb, R. Keynton, and A. El-Baz, "Alzheimer's disease diagnostics by a 3D deeply supervised adaptable convolutional network," *Frontiers in Bioscience (Landmark Edition)*, vol. 23, pp. 584–596, 2018.

158. O. Dekhil, M. Ali, Y. El-Nakieb, A. Shalaby, A. Soliman, A. Switala, A. Mahmoud, M. Ghazal, H. Hajjdiab, M. F. Casanova, A. Elmaghraby, R. Keynton, A. El-Baz, and G. Barnes, "A personalized autism diagnosis CAD system using a fusion of structural MRI and resting-state functional MRI data," *Frontiers in Psychiatry*, vol. 10, p. 392, 2019. [Online]. Available: https://www.frontiersin.org/article/10.3389/fpsyt.2019.00392
159. A. A. Sleman, A. Soliman, M. Ghazal, H. Sandhu, S. Schaal, A. Elmaghraby, and A. El-Baz, "Retinal layers oct scans 3-D segmentation," in *2019 IEEE International Conference on Imaging Systems and Techniques (IST)*. IEEE, 2019, pp. 1–6.
160. N. Eladawi, M. Elmogy, M. Ghazal, O. Helmy, A. Aboelfetouh, A. Riad, S. Schaal, and A. El-Baz, "Classification of retinal diseases based on oct images," *Frontiers in Bioscience (Landmark Edition)*, vol. 23, pp. 247–264, 2018.
161. A. ElTanboly, M. Ismail, A. Shalaby, A. Switala, A. El-Baz, S. Schaal, G. Gimel'farb, and M. El-Azab, "A computer-aided diagnostic system for detecting diabetic retinopathy in optical coherence tomography images," *Medical Physics*, vol. 44, no. 3, pp. 914–923, 2017.
162. H. S. Sandhu, A. El-Baz, and J. M. Seddon, "Progress in automated deep learning for macular degeneration," *JAMA Ophthalmology*, vol. 136, no. 12, pp. 1366–1367, 2018.
163. M. Ghazal, S. S. Ali, A. H. Mahmoud, A. M. Shalaby, and A. El-Baz, "Accurate detection of non-proliferative diabetic retinopathy in optical coherence tomography images using convolutional neural networks," *IEEE Access*, vol. 8, pp. 34387–34397, 2020.
164. K. Hammouda, F. Khalifa, A. Soliman, H. Abdeltawab, M. Ghazal, M. Abou El-Ghar, A. Haddad, H. E. Darwish, R. Keynton, and A. El-Baz, "A 3D CNN with a learnable adaptive shape prior for accurate segmentation of bladder wall using mr images," in *2020 IEEE 17th International Symposium on Biomedical Imaging (ISBI)*. IEEE, 2020, pp. 935–938.
165. A. Naglah, F. Khalifa, A. Mahmoud, M. Ghazal, P. Jones, T. Murray, A. S. Elmaghraby, and A. El-Baz, "Athlete-customized injury prediction using training load statistical records and machine learning," in *2018 IEEE International Symposium on Signal Processing and Information Technology (ISSPIT)*. IEEE, 2018, pp. 459–464.
166. A. H. Mahmoud, "Utilizing radiation for smart robotic applications using visible, thermal, and polarization images." Ph.D. dissertation, University of Louisville, 2014.
167. A. Mahmoud, A. El-Barkouky, J. Graham, and A. Farag, "Pedestrian detection using mixed partial derivative based his togram of oriented gradients," in *2014 IEEE International Conference on Image Processing (ICIP)*. IEEE, 2014, pp. 2334–2337.
168. A. El-Barkouky, A. Mahmoud, J. Graham, and A. Farag, "An interactive educational drawing system using a humanoid robot and light polarization," in *2013 IEEE International Conference on Image Processing*. IEEE, 2013, pp. 3407–3411.

169. A. H. Mahmoud, M. T. El-Melegy, and A. A. Farag, "Direct method for shape recovery from polarization and shading," in *2012 19th IEEE International Conference on Image Processing*. IEEE, 2012, pp. 1769–1772.
170. M. A. Ghazal, A. Mahmoud, A. Aslantas, A. Soliman, A. Shalaby, J. A. Benediktsson, and A. El-Baz, "Vegetation cover estimation using convolutional neural networks," *IEEE Access*, vol. 7, pp. 132563–132576, 2019.
171. M. Ghazal, A. Mahmoud, A. Shalaby, and A. El-Baz, "Automated framework for accurate segmentation of leaf images for plant health assessment," *Environmental Monitoring and Assessment*, vol. 191, no. 8, p. 491, 2019.

CHAPTER 14

Early Classification of Renal Rejection Types: A Deep Learning Approach

Mohamed Shehata, Fahmi Khalifa, Ahmed Soliman, Shams Shaker, Ahmed Shalaby, Maryam El-Baz, Ali Mahmoud, and Amy C. Dwyer

University of Louisville
Louisville, Kentucky

Mohamed Abou El-Ghar

University of Mansoura
Mansoura, Egypt

Mohammed Ghazal

Abu Dhabi University
Abu Dhabi, United Arab Emirates

Jasjit S. Suri

AtheroPoint LLC
Roseville, California

Ayman El-Baz

University of Louisville
Louisville, Kentucky
University of Louisville at AlAlamein
International University (UofL-AIU)
New Alamein City, Egypt

CONTENTS

14.1 INTRODUCTION

In the United States alone, approximately 700,000 of the population suffer from chronic kidney disease (CKD) and if not treated promptly in a timely manner, it will lead to end-stage kidney disease (ESKD) and might lead to death. The optimal solution is to go through a renal transplantation surgery, but given the fact that kidney donors are very rare makes this task more complicated. In addition, these renal allografts might be diagnosed with renal transplantation failure in the first 5-year post-transplantation. One of the most detrimental factors of renal transplantation failure is acute renal rejection. In other words, the body rejects the new kidney due to immunological response [1]. To avoid such things, precautions should be taken during the early stages to prolong the survival rate of the transplanted organ [2,3]. Namely, routine clinical follow-ups, estimation, and correct evaluation of the renal allograft after transplantation are essential to curtail the loss of allograft. This loss of allograft may be due to a few types of kidney rejection such as acute tubular necrosis (ATN), antibody-mediated rejection (AMR), or T-cell mediated rejection (TMR). Other types include immunosuppressive toxicity (IT) and viral infection (VI). Although each type of rejection contains a possible treatment, the possibility of two types of rejections occurring at the same time abates the treatment process [4].

Though biopsy is the gold standard method, it cannot be used for early detection because it is extremely invasive, time-consuming, expensive, and frequently causes injurious events such as bleeding, infections, and more [1]. Therefore, alternatives to biopsy that are safer and noninvasive are important. A precise renal computer-aided diagnostic system (CAD) that is non-invasive holds a reassuring analysis on renal allograft rejection. This system collects information, one kidney at a time, and then combines the information quickly at low cost to increase the patient's survival rate.

A non-invasive method that has been commonly used to determine the status of the renal allograft during the early stage after transplantation is diffusion-weighted magnetic resonance imaging (DW-MRI). This method is often advantageous because it contains both anatomical and functional information about the soft tissue being detected [5]. Also, it averts the use of contrast agents due to the possibility of their toxicity. Many studies have tested the function of DW-MRI by obtaining the cortical apparent diffusion coefficient (CADC) or the medullary ADC (MADC) which provided a variety of results [6]. However, one of the studies by Abou-El-Ghar et al. provided a successful differentiation in DW-MRI [7]. Their experiment included 21 patients with acute graft impairment with ten TMR, seven ATN, and four IT rejection types. They also had a region of interest (ROI) medial of a single cross-section of the kidney with the entire renal parenchyma, suspending the renal sinus. If an area contains a higher signal intensity or abnormal focal area, then a different ROI is obtained. Evidently, the ADC values obtained from ATN are heterogeneous due to them being calculated from three different groups. In other words, it is a mosaic pattern with a tiger stripe appearance. Additionally, the diffusion and blood perfusion played a major role in influencing the ADC values under low *b*-values. On the other hand, under high *b*-values, blood perfusion does not influence the ADC values. Other studies carried out by Eisenberg et al. suggest that a manual placement of individual ROIs can be used to cover a large area of the allograft [8]. Then, the individual ROIs in the upper, mid, and lower poles of the medulla are brought together to provide one ROI for the full cortex and another for the medulla. Of the five patients, four showed acute rejection while the remaining has ATN. Values such as standard deviation and mean were calculated. The issue with this study was the lack of patients who have transplant dysfunction. This is an issue because the trends do not provide a big enough differentiation between AR and ATN patients. Furthermore, other studies [9,10] showed that a major decrement in renal perfusion in AR was due to perfusion MRI. However, studies [7,8] concluded that water diffusion and blood perfusion levels are directly correlated with AR allografts, but only water diffusion with ATN patients.

Furthermore, BOLD MRI (blood oxygen level-dependent MRI) has also been used for renal rejection studies. With BOLD MRI, oxygen diffused blood is used to study the kidney's function. More specifically, the extent of deoxyhemoglobin is calculated from the apparent relation rate (ARR) parameter [6]. Although the medullary values vary, multiple studies concluded that ATN kidneys contain increased medullary ARR in comparison to AR kidneys [6,10–12]. A study [11] stated that ATN kidneys contain higher cortical ARR values rather than AR kidneys. It is safe to say that the general trend is higher ARR values. However, all these experiments contained limitations: subjective delineation using manual delineation of the kidney via 2D ROIs, failure to include kidney motion as a whole, failure to gather the fusion of ADC at high and low *b*-values, or establishing only statistical analysis to differentiate between pairs at certain *b*-values.

Neither of the studies incorporated MRI modalities with clinical biomarkers for an inclusive, computer-aided diagnostic system for early-stage AR identification. Therefore, a system is needed to overcome such limitations. Our work consists of a fully automated system to assess acute rejection at an early stage shown in Figure 14.1. The developed system is able to delineate the entire kidney, which also means that it can handle any motion. Additionally, the system can implement a stacked autoencoder in order to fuse calculated ADC values from the DW-MRI segmentation at low and high *b*-values. In Section 14.3, promising results are indicated from the newly developed CAD system. The results conclude that the system is indeed a non-invasive diagnostic tool.

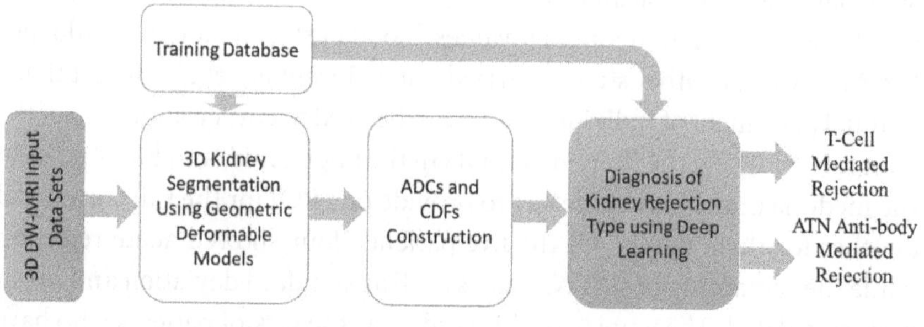

FIGURE 14.1 Shows the framework for the developed CAD system using DW-MRI.

14.2 METHODS

A precise Renal-CAD algorithm (see Figure 14.1) to assess the renal allograft status was developed. This system must contain certain steps to obtain the final evaluation. First, the kidney must be segmented from all other surroundings using DW-MRIs. Then, extraction or calculation was carried out for cumulative distribution functions (CDFs) of the voxel-wise ADC maps section of the kidney (Section 14.2.2). Lastly, TMR is allocated from the ATN kidney status to examine whether the proposed CAD system is a successful diagnostic measure.

14.2.1 Preprocessing/Segmenting Kidneys

Starting with a bias correction step on MR images [13], an intensity histogram equalization to reduce possible noise effect and image heterogeneities in these bias-corrected MR images was applied. As for the kidney motions, non-rigid registration of B-splines [14] was applied to decrease the variability of the subjects in the data using the sum of square difference (SSD). Next, the level sets approach was used to obtain an accurate 3D kidney segmentation [15]. For a precise kidney analysis, a guiding force that includes local appearance, shape, and spatial MRI features is placed in the regional statistics, which come from the kidney as well as the background regions given. Those features are merged using a joint Markov–Gibbs random field (MGRF) image model [16], more specifically, regional appearance [17,18], shape, and spatial DW-MRI features such as in Figure 14.2. Further details may be found in Ref. [15,19].

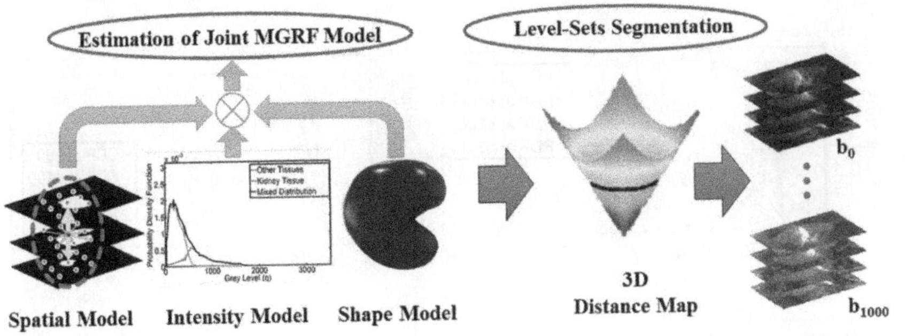

FIGURE 14.2 Represents the joint estimation of the MGRF to guide the level-set segmentation technique.

14.2.2 Diffusion Features Extraction

Post kidney segmentation, discriminatory physiological features must be calculated from images in order to differentiate between ATN and TMR of ARTR types. Using Le Bihan's [20] ADC definition, the rejection status is calculated using the below equation:

$$\mathrm{ADC}_p = \left(1/b_0 - b\right)\ln\left(g_b : p/g_0 : p\right) = \left(\left(\ln g_b - \ln g_0 : p\right)/\left(b_0 - b\right)\right)$$

To better explain this equation, p is (x, y, z) which is a voxel at the position with discrete Cartesian coordinates (x, y, z). As for g_0 and g_b, they are the segmented DW-MRI pictures that were gathered with the b_0 and a given different b-value.

To classify the rejection status of the renal transplant, the data dimensionality must be reduced. To do this, a characterization of the gross 3D ADC maps was gathered for the multiple b-values as illustrated in Figure 14.3.

14.2.3 Deep Learning Classification

A deep neural network technique based on stacking autoencoders (AE) is embedded into the developed CAD system for a more accurate classification of the renal rejection types. Each AE mainly consists of an input layer, hidden layers, and an output layer and is pre-trained separately in an unsupervised manner to extract the most important discriminatory features [21]. Then, these AEs are stacked together along with a supervised softmax classifier to get the final output probabilities of being ATN or TMR. This softmax is fine-tuned to minimize the total loss. It is worth mentioning that a non-negativity constraint (NCAE) [22] is added to the AEs training

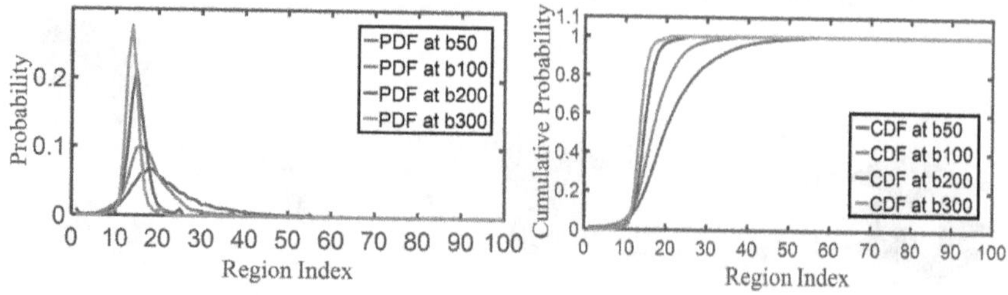

FIGURE 14.3 Illustrated empirical distribution of ADC values as well as their CDFs for a kidney with rejection status at different b-values (b_{50}, b_{100}, and b_{200}) s/mm^2.

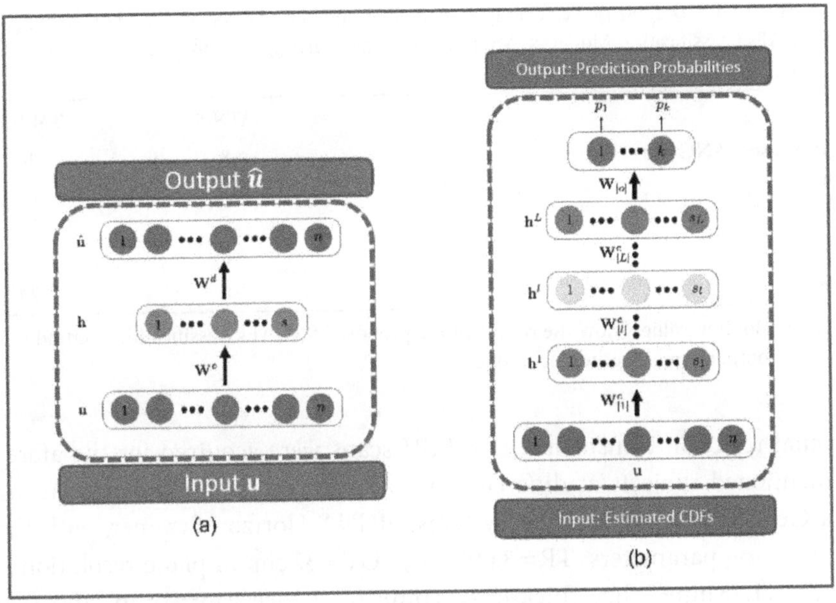

FIGURE 14.4 The AEs with their different layers (a) and the stacked-AES with the non-negativity constraints (SNCAEs) (b). Starting from the input (*u*: estimated CDFs) going through different hidden layers (h^i), each with activation units (S_i) and encoding weights (W^i), the final predicted output can be represented by probabilities of each assigned class (P1 or P2).

to facilitate solution conversion and optimize the classification performance. An illustrative figure about the stand-alone AEs and the stacked AEs with a softmax classifier on top of them is shown in Figure 14.4.

The proposed SNCAE network was trained and tested using a leave-one-out cross-validation (LOOCV). The training and testing processes were repeated using a grid search algorithm to get the optimal set of hyper-parameters. The average accuracy was selected as an optimization metric during the hyper-tuning process. With $s_1=25$, $s_2=5$, $s^{\circ}=2$, non-negativity constraint=0.03, sparsity constraint=3, and hidden units' average activation value=0.5, the developed SNCAE model provided the best classification results and was selected.

14.3 EXPERIMENTAL RESULTS

The developed CAD system was validated and tested on a total of 39 renal allografts, with their biopsy confirmation provided, of which eight subjects were diagnosed as ATN and 31 were diagnosed as TMR

TABLE 14.1 Diagnostic Performance of the Developed CAD System Based on Using SNCAEs Classification Model vs. Multiple Machine Learning Classifiers Using Weka Tool [26]

	Accuracy (%)	ATN/8	TMR/31
Proposed (SNCAEs)	**98**	**8**	**30**
RFs	95	7	30
kNN	90	8	27
LR	85	8	25
RTs	77	6	24

Note: Bolding values show the results of the proposed SNCAEs classification method that outperforms all other techniques.

renal rejection transplants. DW-MRI scans were acquired for the aforementioned subjects at different b-values starting from b_0 to $b_{1,000}$ using a General Electric Medical Systems, SIGNA Horizon Scanner, with the following parameters: TR=8,000 ms; FOV=32 cm; in-plane resolution = $1.25 \times 1.25\,\text{mm}^2$; slice thickness=4 mm; inter-slice gap=0 mm; and two excitations.

Using the estimated CDFs with the developed SNCAE classification model, the proposed CAD system was tested using a LOOCV and it achieved a 98% diagnostic accuracy with 8/8 correctly classified instances of ATN and 30/31 of TMR.

To highlight the advantages of using such an SNCAE classification model, the obtained results were compared to those obtained using multiple well-known conventional machine learning classifiers built-in Weka tool [23]: K-nearest neighbor (kNN), logistic regression (LR), random trees (RTs), and random forests (RFs). All results are compared and summarized in Table 14.1. With an accuracy of 98%, the developed classification system using SNCAE outperformed all other machine learning classifiers, holding a promise for the development as an outstanding diagnostic tool for renal rejection type identification.

14.4 CONCLUSION

To recap, our work offers a Renal-CAD system that estimates whether the renal transplant is acute rejection or non-rejection during early stages of post-transplantation in a non-invasive way through 4D DW-MRI data. Our CAD system uses not only previous techniques but adds new non-rigid image aligning techniques. Additionally, it utilizes kidney segmentation that includes deformable boundary, calculating ADC values, as well as utilized SNCAEs to determine the rejected kidney status through CDFs of the ADCs, as integral status descriptions. In terms of accuracy, we used a biopsy-proven cohort with 39 patients and obtained a 98% overall accuracy in ATN and TMR rejection status. These promising results confirm that the proposed CAD system is a non-invasive diagnostic tool to detect the status of the renal transplant. For future testing, we plan on expanding the ATN and TMR data sets to further estimate the accuracy as well as the robustness of our framework in diagnosis. Furthermore, to take other causes of rejection into account—drug toxicity, viral infection, and so on—we intend on expanding our rejection groups into four to further analyze the robustness of the newly developed CAD system within the four different groups.

In addition to kidney [24–51], this work could also be applied to various other applications in medical imaging, such as the prostate [52–54], the heart [55–71], the lung [72–119], the brain [120–141], the vascular system [142–151], the retina [152–156], the bladder [157], and injury prediction [158] as well as several non-medical applications [159–164].

ACKNOWLEDGMENT

The National Institutes of Health (NIH R15 grant 1R15AI135924-01A1) provided the fund required for this study.

REFERENCES

1. F. Khalifa, A. Soliman, A. El-Baz, M. Abou El-Ghar, T. El-Diasty, G. Gimel'farb, R. Ouseph, and A. C. Dwyer, "Models and methods for analyzing DCE-MRI: A review," *Medical Physics*, vol. 41, no. 12, p. 124301, 2014.
2. S. M. Gieser and A. Z Fenves, "Chronic kidney disease, dialysis, & transplantation, edited by Brian JG Pereira, MD, DM, Mohamed H. Sayegh, MD, and Peter Blake, MD," *Proceedings (Baylor University. Medical Center)*, vol. 19, no. 1, p. 69, 2006.
3. W. J. Chon et al., "Clinical manifestations and diagnosis of acute renal allograft rejection," UpToDate Version, vol. 21, 2014.
4. W. J. Chon et al., "Acute renal allograft rejection: Treatment," UpToDate, Waltham, MA, 2015.
5. H. J. Michaely, K. A. Herrmann, K. Nael, N. Oesingmann, M. F. Reiser, and S. O. Schoenberg, "Functional renal imaging: Nonvascular renal disease," *Abdominal Imaging*, vol. 32, no. 1, pp. 1–16, 2007.
6. G. Liu, F. Han, W. Xiao, Q. Wang, Y. Xu, and J. Chen, "Detection of renal allograft rejection using blood oxygen level-dependent and diffusion weighted magnetic resonance imaging: A retrospective study," *BMC Nephrology*, vol. 15, no. 1, p. 158, 2014.

7. M. E. Abou-El-Ghar, T. A. El-Diasty, A. M. El-Assmy, H. F. Refaie, A. F. Refaie, and M. A. Ghoneim, "Role of diffusion-weighted MRI in diagnosis of acute renal allograft dysfunction: A prospective preliminary study," *The British Journal of Radiology*, vol. 85, no. 1014, pp. 206–211, 2014.
8. U. Eisenberger, H. C. Thoeny, T. Binser, M. Gugger, F. J. Frey, C. Boesch, and P. Vermathen, "Evaluation of renal allograft function early after transplantation with diffusion-weighted MR imaging," *European Radiology*, vol. 20, no. 6, pp. 1374–1383, 2010.
9. L. Nilsson, H. Ekberg, K. F¨alt, H. L.¨ofberg, and G. Sterner, "Renal arteriovenous shunting in rejecting allograft, hydronephrosis, or haemorrhagic hypotension in the rat," *Nephrology Dialysis Transplantation*, vol. 9, no. 11, pp. 1634–1639, 1994.
10. E. A. Sadowski, A. Djamali, A. L. Wentland, R. Muehrer, B. N. Becker, T. M. Grist, and S. B. Fain, "Blood oxygen level-dependent and perfusion magnetic resonance imaging: Detecting differences in oxygen bioavailability and blood flow in transplanted kidneys," *Magnetic Resonance Imaging*, vol. 28, no. 1, pp. 56–64, 2010.
11. F. Han, W. Xiao, Y. Xu, J. Wu, Q. Wang, H. Wang, M. Zhang, and J. Chen, "The significance of BOLD MRI in differentiation between renal transplant rejection and acute tubular necrosis," *Nephrology Dialysis Transplantation*, vol. 23, no. 8, pp. 2666–2672, 2008.
12. A. Djamali, E. A. Sadowski, M. Samaniego- Picota, S. B. Fain, R. J. Muehrer, S. K. Alford, T. M. Grist, and B. N. Becker, "Noninvasive assessment of early kidney allograft dysfunction by blood oxygen level-dependent magnetic resonance imaging," *Transplantation*, vol. 82, no. 5, pp. 621–628, 2006.
13. N. J. Tustison, B. B. Avants, P. A. Cook, Y. Zheng, A. Egan, P. A. Yushkevich, and J. C. Gee, "N4ITK: Improved N3 bias correction," *IEEE Transactions on Medical Imaging*, vol. 29, no. 6, pp. 1310–1320, 2010.
14. B. Glocker, N. Komodakis, N. Paragios, and N. Navab, "Non-rigid registration using discrete MRFs: Application to thoracic CT images," in *Proceedings on MICCAI Workshop on Evaluation of Methods for Pulmonary Image Registration, (MICCAI'10)*, 2010, pp. 147–154.
15. M. Shehata, F. Khalifa, A. Soliman, R.Alrefai, M. A El-Ghar, A. C. Dwyer, R. Ouseph, and A. El-Baz, "A novel framework for automatic segmentation of kidney from DW-MRI," in *IEEE 12th Proceedings on the International Symposium on Biomedical Imaging (ISBI'15)*. IEEE, 2015, pp. 951–954.
16. A. A. Farag, A. S. El-Baz, and G. Gimel'farb, "Precise segmentation of multimodal images," *IEEE Transactions on Image Processing*, vol. 15, no. 4, pp. 952–968, 2006.
17. A. El-Baz, A. Elnakib, F. Khalifa, M. Abou El-Ghar, P. McClure, A. Soliman, and G. Gimel'farb, "Precise segmentation of 3-D magnetic resonance angiography," *IEEE Transactions on Biomedical Engineering*, vol. 59, no. 7, pp. 2019–2029, 2012.

18. F. Khalifa, M. Shehata, A. Soliman, M. A. El-Ghar, T. El-Diasty, A. C. Dwyer, M. El-Melegy, G. Gimel'farb, R. Keynton, A. El-Baz, "A generalized MRI-based CAD system for functional assessment of renal transplant," *in Proceedings on 14th IEEE International Symposium on Biomedical Imaging (ISBI 2017)*, Melbourne, VIC, 2017, pp. 758–761.
19. M. Shehata, F. Khalifa, A. Soliman, A. Takieldeen, M. Abou El-Ghar, A. Shaffie, A. C. Dwyer, R. Ouseph, A. El-Baz, and R. Keynton, "3D diffusion MRI-based CAD system for early diagnosis of acute renal rejection," in *IEEE 13th Proceedings on International Symposium on Biomedical Imaging (ISBI'16)*. IEEE, 2016, pp. 1177–1180.
20. D. Le Bihan and E. Breton, "Imagerie de diffusion invivo par r´esonance magn´etique nucl´eaire," *Comptes-Rendus de l'Acad´emie des Sciences*, vol. 93, no. 5, pp. 27–34, 1985.
21. Y. Bengio et al., "Greedy layer-wise training of deep networks," *Advances in Neural Information Processing Systems*, vol. 19, p. 153, 2007.
22. M. Shehata, F. Khalifa, A. Soliman, M. Ghazal, F. Taher, M. Abou El-Ghar, A. C. Dwyer, G. Gimel'farb, R. Keynton, and A. El-Baz, "Computer-aided diagnostic system for early detection of acute renal transplant rejection using diffusion-weighted MRI," *IEEE Transaction on Biomedical Engineering*, vol. 66, no. 2, pp. 539–552, 2019.
23. M. Hall, E.e. Frank, G. Holmes, B. Pfahringer, P. Reutemann, and I. H. Witten, "The weak data mining software: An update," *ACM SIGKDD Explorations Newsletter*, vol. 11, no. 1, pp. 10–18, 2009.
24. M. Shehata, M. Abou El-Ghar, T. Eldiasty, and A. El-Baz, "An integrated CAD system of DWI-MRI and laboratory biomarkers in diagnosis of kidney transplant dysfunction," in *European Congress of Radiology (ECR 2018)*, Austria Center Vienna, Bruno-Kreisky-Platz 11220, Vienna, Austria, February 28–March 4, 2018.
25. M. Shehata, M. Ghazal, G. M. Beache, M. Abou El-Ghar, A. C. Dwyer, A. Khalil, and A. El-Baz, "Role of integrating diffusion MR image-markers with clinical-biomarkers for early assessment of renal transplants," in *Proceedings of International Conference on Image Processing (ICIP'18)*, Athens, Greece, October 7–10, 2018, pp. 146–150.
26. H. Abdeltawab, M. Shehata, A. Shalaby, S. Mesbah, M. El-Baz, M. Ghazal, Y. Al Khalil, M. Abou El-Ghar, A. C. Dwyer, M. El-Melegy, G. Giridharan, and A. El-Baz, "A new 3D CNN-based CAD system for early detection of acute renal transplant rejection," in *Proceedings of International Conference on Pattern recognition (ICPR'18)*, Beijing, China, August 20–24, 2018, pp. 3898–3903.
27. M. Shehata, M. Abou El-Ghar, T. Eldiasty, and A. El-Baz, "Integrating clinical with diffusion image markers as a noninvasive alternative to renal biopsy," in *European Congress of Radiology (ECR 2019)*, Austria Center Vienna, Bruno-Kreisky-Platz 11220, Vienna, Austria, February 27–March 3, 2019.

28. M. Shehata, M. Ghazal, G. Beache, M. Abou El-Ghar, A. Dwyer, A. Khalil, A. El-maghraby, and A. El-Baz, "Fusion of image and clinical markers for renal transplant rejection assessment: A pilot study", in *Biomedical Engineering Society Annual Scientific Meeting (BMES18)*, Atlanta, GA, October 17–20, 2018.
29. H. Abdeltawab, M. Shehata, A. Shalaby, S. Mesbah, M. El-Baz, M. Ghazal, Y. Al Khalil, M. Abou El-Ghar, A. Dwyer, M. El-Melegy, A. Elmaghraby, and A. El-Baz, "Deep learning based framework for early detection of acute renal transplant rejection", in *Biomedical Engineering Society Annual Scientific Meeting (BMES18)*, Atlanta, Georgia, USA, October 17–20, 2018.
30. M. Shehata, F. Taher, M. Ghazal, A. Mahmoud, G. Beache, M. Abou El-Ghar, A. C. Dwyer, A. Elmaghraby, and A. El-Baz, "Early assessment of acute renal rejection post-transplantation: A combined imaging and clinical biomarkers protocol," in *Proceedings of International Symposium on Signal Processing and Information Technology (ISSPIT'18)*, Louisville, KY, December 9–12, 2018, pp. 297–302.
31. F. Khalifa, G. M. Beache, M. A. El-Ghar, T. El-Diasty, G. Gimel'farb, M. Kong, and A. El-Baz, "Dynamic contrast-enhanced MRI based early detection of acute renal transplant rejection," *IEEE Transactions on Medical Imaging*, vol. 32, no. 10, pp. 1910–1927, 2013.
32. M. Shehata, E. Hollis, M. Abou El-Ghar, M. Ghazal, T. Eldiasty, M. Merchant, A. Switala, A. C. Dwyer, and A. El-Baz, "Possible role of diffusion MRI in diagnosing acute renal rejection," in *Proceedings of 14th Annual Scientific Meeting of American Society for Diagnostics and Interventional Nephrology (ASDIN'18)*, Salt Lake City, UT, February 16–18, 2018.
33. M. Shehata, A. Shalaby, A. Mahmoud, M. Ghazal, H. Hajjdiab, M. A. Badawy, M. Abou El-Ghar, A. M. Bakr, A. C. Dwyer, R. Keynton, A. Elmaghraby, and A. El-Baz, "Towards big data in acute renal rejection," in *Big Data in Multimodal Medical Imaging*, A. El-Baz and J. Suri, Eds. Chapman and Hall/CRC, Boca Raton, 2019, pp. 205–223.
34. F. Khalifa, M. A. El-Ghar, B. Abdollahi, H. Frieboes, T. El-Diasty, and A. El-Baz, "A comprehensive non-invasive framework for automated evaluation of acute renal transplant rejection using DCE-MRI," *NMR in Biomedicine*, vol. 26, no. 11, pp. 1460–1470, 2013.
35. M. Shehata, M. Ghazal, F. Khalifa, M. Abou El-Ghar, A. C. Dwyer, A. El-giziri, M. El-Melegy, and A. El-Baz, "A novel CAD system for detecting acute rejection of renal allografts based on integrating imaging-markers and laboratory biomarkers," in *Proceedings of International Conference on Imaging Systems and Techniques (IST'18)*, Krakow, Poland, October 16–18, 2018, pp. 1–6.
36. F. Khalifa, A. Elnakib, G. M. Beache, G. Gimel'farb, M. A. El-Ghar, G. Sokhadze, S. Manning, P. McClure, and A. El-Baz, "3D kidney segmentation from CT images using a level set approach guided by a novel stochastic speed function," in *Proceedings of International Conference Medical Image Computing and Computer-Assisted Intervention, (MICCAI'11)*, Toronto, Canada, September 18–22, 2011, pp. 587–594.

37. M. Shehata, F. Khalifa, A. Soliman, A. Taki Eldeen, M. Abou El-Ghar, T. ElDiasty, A. El-Baz, and R. Keynton, "An appearance-guided deformable model for 4D kidney segmentation using diffusion MRI," in *Biomedical Image Segmentation: Advances and Trends*, A. El-Baz, X. Jiang, and J. Suri, Eds. Taylor & Francis, Boca Raton, 2016, Ch. 12, pp. 269–283.
38. M. Mostapha, F. Khalifa, A. Alansary, A. Soliman, J. Suri, and A. El-Baz, "Computer-aided diagnosis systems for acute renal transplant rejection: Challenges and methodologies," in *Abdomen and Thoracic Imaging*, A. El-Baz, L. Saba, and J. Suri, Eds. Springer, 2014, pp. 1–35.
39. E. Hollis, M. Shehata, M. Abou El-Ghar, M. Ghazal, T. El-Diasty, M. Merchant, A. Switala, and A. El-Baz, "Statistical analysis of ADCs and clinical biomarkers in detecting acute renal transplant rejection," *The British Journal of Radiology*, vol. 90(1080), p. 20170125, 2017.
40. F. Khalifa, A. Soliman, A. Takieldeen, M. Shehata, M. Mostapha, A. Shaffie, R. Ouseph, A. Elmaghraby, and A. El-Baz, "Kidney segmentation from CT images using a 3D NMF-guided active contour model," in *IEEE 13th International Symposium on Biomedical Imaging (ISBI)*, 2016, pp. 432–435.
41. M. Shehata, A. Shalaby, M. Ghazal, M. Abou El-Ghar, M. A. Badawy, G. M. Beache, A. C. Dwyer, M. El-Melegy, G. Giridharan, R. Keynton, and A. El-Baz, "Early assessment of renal transplants using bold-MRI: Promising results," in *Proceedings of International Conference on Image Processing (ICIP'19)*, Taipei, Taiwan, September 22–25, 2019, pp. 1395–1399.
42. M. Shehata, F. Khalifa, A. Soliman, R. Alrefai, M. A. El-Ghar, A. C. Dwyer, R. Ouseph, and A. El-Baz, "A level set-based framework for 3D kidney segmentation from diffusion MR images," in *IEEE International Conference on Image Processing (ICIP)*, 2015, pp. 4441–4445.
43. M. Shehata, F. Khalifa, A. Soliman, M. A. El-Ghar, A. C. Dwyer, G. Gimel'farb, R. Keynton, and A. El-Baz, "A promising non-invasive cad system for kidney function assessment," in *International Conference on Medical Image Computing and Computer-Assisted Intervention*. Springer, 2016, pp. 613–621.
44. F. Khalifa, A. Soliman, A. Elmaghraby, G. Gimel'farb, and A. El-Baz, "3D kidney segmentation from abdominal images using spatial-appearance models," *Computational and Mathematical Methods in Medicine*, vol. 2017, pp. 1–10, 2017.
45. E. Hollis, M. Shehata, F. Khalifa, M. A. El-Ghar, T. El-Diasty, and A. El-Baz, "Towards non-invasive diagnostic techniques for early detection of acute renal transplant rejection: A review," *The Egyptian Journal of Radiology and Nuclear Medicine*, vol. 48, no. 1, pp. 257–269, 2016.
46. M. Shehata, F. Khalifa, A. Soliman, M. A. El-Ghar, A. C. Dwyer, and A. El-Baz, "Assessment of renal transplant using image and clinical-based biomarkers," in *Proceedings of 13th Annual Scientific Meeting of American Society for Diagnostics and Interventional Nephrology (ASDIN'17)*, New Orleans, LA, February 10–12, 2017.

47. ——, "Early assessment of acute renal rejection," in *Proceedings of 12th Annual Scientific Meeting of American Society for Diagnostics and Interventional Nephrology (ASDIN'16)*, Pheonix, AZ, February 19–21, 2016, 2017.
48. M. Shehata, M. Ghazal, H. Abu Khalifeh, A. Khalil, A. Shalaby, A. C. Dwyer, A. M. Bakr, R. Keynton, and A. El-Baz, "A deep learning-based CAD system for renal allograft assessment: Diffusion, BOLD, and clinical biomarkers," in *Proceedings of International Conference on Image Processing (ICIP'20)*, Abu Dhabi, UAE, October 25–28, 2020, pp. 355–359.
49. M. Shehata, A. Mahmoud, A. Soliman, F. Khalifa, M. Ghazal, M. A. El-Ghar, M. El-Melegy, and A. El-Baz, "3D kidney segmentation from abdominal diffusion MRI using an appearance-guided deformable boundary," *PLoS One*, vol. 13, no. 7, p. e0200082, 2018.
50. H. Abdeltawab et al., "A novel CNN-based CAD system for early assessment of transplanted kidney dysfunction," *Scientific Reports*, vol. 9, no. 1, p. 5948, 2019.
51. M. Shehata, A. Shalaby, A. E. Switala, M. El-Baz, M. Ghazal, L. Fraiwan, A. Khalil, M. Abou El-Ghar, M. Badawy, A. M. Bakr, A. C. Dwyer, A. Elmagraby, G. Giridharan, R. Keynton, and A. El-Baz," A multimodal computer-aided diagnostic system for precise identification of renal allograft rejection: Preliminary results," *Medical Physics*, vol. 47, no. 6, pp. 2427–2440, 2020.
52. I. Reda, M. Ghazal, A. Shalaby, M. Elmogy, A. AbouEl-Fetouh, B. O. Ayinde, M. Abou El Ghar, A. Elmaghraby, R. Keynton, and A. El-Baz, "A Novel ADCs-Based CNN classification system for precise diagnosis of prostate cancer," in *2018 24th International Conference on Pattern Recognition (ICPR)*. IEEE, 2018, pp. 3923–3928.
53. I. Reda, A. Khalil, M. Elmogy, A. Abou El-Fetouh, A. Shalaby, M. Abou El-Ghar, A. Elmaghraby, M. Ghazal, and A. El-Baz, "Deep learning role in early diagnosis of prostate cancer," *Technology in Cancer Research & Treatment*, vol. 17, p. 1533034618775530, 2018.
54. I. Reda, B. O. Ayinde, M. Elmogy, A. Shalaby, M. El-Melegy, M. A. El-Ghar, A. A. El-fetouh, M. Ghazal, and A. El-Baz, "A new CNN-based system for early diagnosis of prostate cancer," in *2018 IEEE 15th International Symposium on Biomedical Imaging (ISBI 2018)*. IEEE, 2018, pp. 207–210.
55. F. Khalifa, G. Beache, A. El-Baz, and G. Gimel'farb, "Deformable model guided by stochastic speed with application in cine images segmentation," in *Proceedings of IEEE International Conference on Image Processing, (ICIP'10)*, Hong Kong, September 26–29, 2010, pp. 1725–1728.
56. F. Khalifa, G. M. Beache, A. Elnakib, H. Sliman, G. Gimel'farb, K. C. Welch, and A. El-Baz, "A new shape-based framework for the left ventricle wall segmentation from cardiac first-pass perfusion MRI," in *Proceedings of IEEE International Symposium on Biomedical Imaging: From Nano to Macro, (ISBI'13)*, San Francisco, CA, April 7–11, 2013, pp. 41–44.

57. ——, "A new nonrigid registration framework for improved visualization of transmural perfusion gradients on cardiac first-pass perfusion MRI," in *Proceedings of IEEE International Symposium on Biomedical Imaging: From Nano to Macro, (ISBI'12)*, Barcelona, Spain, May 2–5, 2012, pp. 828–831.
58. F. Khalifa, G. M. Beache, A. Firjani, K. C. Welch, G. Gimel'farb, and A. El-Baz, "A new nonrigid registration approach for motion correction of cardiac first-pass perfusion MRI," in *Proceedings of IEEE International Conference on Image Processing, (ICIP'12)*, Lake Buena Vista, FL, September 30–October 3, 2012, pp. 1665–1668.
59. F. Khalifa, G. M. Beache, G. Gimel'farb, and A. El-Baz, "A novel CAD system for analyzing cardiac first-pass MR images," in *Proceedings of IAPR International Conference on Pattern Recognition (ICPR'12)*, Tsukuba Science City, Japan, November 11–15, 2012, pp. 77–80.
60. ——, "A novel approach for accurate estimation of left ventricle global indexes from short-axis cine MRI," in *Proceedings of IEEE International Conference on Image Processing, (ICIP'11)*, Brussels, Belgium, September 11–14, 2011, pp. 2645–2649.
61. F. Khalifa, G. M. Beache, G. Gimel'farb, G. A. Giridharan, and A. El-Baz, "A new image-based framework for analyzing cine images," in *Handbook of Multi-Modality State-of-the-Art Medical Image Segmentation and Registration Methodologies*, A. El-Baz, U. R. Acharya, M. Mirmedhdi, and J. S. Suri, Eds. Springer, New York, NY, 2011, vol. 2, Ch. 3, pp. 69–98.
62. ——, "Accurate automatic analysis of cardiac cine images," *IEEE Transactions on Biomedical Engineering*, vol. 59, no. 2, pp. 445–455, 2012.
63. F. Khalifa, G. M. Beache, M. Nitzken, G. Gimel'farb, G. A. Giridharan, and A. El-Baz, "Automatic analysis of left ventricle wall thickness using short-axis cine CMR images," in *Proceedings of IEEE International Symposium on Biomedical Imaging: From Nano to Macro, (ISBI'11)*, Chicago, IL, March 30–April 2, 2011, pp. 1306–1309.
64. M. Nitzken, G. Beache, A. Elnakib, F. Khalifa, G. Gimel'farb, and A. El-Baz, "Accurate modeling of tagged CMR 3D image appearance characteristics to improve cardiac cycle strain estimation," in *Image Processing (ICIP), 2012 19th IEEE International Conference on*. Orlando, FL: IEEE, Sep. 2012, pp. 521–524.
65. ——, "Improving full-cardiac cycle strain estimation from tagged cmr by accurate modeling of 3D image appearance characteristics," in *Biomedical Imaging (ISBI), 2012 9th IEEE International Symposium on*. Barcelona, Spain: IEEE, May 2012, pp. 462–465, (Selected for oral presentation).
66. M. J. Nitzken, A. S. El-Baz, and G. M. Beache, "Markov-Gibbs random field model for improved full-cardiac cycle strain estimation from tagged CMR," *Journal of Cardiovascular Magnetic Resonance*, vol. 14, no. 1, pp. 1–2, 2012.
67. H. Sliman, A. Elnakib, G. Beache, A. Elmaghraby, and A. El-Baz, "Assessment of myocardial function from cine cardiac MRI using a novel 4D tracking approach," *Journal of Computer Science and Systems Biology*, vol. 7, pp. 169–173, 2014.

68. H. Sliman, A. Elnakib, G. M. Beache, A. Soliman, F. Khalifa, G. Gimel'farb, A. Elmaghraby, and A. El-Baz, "A novel 4D PDE-based approach for accurate assessment of myocardium function using cine cardiac magnetic resonance images," in *Proceedings of IEEE International Conference on Image Processing (ICIP'14)*, Paris, France, October 27–30, 2014, pp. 3537–3541.
69. H. Sliman, F. Khalifa, A. Elnakib, G. M. Beache, A. Elmaghraby, and A. El-Baz, "A new segmentation-based tracking framework for extracting the left ventricle cavity from cine cardiac MRI," in *Proceedings of IEEE International Conference on Image Processing, (ICIP'13)*, Melbourne, Australia, September 15–18, 2013, pp. 685–689.
70. H. Sliman, F. Khalifa, A. Elnakib, A. Soliman, G. M. Beache, A. Elmaghraby, G. Gimel'farb, and A. El-Baz, "Myocardial borders segmentation from cine MR images using bi-directional coupled parametric deformable models," *Medical Physics*, vol. 40, no. 9, pp. 1–13, 2013.
71. H. Sliman, F. Khalifa, A. Elnakib, A. Soliman, G. M. Beache, G. Gimel'farb, A. Emam, A. Elmaghraby, and A. El-Baz, "Accurate segmentation framework for the left ventricle wall from cardiac cine MRI," in *Proceedings of International Symposium on Computational Models for Life Science, (CMLS'13)*, Sydney, Australia, November 27–29, 2013, vol. 1559, pp. 287–296.
72. B. Abdollahi, A. C. Civelek, X.-F. Li, J. Suri, and A. El-Baz, "PET/CT nodule segmentation and diagnosis: A survey," in *Multi Detector CT Imaging*, L. Saba and J. S. Suri, Eds. Taylor & Francis, Boca Raton, 2014, Ch. 30, pp. 639–651.
73. B. Abdollahi, A. El-Baz, and A. A. Amini, "A multi-scale non-linear vessel enhancement technique," in *Engineering in Medicine and Biology Society, EMBC, 2011 Annual International Conference of the IEEE*. IEEE, 2011, pp. 3925–3929.
74. B. Abdollahi, A. Soliman, A. Civelek, X.-F. Li, G. Gimel'farb, and A. El-Baz, "A novel gaussian scale space-based joint MGRF framework for precise lung segmentation," in *Proceedings of IEEE International Conference on Image Processing, (ICIP'12)*. IEEE, 2012, pp. 2029–2032.
75. Abdollahi, B., Soliman, A., Civelek, A. C., Li, X. F., Gimel'farb, G., & El-Baz, A. (2012, October). A novel 3D joint MGRF framework for precise lung segmentation. In *International Workshop on Machine Learning in Medical Imaging* (pp. 86–93). Springer, Berlin, Heidelberg.3.
76. A. M. Ali, A. S. El-Baz, and A. A. Farag, "A novel framework for accurate lung segmentation using graph cuts," in *Proceedings of IEEE International Symposium on Biomedical Imaging: From Nano to Macro, (ISBI'07)*. IEEE, 2007, pp. 908–911.
77. A. El-Baz, G. M. Beache, G. Gimel'farb, K. Suzuki, and K. Okada, "Lung imaging data analysis," *International Journal of Biomedical Imaging*, vol. 2013, pp. 1–2, 2013.
78. A. El-Baz, G. M. Beache, G. Gimel'farb, K. Suzuki, K. Okada, A. Elnakib, A. Soliman, and B. Abdollahi, "Computer-aided diagnosis systems for lung cancer: Challenges and methodologies," *International Journal of Biomedical Imaging*, vol. 2013, pp. 1–46, 2013.

79. A. El-Baz, A. Elnakib, M. Abou El-Ghar, G. Gimel'farb, R. Falk, and A. Farag, "Automatic detection of 2D and 3D lung nodules in chest spiral CT scans," *International Journal of Biomedical Imaging*, vol. 2013, pp. 1–11, 2013.
80. A. El-Baz, A. A. Farag, R. Falk, and R. La Rocca, "*A Unified Approach for Detection, Visualization, and Identification of Lung Abnormalities in Chest Spiral CT Scans*," in International Congress Series. Elsevier, Amsterdam, Netherlands, 2003, vol. 1256, pp. 998–1004.
81. ——, "Detection, visualization and identification of lung abnormalities in chest spiral CT scan: Phase-I," in *Proceedings of International conference on Biomedical Engineering*, Cairo, Egypt, 2002, vol. 12, no. 1.
82. A. El-Baz, A. Farag, G. Gimel'farb, R. Falk, M. A. El-Ghar, and T. Eldiasty, "A framework for automatic segmentation of lung nodules from low dose chest CT scans," in *Proceedings of International Conference on Pattern Recognition, (ICPR'06)*. IEEE, 2006, vol. 3, pp. 611–614.
83. A. El-Baz, A. Farag, G. Gimel'farb, R. Falk, and M. A. El-Ghar, "A novel level set-based computer-aided detection system for automatic detection of lung nodules in low dose chest computed tomography scans," *Lung Imaging and Computer Aided Diagnosis*, vol. 10, pp. 221–238, 2011.
84. A. El-Baz, G. Gimel'farb, M. Abou El-Ghar, and R. Falk, "Appearance-based diagnostic system for early assessment of malignant lung nodules," in *Proceedings of IEEE International Conference on Image Processing, (ICIP'12)*. IEEE, 2012, pp. 533–536.
85. A. El-Baz, G. Gimel'farb, and R. Falk, "A novel 3D framework for automatic lung segmentation from low dose CT images," in *Lung Imaging and Computer Aided Diagnosis*, A. El-Baz and J. S. Suri, Eds. Taylor & Francis, Boca Raton, 2011, Ch. 1, pp. 1–16.
86. A. El-Baz, G. Gimel'farb, R. Falk, and M. El-Ghar, "Appearance analysis for diagnosing malignant lung nodules," in *Proceedings of IEEE International Symposium on Biomedical Imaging: From Nano to Macro (ISBI'10)*. IEEE, 2010, pp. 193–196.
87. A. El-Baz, G. Gimel'farb, R. Falk, and M. A. El-Ghar, "A novel level set-based CAD system for automatic detection of lung nodules in low dose chest CT scans," in *Lung Imaging and Computer Aided Diagnosis*, A. El-Baz and J. S. Suri, Eds. Taylor & Francis, Boca Raton, 2011, vol. 1, Ch. 10, pp. 221–238.
88. ——, "A new approach for automatic analysis of 3D low dose CT images for accurate monitoring the detected lung nodules," in *Proceedings of International Conference on Pattern Recognition, (ICPR'08)*. IEEE, 2008, pp. 1–4.
89. ——, "A novel approach for automatic follow-up of detected lung nodules," in *Proceedings of IEEE International Conference on Image Processing, (ICIP'07)*, vol. 5. IEEE, 2007, pp. V–501.
90. ——, "A new CAD system for early diagnosis of detected lung nodules," in *Image Processing, 2007. ICIP 2007. IEEE International Conference on*. IEEE, 2007, vol. 2, pp. II–461.

91. A. El-Baz, G. Gimel'farb, R. Falk, M. A. El-Ghar, and H. Refaie, "Promising results for early diagnosis of lung cancer," in *Proceedings of IEEE International Symposium on Biomedical Imaging: From Nano to Macro, (ISBI'08)*. IEEE, 2008, pp. 1151–1154.
92. A. El-Baz, G. L. Gimel'farb, R. Falk, M. Abou El-Ghar, T. Holland, and T. Shaffer, "A new stochastic framework for accurate lung segmentation," in *Proceedings of Medical Image Computing and Computer-Assisted Intervention, (MICCAI'08)*, 2008, pp. 322–330.
93. A. El-Baz, G. L. Gimel'farb, R. Falk, D. Heredis, and M. Abou El-Ghar, "A novel approach for accurate estimation of the growth rate of the detected lung nodules," in *Proceedings of International Workshop on Pulmonary Image Analysis*, 2008, pp. 33–42.
94. A. El-Baz, G. L. Gimel'farb, R. Falk, T. Holland, and T. Shaffer, "A framework for unsupervised segmentation of lung tissues from low dose computed tomography images," in *Proceedings of British Machine Vision, (BMVC'08)*, 2008, pp. 1–10.
95. A. El-Baz, G. Gimel'farb, R. Falk, and M. A. El-Ghar, "3D MGRF-based appearance modeling for robust segmentation of pulmonary nodules in 3D LDCT chest images," in *Lung Imaging and Computer Aided Diagnosis*, A. El-Baz and J. S. Suri, Eds. Taylor & Francis, Boca Raton, 2011, Ch. 3, pp. 51–63.
96. ——, "Automatic analysis of 3D low dose CT images for early diagnosis of lung cancer," *Pattern Recognition*, vol. 42, no. 6, pp. 1041–1051, 2009.
97. A. El-Baz, G. Gimel'farb, R. Falk, M. A. El-Ghar, S. Rainey, D. Heredia, and T. Shaffer, "Toward early diagnosis of lung cancer," in *Proceedings of Medical Image Computing and Computer-Assisted Intervention, (MICCAI'09)*. Springer, 2009, pp. 682–689.
98. A. El-Baz, G. Gimel'farb, R. Falk, M. A. El-Ghar, and J. Suri, "Appearance analysis for the early assessment of detected lung nodules," in *Lung Imaging and Computer Aided Diagnosis*, A. El-Baz and J. S. Suri, Eds. Taylor & Francis, Boca Raton, 2011, Ch. 17, pp. 395–404.
99. A. El-Baz, F. Khalifa, A. Elnakib, M. Nitkzen, A. Soliman, P. McClure, G. Gimel'farb, and M. A. El-Ghar, "A novel approach for global lung registration using 3D Markov Gibbs appearance model," in *Proceedings of International Conference Medical Image Computing and Computer-Assisted Intervention, (MICCAI'12)*, Nice, France, October 1–5, 2012, pp. 114–121.
100. A. El-Baz, M. Nitzken, A. Elnakib, F. Khalifa, G. Gimel'farb, R. Falk, and M. A. El-Ghar, "3D shape analysis for early diagnosis of malignant lung nodules," in *Proceedings of International Conference Medical Image Computing and Computer-Assisted Intervention, (MICCAI'11)*, Toronto, Canada, September 18–22, 2011, pp. 175–182.
101. A. El-Baz, M. Nitzken, G. Gimel'farb, E. Van Bogaert, R. Falk, M. A. El-Ghar, and J. Suri, "Three-dimensional shape analysis using spherical harmonics for early assessment of detected lung nodules," in *Lung Imaging and Computer Aided Diagnosis*, A. El-Baz and J. S. Suri, Eds. Taylor & Francis, 2011, Ch. 19, pp. 421–438.

102. A. El-Baz, M. Nitzken, F. Khalifa, A. Elnakib, G. Gimel'farb, R. Falk, and M. A. El-Ghar, "3D shape analysis for early diagnosis of malignant lung nodules," in *Proceedings of International Conference on Information Processing in Medical Imaging, (IPMI'11)*, Monastery Irsee, Germany (Bavaria), July 3–8, 2011, pp. 772–783.
103. A. El-Baz, M. Nitzken, E. Vanbogaert, G. Gimel'Farb, R. Falk, and M. Abo El-Ghar, "A novel shape-based diagnostic approach for early diagnosis of lung nodules," in *Biomedical Imaging: From Nano to Macro, 2011 IEEE International Symposium on*. IEEE, 2011, pp. 137–140.
104. A. El-Baz, P. Sethu, G. Gimel'farb, F. Khalifa, A. Elnakib, R. Falk, and M. A. El-Ghar, "Elastic phantoms generated by microfluidics technology: Validation of an imaged-based approach for accurate measurement of the growth rate of lung nodules," *Biotechnology Journal*, vol. 6, no. 2, pp. 195–203, 2011.
105. ——, "A new validation approach for the growth rate measurement using elastic phantoms generated by state-of-the-art microfluidics technology," in *Proceedings of IEEE International Conference on Image Processing, (ICIP'10)*, Hong Kong, September 26–29, 2010, pp. 4381–4383.
106. A. El-Baz, P. Sethu, G. Gimel'farb, F. Khalifa, A. Elnakib, R. Falk, and M. A. E.-G. J. Suri, "Validation of a new imaged-based approach for the accurate estimating of the growth rate of detected lung nodules using real CT images and elastic phantoms generated by state-of-the-art microfluidics technology," in *Handbook of Lung Imaging and Computer Aided Diagnosis*, A. El-Baz and J. S. Suri, Eds. Taylor & Francis, New York, NY, 2011, vol. 1, Ch. 18, pp. 405–420.
107. A. El-Baz, A. Soliman, P. McClure, G. Gimel'farb, M. A. El-Ghar, and R. Falk, "Early assessment of malignant lung nodules based on the spatial analysis of detected lung nodules," in *Proceedings of IEEE International Symposium on Biomedical Imaging: From Nano to Macro, (ISBI'12)*. IEEE, 2012, pp. 1463–1466.
108. A. El-Baz, S. E. Yuksel, S. Elshazly, and A. A. Farag, "Non-rigid registration techniques for automatic follow-up of lung nodules," in *Proceedings of Computer Assisted Radiology and Surgery, (CARS'05)*. Elsevier, 2005, vol. 1281, pp. 1115–1120.
109. A. S. El-Baz and J. S. Suri, "*Lung Imaging and Computer Aided Diagnosis*," CRC Press, Boca Raton, 2011.
110. A. Soliman, F. Khalifa, N. Dunlap, B. Wang, M. El-Ghar, and A. El-Baz, "An iso-surfaces based local deformation handling framework of lung tissues," in *Biomedical Imaging (ISBI), 2016 IEEE 13th International Symposium on*. IEEE, 2016, pp. 1253–1259.
111. A. Soliman, F. Khalifa, A. Shaffie, N. Dunlap, B. Wang, A. Elmaghraby, and A. El-Baz, "Detection of lung injury using 4d-ct chest images," in *Biomedical Imaging (ISBI), 2016 IEEE 13th International Symposium on*. IEEE, 2016, pp. 1274–1277.

112. A. Soliman, F. Khalifa, A. Shaffie, N. Dunlap, B. Wang, A. Elmaghraby, G. Gimel'farb, M. Ghazal, and A. El-Baz, "A comprehensive framework for early assessment of lung injury," in *Image Processing (ICIP), 2017 IEEE International Conference on*. IEEE, 2017, pp. 3275–3279.
113. A. Shaffie, A. Soliman, M. Ghazal, F. Taher, N. Dunlap, B. Wang, A. Elmaghraby, G. Gimel'farb, and A. El-Baz, "A new framework for incorporating appearance and shape features of lung nodules for precise diagnosis of lung cancer," in *Image Processing (ICIP), 2017 IEEE International Conference on*. IEEE, 2017, pp. 1372–1376.
114. A. Soliman, F. Khalifa, A. Shaffie, N. Liu, N. Dunlap, B. Wang, A. Elmaghraby, G. Gimel'farb, and A. El-Baz, "Image-based cad system for accurate identification of lung injury," in *Image Processing (ICIP), 2016 IEEE International Conference on*. IEEE, 2016, pp. 121–125.
115. A. Soliman, A. Shaffie, M. Ghazal, G. Gimel'farb, R. Keynton, and A. El-Baz, "A novel CNN segmentation framework based on using new shape and appearance features," in *2018 25th IEEE International Conference on Image Processing (ICIP)*. IEEE, 2018, pp. 3488–3492.
116. A. Shaffie, A. Soliman, H. A. Khalifeh, M. Ghazal, F. Taher, R. Keynton, A. Elmaghraby, and A. El-Baz, "On the integration of CT- derived features for accurate detection of lung cancer," in *2018 IEEE International Symposium on Signal Processing and Information Technology (ISSPIT)*. IEEE, 2018, pp. 435–440.
117. A. Shaffie, A. Soliman, H. A. Khalifeh, M. Ghazal, F. Taher, A. Elmaghraby, R. Keynton, and A. El-Baz, "Radiomic-based framework for early diagnosis of lung cancer," in *2019 IEEE 16th International Symposium on Biomedical Imaging (ISBI 2019)*. IEEE, 2019, pp. 1293–1297.
118. A. Shaffie, A. Soliman, M. Ghazal, F. Taher, N. Dunlap, B. Wang, V. Van Berkel, G. Gimelfarb, A. Elmaghraby, and A. El-Baz, "A novel autoencoder-based diagnostic system for early assessment of lung cancer," in *2018 25th IEEE International Conference on Image Processing (ICIP)*. IEEE, 2018, pp. 1393–1397.
119. A. Shaffie et al., "A generalized deep learning-based diagnostic system for early diagnosis of various types of pulmonary nodules," *Technology in Cancer Research & Treatment*, vol. 17, p. 1533033818798800, 2018.
120. Y. ElNakieb et al., "Autism spectrum disorder diagnosis framework using diffusion tensor imaging," in *2019 IEEE International Conference on Imaging Systems and Techniques (IST)*. IEEE, 2019, pp. 1–5.
121. R. Haweel, O. Dekhil, A. Shalaby, A. Mahmoud, M. Ghazal, R. Keynton, G. Barnes, and A. El-Baz, "A machine learning approach for grading autism severity levels using task-based functional MRI," in *2019 IEEE International Conference on Imaging Systems and Techniques (IST)*. IEEE, 2019, pp. 1–5.
122. O. Dekhil et al., "A comprehensive framework for differentiating autism spectrum disorder from neurotypicals by fusing structural MRI and resting state functional MRI," in *Seminars in Pediatric Neurology*. Elsevier, 2020, p. 100805.

123. R. Haweel, O. Dekhil, A. Shalaby, A. Mahmoud, M. Ghazal, A. Khalil, R. Keynton, G. Barnes, and A. El-Baz, "A novel framework for grading autism severity using task-based fMRI," in *2020 IEEE 17th International Symposium on Biomedical Imaging (ISBI)*. IEEE, 2020, pp. 1404–1407.
124. B. Dombroski, M. Nitzken, A. Elnakib, F. Khalifa, A. El-Baz, and M. F. Casanova, "Cortical surface complexity in a population-based normative sample," *Translational Neuroscience*, vol. 5, no. 1, pp. 17–24, 2014.
125. A. El-Baz, M. Casanova, G. Gimel'farb, M. Mott, and A. Switala, "An MRI-based diagnostic framework for early diagnosis of dyslexia," *International Journal of Computer Assisted Radiology and Surgery*, vol. 3, no. 3–4, pp. 181–189, 2008.
126. A. El-Baz, M. Casanova, G. Gimel'farb, M. Mott, A. Switala, E. Vanbogaert, and R. McCracken, "A new CAD system for early diagnosis of dyslexic brains," in *Proceedings on International Conference on Image Processing (ICIP'2008)*. IEEE, 2008, pp. 1820–1823.
127. A. El-Baz, M. F. Casanova, G. Gimel'farb, M. Mott, and A. E. Switwala, "A new image analysis approach for automatic classification of autistic brains," in *Proceedings on IEEE International Symposium on Biomedical Imaging: From Nano to Macro (ISBI'2007)*. IEEE, 2007, pp. 352–355.
128. A. El-Baz, A. Elnakib, F. Khalifa, M. A. El-Ghar, P. McClure, A. Soliman, and G. Gimel'farb, "Precise segmentation of 3-D magnetic resonance angiography," *IEEE Transactions on Biomedical Engineering*, vol. 59, no. 7, pp. 2019–2029, 2012.
129. A. El-Baz, A. A. Farag, G. Gimel'farb, and S. G. Hushek, "Automatic cerebrovascular segmentation by accurate probabilistic modeling of tof-MRA images," in *Medical Image Computing and Computer-Assisted Intervention–MICCAI 2005*. Springer, 2005, pp. 34–42.
130. A. El-Baz, A. Farag, A. Elnakib, M. F. Casanova, G. Gimel'farb, A. E. Switala, D. Jordan, and S. Rainey, "Accurate automated detection of autism related corpus callosum abnormalities," *Journal of Medical Systems*, vol. 35, no. 5, pp. 929–939, 2011.
131. El-Baz, A., Farag, A., & Gimelfarb, G. (2005, June). Cerebrovascular segmentation by accurate probabilistic modeling of TOF-MRA images. In *Scandinavian Conference on Image Analysis* (pp. 1128–1137). Springer, Berlin, Heidelberg.
132. A. El-Baz, G. Gimel'farb, R. Falk, M. A. El-Ghar, V. Kumar, and D. Heredia, "A novel 3D joint Markov–Gibbs model for extracting blood vessels from PC–MRA images," in *Medical Image Computing and Computer-Assisted Intervention–MICCAI 2009*. Springer, 2009, vol. 5762, pp. 943–950.
133. A. Elnakib, A. El-Baz, M. F. Casanova, G. Gimel'farb, and A. E. Switala, "Image-based detection of corpus callosum variability for more accurate discrimination between dyslexic and normal brains," in *Proceedings on IEEE International Symposium on Biomedical Imaging: From Nano to Macro (ISBI'2010)*. IEEE, 2010, pp. 109–112.

134. A. Elnakib, M. F. Casanova, G. Gimel'farb, A. E. Switala, and A. El-Baz, "Autism diagnostics by centerline-based shape analysis of the corpus callosum," in *Proceedings on IEEE International Symposium on Biomedical Imaging: From Nano to Macro (ISBI'2011)*. IEEE, 2011, pp. 1843–1846.
135. A. Elnakib, M. Nitzken, M. Casanova, H. Park, G. Gimel'farb, and A. El-Baz, "Quantification of age-related brain cortex change using 3D shape analysis," in *Pattern Recognition (ICPR), 2012 21st International Conference on*. IEEE, 2012, pp. 41–44.
136. M. Nitzken, M. Casanova, G. Gimel'farb, A. Elnakib, F. Khalifa, A. Switala, and A. El-Baz, "3D shape analysis of the brain cortex with application to dyslexia," in *Image Processing (ICIP), 2011 18th IEEE International Conference on*. Brussels, Belgium: IEEE, Sep. 2011, pp. 2657–2660, (Selected for oral presentation. Oral acceptance rate is 10% and the overall acceptance rate is 35%).
137. F. E.-Z. A. El-Gamal, M. M. Elmogy, M. Ghazal, A. Atwan, G. N. Barnes, M. F. Casanova, R. Keynton, and A. S. El-Baz, "A novel CAD system for local and global early diagnosis of Alzheimer's disease based on pib-pet scans," in *2017 IEEE International Conference on Image Processing (ICIP)*. IEEE, 2017, pp. 3270–3274.
138. M. M. Ismail, R. S. Keynton, M. M. Mostapha, A. H. ElTanboly, M. F. Casanova, G. L. Gimel'farb, and A. El-Baz, "Studying autism spectrum disorder with structural and diffusion magnetic resonance imaging: a survey," *Frontiers in Human Neuroscience*, vol. 10, p. 211, 2016.
139. A. Alansary et al., "Infant brain extraction in t1-weighted mr images using bet and refinement using LCDG and MGRF models," *IEEE Journal of Biomedical and Health Informatics*, vol. 20, no. 3, pp. 925–935, 2016.
140. E. H. Asl, M. Ghazal, A. Mahmoud, A. Aslantas, A. Shalaby, M. Casanova, G. Barnes, G. Gimel'farb, R. Keynton, and A. El-Baz, "Alzheimer's disease diagnostics by a 3D deeply supervised adaptable convolutional network," *Frontiers in Bioscience (Landmark Edition)*, vol. 23, pp. 584–596, 2018.
141. O. Dekhil, M. Ali, Y. El-Nakieb, A. Shalaby, A. Soliman, A. Switala, A. Mahmoud, M. Ghazal, H. Hajjdiab, M. F. Casanova, A. Elmaghraby, R. Keynton, A. El-Baz, and G. Barnes, "A personalized autism diagnosis cad system using a fusion of structural MRI and resting-state functional MRI data," *Frontiers in Psychiatry*, vol. 10, p. 392, 2019. [Online]. Available: https://www.frontiersin.org/article/10.3389/fpsyt.2019.00392
142. A. Mahmoud, A. El-Barkouky, H. Farag, J. Graham, and A. Farag, "A non-invasive method for measuring blood flow rate in superficial veins from a single thermal image," in *Proceedings of the IEEE Conference on Computer Vision and Pattern Recognition Workshops*, 2013, pp. 354–359.
143. A. El-Baz, A. Farag, G. Gimel'farb, M. A. El-Ghar, and T. Eldiasty, "Probabilistic modeling of blood vessels for segmenting MRA images," in *18th International Conference on Pattern Recognition (ICPR'06)*, vol. 3. IEEE, 2006, pp. 917–920.

144. A. El-Baz, A. A. Farag, G. Gimel'farb, M. A. El-Ghar, and T. Eldiasty, "A new adaptive probabilistic model of blood vessels for segmenting MRA images," in *Medical Image Computing and Computer-Assisted Intervention–MICCAI 2006*. Springer, 2006, vol. 4191, pp. 799–806.
145. A. El-baz, A. Shalaby, F. Taher, M. El-Baz, M. Ghazal, M. A. El-Ghar, A. Takieldeen, and J. Suri, "Probabilistic modeling of blood vessels for segmenting magnetic resonance angiography images," *Medical Research Archives*, 2017, vol. 5, no. 3, pp. 34–42.
146. A. S. Chowdhury, A. K. Rudra, M. Sen, A. Elnakib, and A. El-Baz, "Cerebral white matter segmentation from MRI using probabilistic graph cuts and geometric shape priors," in *ICIP*, 2010, pp. 3649–3652.
147. Y. Gebru, G. Giridharan, M. Ghazal, A. Mahmoud, A. Shalaby, and A. El-Baz, "Detection of cerebrovascular changes using magnetic resonance angiography," in *Cardiovascular Imaging and Image Analysis*. CRC Press, Boca Raton, 2018, pp. 1–22.
148. A. Mahmoud, A. Shalaby, F. Taher, M. El-Baz, J. S. Suri, and A. El-Baz, "Vascular tree segmentation from different image modalities," in *Cardiovascular Imaging and Image Analysis*. CRC Press, 2018, pp. 43–70.
149. F. Taher, A. Mahmoud, A. Shalaby, and A. El-Baz, "A review on the cerebrovascular segmentation methods," in *2018 IEEE International Symposium on Signal Processing and Information Technology (ISSPIT)*. IEEE, 2018, pp. 359–364.
150. H. Kandil, A. Soliman, L. Fraiwan, A. Shalaby, A. Mahmoud, A. ElTanboly, A. Elmaghraby, G. Giridharan, and A. El-Baz, "A novel MRA framework based on integrated global and local analysis for accurate segmentation of the cerebral vascular system," in *2018 IEEE 15th International Symposium on Biomedical Imaging (ISBI 2018)*. IEEE, 2018, pp. 1365–1368.
151. F. Taher, A. Soliman, H. Kandil, A. Mahmoud, A. Shalaby, G. Gimel'farb, and A. El-Baz, "Accurate segmentation of cerebrovasculature from TOF-MRA images using appearance descriptors," *IEEE Access*, 2020.
152. A. A. Sleman, A. Soliman, M. Ghazal, H. Sandhu, S. Schaal, A. Elmaghraby, and A. El-Baz, "Retinal layers oct scans 3-D segmentation," in *2019 IEEE International Conference on Imaging Systems and Techniques (IST)*. IEEE, 2019, pp. 1–6.
153. N. Eladawi, M. Elmogy, M. Ghazal, O. Helmy, A. Aboelfetouh, A. Riad, S. Schaal, and A. El-Baz, "Classification of retinal diseases based on OCT images," *Frontiers in Bioscience (Landmark Edition)*, vol. 23, pp. 247–264, 2018.
154. A. ElTanboly, M. Ismail, A. Shalaby, A. Switala, A. El-Baz, S. Schaal, G. Gimel'farb, and M. El-Azab, "A computer-aided diagnostic system for detecting diabetic retinopathy in optical coherence tomography images," *Medical Physics*, vol. 44, no. 3, pp. 914–923, 2017.
155. H. S. Sandhu, A. El-Baz, and J. M. Seddon, "Progress in automated deep learning for macular degeneration," *JAMA Ophthalmology*, vol. 136, no. 12, pp. 1366–1367, 2018.

156. M. Ghazal, S. S. Ali, A. H. Mahmoud, A. M. Shalaby, and A. El-Baz, "Accurate detection of non-proliferative diabetic retinopathy in optical coherence tomography images using convolutional neural networks," *IEEE Access*, vol. 8, pp. 34387–34397, 2020.
157. K. Hammouda, F. Khalifa, A. Soliman, H. Abdeltawab, M. Ghazal, M. Abou El-Ghar, A. Haddad, H. E. Darwish, R. Keynton, and A. El-Baz, "A 3D CNN with a learnable adaptive shape prior for accurate segmentation of bladder wall using MR images," in *2020 IEEE 17th International Symposium on Biomedical Imaging (ISBI)*. IEEE, 2020, pp. 935–938.
158. A. Naglah, F. Khalifa, A. Mahmoud, M. Ghazal, P. Jones, T. Murray, A. S. Elmaghraby, and A. El-Baz, "Athlete-customized injury prediction using training load statistical records and machine learning," in *2018 IEEE International Symposium on Signal Processing and Information Technology (ISSPIT)*. IEEE, 2018, pp. 459–464.
159. A. H. Mahmoud, "Utilizing radiation for smart robotic applications using visible, thermal, and polarization images." Ph.D. dissertation, University of Louisville, 2014.
160. A. Mahmoud, A. El-Barkouky, J. Graham, and A. Farag, "Pedestrian detection using mixed partial derivative based his togram of oriented gradients," in *2014 IEEE International Conference on Image Processing (ICIP)*. IEEE, 2014, pp. 2334–2337.
161. A. El-Barkouky, A. Mahmoud, J. Graham, and A. Farag, "An interactive educational drawing system using a humanoid robot and light polarization," in *2013 IEEE International Conference on Image Processing*. IEEE, 2013, pp. 3407–3411.
162. A. H. Mahmoud, M. T. El-Melegy, and A. A. Farag, "Direct method for shape recovery from polarization and shading," in *2012 19th IEEE International Conference on Image Processing*. IEEE, 2012, pp. 1769–1772.
163. M. A. Ghazal, A. Mahmoud, A. Aslantas, A. Soliman, A. Shalaby, J. A. Benediktsson, and A. El-Baz, "Vegetation cover estimation using convolutional neural networks," *IEEE Access*, vol. 7, pp. 132563–132576, 2019.
164. M. Ghazal, A. Mahmoud, A. Shalaby, and A. El-Baz, "Automated framework for accurate segmentation of leaf images for plant health assessment," *Environmental Monitoring and Assessment*, vol. 191, no. 8, p. 491, 2019.

Index

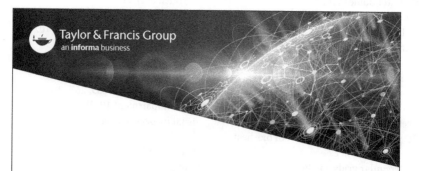